Engineering Chemistry

Ajay Singh

PhD. (H.N.B.Garhwal University, Srinagar)
CSIR-NET (Chemical Sciences, 2001)
Associate Professor and Head
Deptt. of Chemistry and Env. Sc.
Uttaranchal Institute of Technology
(Uttarakhand Technical University)
Dehradun, Uttarakhand, India

IKON BOOKS
Publishers and Distributors

CBS

CBS Publishers & Distributors Pvt Ltd

New Delhi • Bengaluru • Chennai • Kochi • Pune
Hyderabad • Kolkata • Mumbai • Nagpur • Patna

CBS Publishers & Distributors Pvt Ltd
4819//XI, 24 Ansari Road, Daryaganj
New Delhi-110 002 (India)

IKON BOOKS, Publishers and Distributors
B-37, First Floor, Office No. 105
Street No. 14, Madhu Vihar
I.P. Extention, Delhi - 110 092
Telephone: 91-11-43618579
Email: ikonbooks@gmail.com
           cs@ikonbooks.com
           Website: www.ikonbooks.com

© 2013 IKON BOOKS and CBS Publishers & Distributors

| **Engineering** |
| **Chemistry** |

First Edition: 2013

ISBN: 978-81-239-2287-4

CBS Publishers & Distributors Pvt Ltd
Ph: 23289259, 23266861, 23266867
Website: www.cbspd.com

Fax: 011-23243014
e-mail: delhi@cbspd.com;
cbspubs@airtelmail.in

Corporate Office: 204 FIE, Industrial Area, Patparganj, Delhi 110 092
Ph: 4934 4934   Fax: 4934 4935   e-mail: publishing@cbspd.com;
publicity@cbspd.com

Branches

- **Bengaluru:** Seema House 2975, 17th Cross, K.R. Road,
  Banasankari 2nd Stage, Bengaluru 560 070, Karnataka
  Ph: +91-80-26771678/79   Fax: +91-80-26771680   e-mail: bangalore@cbspd.com

- **Chennai:** 20, West Park Road, Shenoy Nagar, Chennai 600 030, Tamil Nadu
  Ph: +91-44-26260666, 26208620   Fax: +91-44-42032115   e-mail: chennai@cbspd.com

- **Kochi:** 36/14 Kalluvilakam, Lissie Hospital Road, Kochi 682 018, Kerala
  Ph: +91-484-4059061-65   Fax: +91-484-4059065   e-mail: kochi@cbspd.com

- **Pune:** Bhuruk Prestige, Sr. No. 52/12/2+1+3/2 Narhe, Haveli
  (Near Katraj-Dehu Road Bypass), Pune 411 041, Maharashtra
  Ph: +91-20-64704058, 64704059, 32342277 Fax: +91-20-24300160   e-mail: pune@cbspd.com

Representatives

- **Hyderabad** 0-9885175004   • **Kolkata** 0-9831437309, 0-9051152362
- **Mumbai**   0-9833017933   • **Nagpur** 0-9021734563   • **Patna**   0-9334159340

Printed at India Binding House Noida

This book is dedicated
to
Shri Shirdi Sai Baba

PREFACE

This book of Engineering Chemistry is primarily intended to be a text book for B.Tech 1st year student of Engineering and Technology. Efforts have been made to cover almost all syllabus of Engineering Chemistry of all Indian universities, especially as prescribed by Uttarakhand Technical University, Dehradun and UP Technical University, Punjab Technical University etc.

This book is the outcome of many years of research and teaching experience based on the class notes as well as suggestions given by experts in the field. This book is divided into 15 chapters, each of which is complete in itself and has been discussed with sufficient information of the topic including basic concepts, however some topics have been discussed concisely as per requirement of I and II semester students of B.Tech.

Chapters like Liquid crystals, phase rule, Chemical Kinetics, Water chemistry, Analytical Chemistry, Spectroscopy, Lubricants have been discussed with a different kind of approach so that students may understand easily and information provided by these chapters will be also helpful in enhancing the basic concept, level of the students. A different and easy approach has been done for some difficult numerical problems in the topics like water chemistry, analytical chemistry, Chemical kinetics and fuels. At the end question bank of important questions have been provided.

We hope this book will serve the purpose. Although we have tried to accommodate the study material in a phased manner with accuracy, however there may be unintentional errors. We will appreciate the information and suggestions provided by the readers of the book regarding the error or improvements in the book, which would be helpful for making this text book useful for all concerned.

(Dr. Ajay Singh)

Email- ajay21singh@yahoo.com

ACKNOWLEDGEMENT

I wish to express my deep sense of gratitude to Prof. M.S.M Rawat (H.N.B. Garhwal Central University, Srinagar, UK) my guide of Ph.D for his encouragement and blessings.

I am extremely thankful to my friends Mr. S.K. Joshi, Mr. S.K. Shah, Mr. V.K. Srivastava, Dr. Santosh Kumar, Mr. Vinod Joshi, Dr. Harish Chandra (GBPEC-Pauri), Dr. Vrij Bhusan, Mr. Kuldeep Garg, Mr. Umendra Kumar, Mr. Hrishikesh Dhasmana Dr. Ashwani Sanghi, Dr. Manoj Gehlot (SGRITS-DUN), Dr. Poonam Negi, Mrs. Bharti Ramola, Mr. Deepak Kumar and other colleagues of UIT-Dehradun for helping and encouraging during this work.

I am thankful to Prof V.K. Singh, Prof V.K. Mehta (COER-Roorkee), Prof. Naveen Singhal (DIT), Prof. Chhiber (Shivalik-Ddun) Dr. Ajay Pali (Amrapai–Haldwani), Dr. Tarn Kumar (Tula-Ddun), Dr. Mishra (Birla-Bhimtal), Dr. Raghvendra Chauhan (Phonics-Roorkee), Mr. Amit Gautam (Phonics) UVS Teotia (Res Director-Venkteshwar Univ, Meerut), Dr. Mahavir Singh (Director-Beehive), Mr. Durgesh Pandey (HDR), Mr. Kapil Ghai (Graphic Era Univ), Dr. Ekta Chitkara (LPU) and Dr. A.K. Seth (Quantum) their time to time support and encouragement.

I record my indebtedness to Chairman (Mr. Jitendra Joshi) of UIT, Advisor (Mr H.C. Devrani), Director (Dr. Vijay Raj), VC of UTU (Prof. D.S. Chauhan) and COE-UTU (Mr. R.K. Singh) for their blessings.

I am overwhelmed to express my heartful thanks to my parents, wife, brother, sister, my lovely sons-Akarsh and Aryash, inlaws and other members of the family, who inspired and boosted me during completion of this book.

At the last but not the least, I am highly thankful to the Publishers of this book, who cooperated and provided support constantly for writing this book.

(Dr. Ajay Singh)

CONTENTS

Preface (*v*)

Acknowledgement (*vii*)

1. Analytical Chemistry: Vol. Analysis 1-37
Basic Terms 1

Acid-Alkalimetry 8

Complexometry 11

Redox Titrations 18

Precipitation Titrations 21

Numerical Problems 25

2. Spectroscopic methods of Analysis 38-106
Laws of spectroscopy 40

UV-Visible Spectroscopy 41

Woodword Fieser rules 45

NMR Principle 53

NMR Signals 62

Infra-red Spectroscopy 74

Mass Spectroscopy 100

3. Chemical Kinetics 107-146
Rate of reaction 108

Zero order 126

1st Order 128

2nd Order   132

Order determination methods   133

Activation Energy   140

Surface chemistry   141

4. Phase Rule   **147-169**

Phase rule and derivation   148

One Component System   153

Two Component System   163

5. Electrochemistry   **170-228**

General Introduction   170

Laws of Electrochemistry   172

Conductivity   175

Kohlrausch Law   182

Electrochemical Cell   185

Electrochemical series   205

Battery and Fuel Cell   215

Buffer Solutions   223

Solubility and Solubility Product   225

Hydrolysis of Salts   225

6. Corrosion   **229-240**

Dry Corrosion   229

Wet Corrosion   230

Electrochemical theory   230

Corrosion Control   234

7. Water Chemistry   **241-267**

Hardness of Water   242

Boiler Problem   248

Internal Treatment of Water   250

Lime Soda process   252

Zeolite process 256
Ion Exchange Process 260
Reverse Osmosis 262

8. Polymer Chemistry   **268-310**
Polymers 268
Classification of Polymers 269
Polymerisation mechanism 276
Polymerization techniques 282
Biodegradable Polymers 304
Conducting Polymers 306

9. Engineering Materials   **311-338**
Alloys 311
Nanocomposites 317
Refractory 318
Ceramics-Glass 326
Organometallics 334

10. Lubricants   **339-361**
General Introduction 331
Functions of Lubricants 340
Classification of Lubricant 343
Synthetic lubricant 351
Mechanism of Lubricants 353
Properties of Lubricant 356

11. Petroleum Chemistry: Fuels   **362-387**
Fuel:classification 362
Solid fuel: Coal 366
Liquid fuel: Petroleum 369
Gaseous fuel 371
Calorific Value: GCV 374

Biofuel   378

Esterification and Transesterification   380

Biomass   381

Biogas   384

12. Chemical Bonding   **388-422**

Introduction   380

Metallic Bonding   393

Hydrogen Bonding   397

VBT   400

VSEPR   401

MOT   410

13. States of Matter   **423-448**

Introduction: Unit Cell   423

Density of unit cell   427

Bragg's law   436

Liquid Crystal   439

Fullerene   446

14. Organic Chemistry   **449-464**

Electronic Effects   449

Reaction Intermediates   453

Types of Attacking Reagents   454

Types of Reactions   456

Special Name Reactions   460

15. Stereo Chemistry of Carbon   **465-483**

Structural Isomerism   465

Geometrical Isomerism   466

Optical Isomerism   469

Conformations   477

Important Questions: Question bank   **484-493**

Index   **494-495**

Chapter 1
ANALYTICAL CHEMISTRY: VOLUMETRIC ANALYSIS

> ➤ **Basic terms**
> ➤ **Volumetric Analysis—Acid alkalimetry**
> ➤ **Complexometric**
> ➤ **Redox and Precipitation Titrations**
> ➤ **Numerical Problems**

INTRODUCTION

Generally chemical analysis of a compound can be done by qualitative method and quantitative analysis. Qualitative methods are used to detect the presence of particular element, ion or molecule while amount or quantity is determined by using quantitative analysis.

Titrimetric analysis (Titration) is one of the most useful analytical procedures that make up quantitative techniques in analytical chemistry. It is fairly rapid with good degree of accuracy. It involves measuring the volume of the reagent (titrant) needed to react with the analyte (test substance or titrand).This unit examines the general principle of volumetric analysis which include technical terms used in describing the analytical procedure, various types of volumetric titrations and calculation in volumetric analysis.

DEFINITION OF VOLUMETRIC ANALYSIS

Volumetric analysis is an analytical technique that deals with reactions between measured volumes of a regent known as titrant or known (std) solution against the test substance called analyte or unknow solutions in a stochiometric manner. It is a quantitative study.

PRINCIPLES AND TECHNICAL TERMS INVOLVED IN VOLUMETRIC ANALYSIS

In a titration the addition of the reagent solution (titrant) of known concentration to analyte continues until their reaction is complete and end point is detected by using suitable indicator. At the equivalent point number of gm equivalents of titrant (generally known substance) are equal to the number of gm equivalents of analyte (unkown compound).

Volumetric analysis is also called as titrimetiric analysis.

GENERAL (BASIC) REQUIREMENTS FOR TITRATION

i. The titration reaction should have large equilibrium constant i.e. each addition of titrant must be completely used up by the analyte

ii. The reaction should be rapid

iii. There should be known reaction pattern between the known and unkown solutions.

iv. There should be no side or parallel reaction i.e. the reaction should be specificwith no interference.

v. There should be distinct features in some property of the solution when the reaction is complete

vi. The end point should coincide with the equivalence point and be reproducible

Titrate: Substance to be analyzed or to be determined.

Titrant: Reagent of known concentration.

Titration: The process of determining the volume.

Equivalence point: The point at which complete chemical reaction takes place and equivalent quantities of reagents are used.

End Point: The point at which the indicator changes its color. This is the actual point when a reaction is observed to be complete.

Normality equation: For unknown(N_1V_1) and known (N_2V_2) solutions

$$N_1V_1 = N_2V_2$$

Indicator: Auxiliary agents used to determine the end point of titration. It is a compound with a physical property (colour) which changes abruptly near the equivalence end point. The change is colour is due complete consumption of analyse near the equivalence point whose concentration is known

Strength or Concentration: A defined quantity of substance in a defined volume of solution. Generally expressed as gm/litre or N or M.

Relation between Strength and Normality

$$S = N.E$$

(where S in gm/litre, N-normality and E is equivalent weight)

Normality: The number of gram equivalents of solute present in one liter of solution and represented by "N".

Molarity: The number of moles of solute presents in one liter of solution and represented by "M".

Relation between N and M

$$N = M \cdot X$$

(where x is a factor = basicity for acid,acidity for base, charge present on ion, change in Oxidation number of reducing or oxidizing agent)

Molality: The number of moles of solute per 1000gm of solvent and represented by "m".

Mole fraction of solute: No of moles of solute divided by total moles of solute and solvents.

Calculation of Equivalent Weight

Equivalent weight of any compound = Formula or molecular weight/x

(where x is a factor = basicity for acid,acidity for base, charge present on ion, change in Oxidation number for reducing or oxidizing agent)

Standardisation: It is a process by which the precise concentration of a solution is determined or fixed.

Primary Standard: It is the purest form of reagent which is used to prepare astandard solution. The purity is above 99.9%v. It shows stable weight at room temperature.It does not absorb moisture.

Secondary standard reagent: The reagents which can not be obtained in the 100% pure form, they show weight variation with change in time and temperature. They are hygroscopic in nature.

Titration Error: The difference between the equivalence point and end point. It is sometimes called indicator error, if indicator is used as a means of detecting end point.

Blank Titration: It is the type of titration in which the solution does notcontain the analyte of interest. It is always carried out to estimate the amountof titration error

Direct titration: Is the most common form of titration in which titrant is added to the analyte until reaction is complete

Back titration: It is the type of titration necessary when direct titration does not give clear or sharp end point. It involves adding a known excess of the standard reagent to the analyte. Then a second standard reagent is used to titrate the excess of the first reagent so as known the amount of first standard reagent that is consumed by the analyte.

Importance of Volumetric Analysis
1. High precision is obtained
2. Simple apparatus is required
3. Easy process and fast result
4. Different methods for different types of substance

Mole Concept

A mole (abbreviated mol) is the amount of substance which contains the same number of specified units as there are atoms in 12grams of carbon (C_{12}). These specified or elementary units could be atoms, molecules, ions etc.

Results show that 12grams of carbon–12 contains 6.02×10^{23} atoms.

One mole each of different compounds or elements or molecules contains the same number of fundamental units which is the constant 6.02×10^{23} referred to as the Avogadro's constant though they have different masses.

Molar Mass (M)

The molar mass, M of a substance is it's relative atomic, molecular or formular mass expressed in grams. It is the mass of one mole of that substance. It is expressed in grams per mole. (e.g. the molar mass M of NaCl is 58.5g/mol)

Exercise: use the above derivation to find the mass of 0.015mol of Baking soda ($NaHCO_3$) given that the molar mass of baking soda is 84g/mol [23 + 1 + 12 + (16 × 3)]

Percentage by mass of an Element in a Compound

Here, the knowledge of molar mass and atomic mass of various elements is employed to find the % by mass of any element in a compound.

Example: Find the % by mass of sodium and Oxygen in baking soda ($NAHCO_3$)

Solution: mass of NaHCO3 is $23 + 1 + 12 + (16 \times 3) = 84$

   i. % by mass of sodium $= 23/84 \times 100\% = 27.38$

   ii. % by mass of Oxygen $= 48/84 \times 100\% = 57.14$

ACIDS

Acid is defined in different ways.

An acid could be defined as substance that reacts with water to produce excess hydroxonium ions (H_3O^+).

It is also defined as a substance that ionizes in water to produce H^+ or H_3O^+ as the only positive ions in solution.

Strong and Weak Acids

A strong acid is one that ionizes almost completely in water. A strong acid releases a large number of H+ when in solution.(like HCl)

On the other hand, a weak acid is one that ionizes only slightly. It releases only very few hydrogen ions in solution. (CH_3COOH)

Examples of ACIDS (Daily Life): Hydrochloric acid (HCl) in gastric juice, Sulphuric acid (H_2SO4), Nitric acid (HNO_3), Carbonic acid in soft drink (H_2CO_3), Uric acid in urine, Ascorbic acid (Vitamin C) in fruit, Citric acid in oranges and lemons, Acetic acid in vinegar, Tannic acid (in tea and wine), Tartaric acid (in grapes)

Basicity: The basicity of an acid is the number of ionizable hydrogen in one mole of the acid.

Acid	Formula	Ionizatin	Basicity
Hydrochloric acid	HCl	$HCl + H_2O = H_3O + (aq) + Cl^- (aq)$	1
Nitric acid	HNO_3	$HNO_3 + H_2O = H_3O+(aq)\ NO_3\text{-}(aq) +$	1
Sulphuric acid	H_2SO_4	$H_2SO_4 + 2H_2O = 2H_3O + (aq) + SO_4^- (aq)$	2

Concentrated and Dilute Acids

If there is only a little water present with the acid, the solution is concentrated. And if a lot of water is present, the acid is said to be dilute.

Caution: It is dangerous to add water to concentrated acids. A dilute solution can be made by pouring the acid carefully into water.

Physical Properties of Acids

- Corrosive ('burns' your skin)
- Sour taste (e.g. lemons, vinegar)

- Contains hydrogen ions (H+) when dissolved in water and has a pH less than 7
- Turns blue litmus paper to a red colour

BASES

Bases are substances that cancel the effect of an acid. More appropriately, a base is defined as a substance that neutralizes the effect of an acid to form a salt and water. Bases are usually metal oxides or metal hydroxides.

Examples of Bases and Alkalis (daily life)

- Sodium hydroxide (NaOH) or caustic soda
- Calcium hydroxide ($Ca(OH)_2$) or limewater
- Ammonium hydroxide (NH_4OH) or ammonia water
- Magnesium hydroxide ($Mg(OH)_2$) or milk of magnesia
- Many bleaches, soaps, toothpastes and cleaning agents have base

Alkalis: Alkalis are bases that are soluble in water. Examples of alkalis are sodium hydroxide NaOH, Potassium hydroxide KOH, Calcium hydroxide $Ca(OH)_2$ and Ammonia NH_3. Alkalis release hydroxide ions (OH^-) in solution. On this note then, when acid (which release H^+ or H_3O^+) and alkalis are mixed, the following reaction takes place.

$$H^+ + OH^- = H_2O$$

OR

$$H_3O^+ + OH^- = 2H_2O$$

Strong and Weak Alkalis

Strong alkalis are those that ionize completely in water to release many hydroxide ions into solution. E.g. NaOH and KOH.

Ammonia and calcium hydroxide are said to be weak acids because they ionize to form only few hydroxide ions in solution.

$$NH_3(aq) + H_2O = NH^+_4(aq) + OH^- (aq)$$

Properties of Bases and Alkalis

- Corrosive ('burns' your skin), Soapy feel, Has a pH more than 7, Turns red litmus paper to a blue colour,Many alkalis (soluble bases) contain hydroxyl ions (OH^-), Reacts with acids to form salt and water.

pH Measurement

pH is a measure of the acidity or alkalinity of a substance. pH is measured using the pH meter. The pH scale ranges from 0 to 14 and it is a convenient

way to express hydrogen ion concentration in a given solution.
Mathematically, $\qquad$ pH $= - \log(H^+)$

Summary Table of Common ACIDS/BASES with pH

Common Acids	pH	Common Bases	pH
Hydrochloric acid	0.1	Human saliva	6-8
Sulphuric acid	0.3	Distilled water	7
Stomach juice	1-3	Blood plasma	7.4
Lemons	2.3	Eggs	7.8
Vinegar	2.9	Seawater	7.9
Apples	3.1	Borax	9.2
Oranges	3.5	Milk of magnesia	10.5
Grapes	4	Ammonia water	11.6
Sour milk	4.4	Limewater	12.4
White bread	5.5	Caustic soda	14
Fresh milk	6.5		

Indicators

Indicators are substances which change colour when acids or alkalis are added to them. They are often made from vegetables or flowers.

The table below shows common indicators

Indicator	Colour in alkaline solution	Colour in neutral solution	Colour in acidic solution	Type of titration
Methyl orange	Yellow	Orange	Pink	Strong acid vs. strong base
Phenolphthalein	Pink	Colourless	Colourless	Weak acid vs. strong base
Litmus	Blue	Purple	Red	

- Universal indicator-Universal indicator is a mixture of different indicators which gives a range of colours. These colours indicate a degree of acidity on a numerical scale called the pH scale. This means that when universal indicator is added to a solution, one of the colours above will be observed. For instance if the solution changes blue, it implies the pH of that particular solution is either 9, 10 or 11 and so on.

Types of Volumetric analysis

There are four common types of titration

- Acid-Base titration
- Complexometric titration
- Oxidation-Reduction(Redox) titration.
- Precipitation titration

Acid-Base titration

The chemical reaction involved in acid-base titration is known as neutralisation reaction. It involves the combination of H_3O^+ ions with OH^- ions to form water. In acid – base titrations, solutions of alkali are titrated against standard acid solutions. The estimation of an alkali solution using a standard solution is called *acidimetry*. Similarly, the estimation of an acid solution using a standard alkali solution is called *alkalimetry*. Determination of alkalinity(alkaline nature) of water sample by titration against standard HCl solution is the example of this type.

For alkalinity of water, unknown water sample is taken with the help of pipette (say-20ml) in the conical flask and then 2-3 drops of indicator (phenolphthalein/methy orange) is added.standard (N/10) HCl solution is taken in the burette and titrated till the end point is reached. Volume of std solution is measured from burette (say 1ml is used) and then calclulation is done by using normality equation

(No. of gm eqwts of unknown solution) = (No.of gm eqwts of
                                                                        known (std) solution)

$$N_1V_1 = N_2V_2$$
$$N \times 20 = 1 \times 1/10$$
$$N = 1/200$$

Strength of alkalinity $S = N \cdot E$

$$= 1/200 \times 61 \quad \text{(as a } HCO_3^-\text{), gm/l}$$
$$= 1000 \times 61/200 = 305 \text{ mg/l or ppm}$$

In acid base titrations, a base is added to an acid successively (or vice versa) and the pH of the solution is noted after every addition. The plot of pH against the amount of base (or acid) added is called a titration curve. Titration curves can be studied for various types of acid base titrations.

Titration of weak acid and weak base—

This type of titration is carried out between a weak acid such as acetic acid ($CH_3 COOH$) and weak base such as ammonium hydroxide (NH_4OH). There is no sharp change in the pH during the titration. Hence, no sharp equivalence point can be obtained with common indicators.

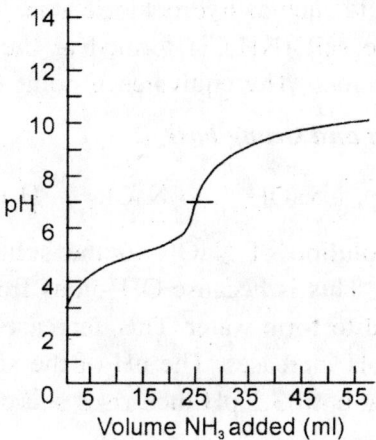

Fig. 1.1: Titration curve of weak base (NH₄OH) and weak acid (CH₂COOH)

Titration of weak acid and a strong base—

$$CH_3COOH_{(aq)} + NaOH_{(aq)} \rightarrow CH_3COONa_{(aq)} + H_2O(I)$$

This type of titration is carried out between acetic acid and sodium hydroxide. The free H+ion from the weak acid is neutralized by OH–ions from the base and there is a small increase in pH. Around the equivalence point large increase in pH is observed.

Titration of weak base and a strong acid—

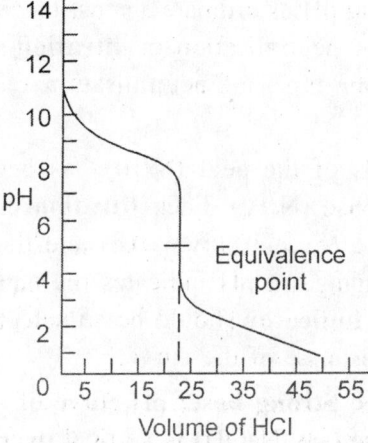

Fig. 1.2: The pH titration curve of weak base (NH₄OH) and strong acid (HCl)

This type of titration is carried out between a weak base such as ammonium hydroxide and strong acid such as hydrochloric acid. The equivalence point is below 7 because the salt (NH₄Cl) formed at the neutralization reacts with water to give H + ions. The equivalence point lies at about pH 5.3.

Titration of strong acid and strong base–

$$HCl_{(aq)} + NaOH_{(aq)} \rightarrow NaCl_{(aq)} + H_2O(l)$$

When we add a solution of NaOH to the solution of HCl, the pH progressively increases. This is because OH - ions from the base will react with H⁺ ions of the acid to form water. This decreases the concentration of H⁺ ions and therefore pH increases. The pH of the solution increases only slightly in the beginning until 3.3 pH then rises sharply upto near 10.5 pH.

Indicators:

Selection of suitable indicator or choice of indicator for acid–base titrations

The neutralisation reactions are of the following four types:

    (i)   A strong acid versus a strong base.

    (ii) A weak acid versus a strong base.

    (iii) A strong acid versus a weak base.

    (iv) A weak acid versus a weak base.

In order to choose a suitable **indicator,** it is necessary to understand the pH changes in the above four types of **titrations**. The change in pH in the vicinity of theequivalence point is most important for this purpose. The curve obtained by plotting pH as ordinate against the volume of alkali added as abscissa is known as neutralisation or **titration curve**. The **titration curves** of the above four types of neutralisation reactions are shown in Fig. 1.3.

In each case 25 mL of the acid (N/10) has been **titrated** against a standard solution of a base (N/10). Each **titration curve** becomes almost vertical for somedistance (except curve 10.4) and then bends away again. This region of abrupt change in pH indicates the equivalence point. For a particular **titration**, the **indicator** should be so selected that it changes its colour within vertical distance of the curve.

    (i) Strong acid vs. Strong base: pH curve of strong acid (say HCl) and strong base (say NaOH) is vertical over almost the pH range 4-10. So the indicators **phenolphthalein** (pH range 8.3 to 10.5), methyl red (pH range 4.4-6.5) and **methyl orange** (pH range 3.2-4.5) are suitable for such a **titration**.

(ii) Weak acid vs. Weak base: pH curve of weak acid (say CH_3COOH of oxalic acid) and strong base (say NaOH) is vertical over the approximate pH range 7 to 11. So phenolphthalein is the suitable indicator for such a titration.

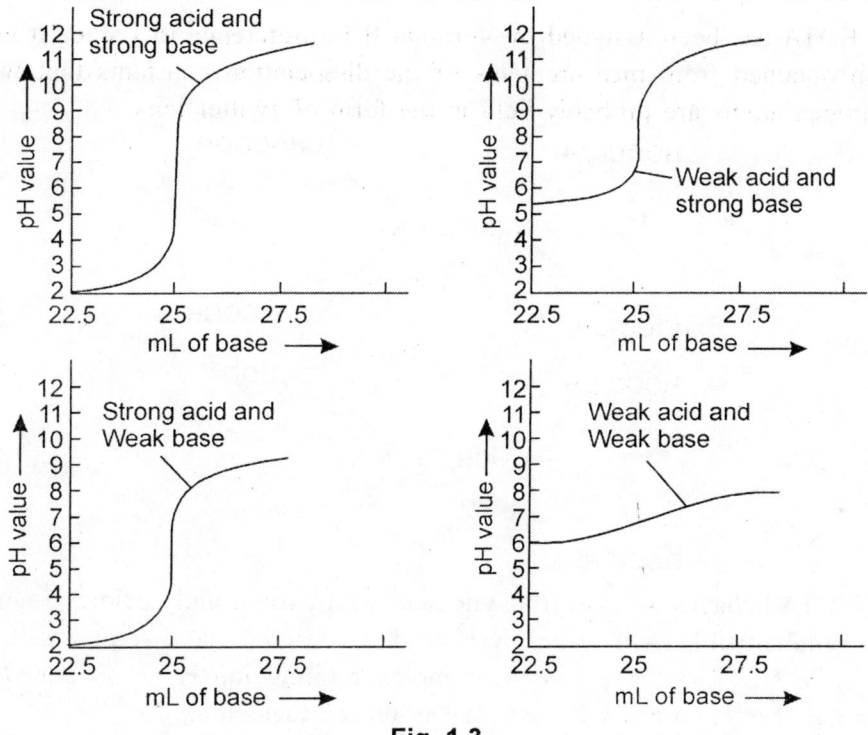

Fig. 1.3

Complexometric Titration

Principle and theory: Complexometric titration (sometimes chelatometry) is a form of *volumetric analysis* in which the formation of a colored complex is used to indicate the end point of a titration. Complexometric titrations are particularly useful for the determination of different metal ions in the solution. In this type of titration, chelating or complexing agent is used as a standard solution, which forms complex/chelate with the metal ions present in the solution at particular pH. An *indicator* capable of producing an unambiguous color change is usually used to detect the end-point of the titration. Ca++/Mg++ ions or hardness determination is the common example of this type.

Ethylene diamine tetra acetic acid (EDTA) is a very common chelating or complexing agent which has four carboxyl groups and two amine groups that can act as electron pair donors, or Lewis bases. The ability of EDTA to potentially donate its six lone pairs of electrons for the formation of coordinate covalent bonds to metal cations makes EDTA a hexadentate ligand. However, in practice EDTA is usually only partially ionized, and thus forms fewer than six coordinate covalent bonds with metal cations.

EDTA has been assigned the formula II in preference to I since it has been obtained from measurements of the dissociation constants that two hydrogen atoms are probably held in the form of zwitter ions.

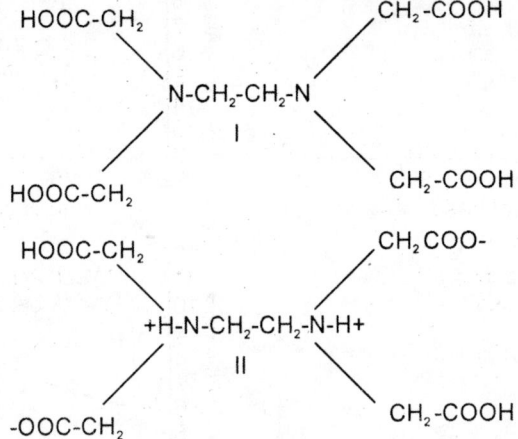

EDTA behaves as a dicarboxylic acid with two strongly acidic groups. For simplicity EDTA may be given the formula H_4Y, the disodium salt is therefore Na_2H_2Y and it has the complex forming ion H_2Y^{2-} in aqueous solution. The reactions with cationsmay be represented as;

$$M^{2+} + H_2Y_2^- \rightarrow MY^{2-} + 2H^+$$

$$M^{3+} + H_2Y_2^- \rightarrow MY^- + 2H^+$$

$$M^{4+} + H_2Y_2^- \rightarrow MY + 2H^+$$

One gram ion of the complex-forming ion H_2Y^{2-} reacts in all cases with one gram ion of the metal. EDTA forms complexes with metal ions in basic solutions. In acid-base titrations the end point is detected by a pH sensitive indicator. In the EDTA titration metal ion indicator is used to detect changes of pM. It is the negative logarithm of the free metal ion concentration, i.e., $pM = -\log[M^{2+}]$. Metal ion complexes form complexes with specific metal ions. These differ in colour from the free indicator and a sudden colour change occurs at the end point. End point can be detected usually with an indicator or instrumentally by potentiometric or conductometric (electrometric) method.

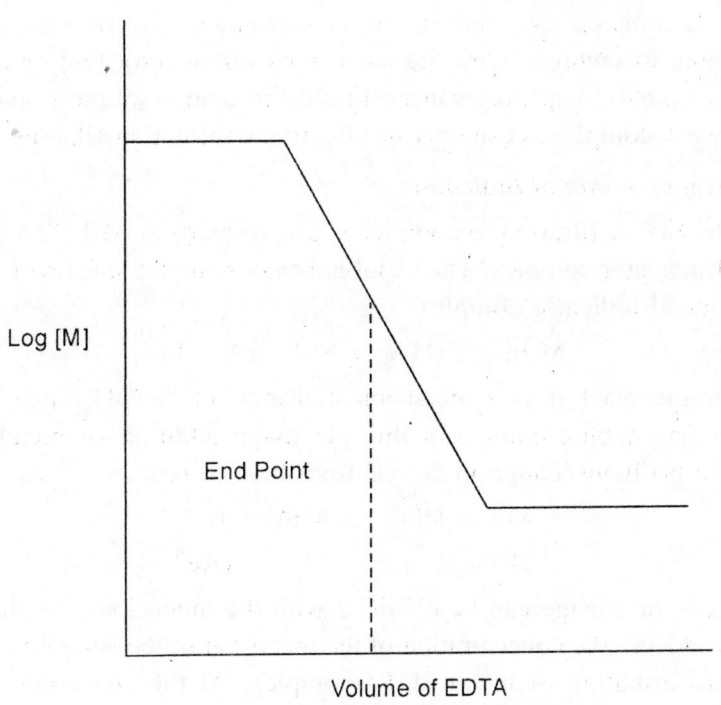

Log [M]

End Point

Volume of EDTA

Fig. 1.4

There are three factors that are important in determining the magnitude of break in titration curve at end point.

- **The stability of complex formed:** The greater the stability constant for complex formed, larger the charge in free metal concentration (pM) at equivalent point and more clear would be the end point.
- **The number of steps involved in complex formation:** Fewer the number of steps required in the formation of the complex, greater would be the break in titration curve at equivalent point and clearer would be the end point.
- **Effect of pH:** During a complexometric titration, the pH must be constant by use of a buffer solution. Control of pH is important since the H^+ ion plays an important role in chelation. Most ligands are basic and bind to H^+ ions throughout a wide range of pH. Some of these H^+ ions are frequently displaced from the ligands (chelating agents) by the metal during chelate formation.
- Equation below shows complexation between metal ion and H^+ ion for ligand:

$$M_2^+ + H_2\text{-EDTA} \rightarrow \text{M-EDTA} + 2H^+$$

Thus, stability of metal complex is pH dependent. Lower the pH of the solution, lesser would be the stability of complex (because more H^+ ions are available to compete with the metal ions for ligand). Only metals that form very stable complexes can be titrated in acidic solution, and metals forming weak complexes can only be effectively titrated in alkaline solution.

Mechanism of action of indicator:

During an EDTA titration 2 complexes are formed: i) M-EDTA complex and ii) M-indicator complex. The metal-indicator complex must be less stable than the metal-indicator complex.

$$M\text{-}In + EDTA \rightarrow M\text{-}EDTA + In$$

Erichrome black T is a metal ion indicator. In the pH range 7-11 the dye itself has a blue colour. In this pH range addition of metallic salts produces a brilliant change in colour from blue to red.

$$M^{2+} + HIn^{2-} \rightarrow MIn^- + H^+$$

$$\text{(Blue)} \qquad\qquad \text{(Red)}$$

This colour change can be obtained with the metal ions. As the EDTA solution is added, the concentration of the metal ion in the solution decreases due to the formation of metal-EDTA complex. At the end point no more free metal ions are present in the solution. At this stage, the free indicator is liberated and hence the colour changes from red to blue.

Indicators used in complexometric titrations are as follows:

S.No.	Name of indicator	Colour change	pH range	Metals detected
1.	Mordant black II Eriochrome black T Solochrome black T	Red to Blue	6-7	Ca,Ba Mg,Zn,Cd,Mn,Pb,Hg
2.	Murexide or Ammonium purpurate	Violet to Blue	12	Ca,cu,Co
3.	Catechol-violet	Violet to Red	8-10	Mn,Mg,Fe,Co,Pb
4.	Methyl Blue Thymol Blue	Blue to Yellow Blue to Grey	4-5 10-12	Pb,Zn,Cd,Hg
5.	Alizarin	Red to Yellow	4.3	Pb,Zn,Co,Mg,Cu
6.	Sodium Alizarin sulphonate	Blue to Red	4	Al, Thorium
7·	Xylenol range	Lemon to Yellow	1-3	Bi, Thorium
			4-5	Pb, Zn
			5-6	Cd, Hg

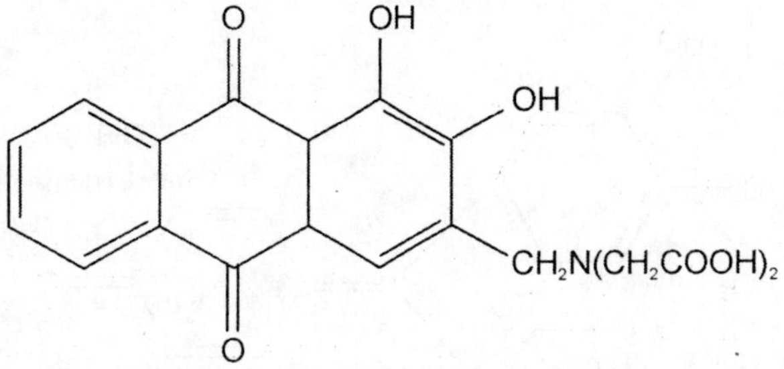

Alzarin fluorine blue (alizarin complexone)

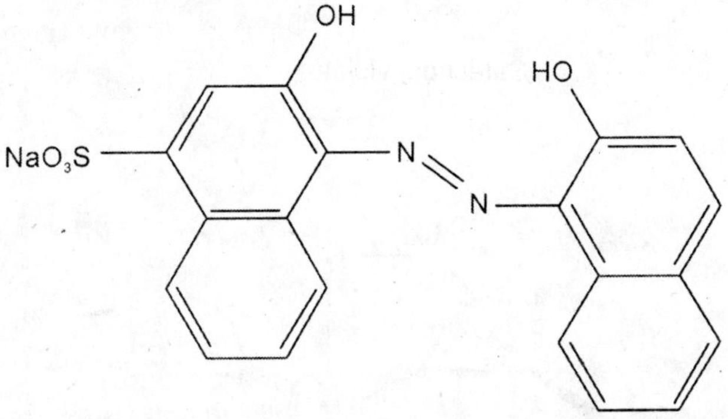

Calcone (mordant black 17)
Eriochrome Blue Black R

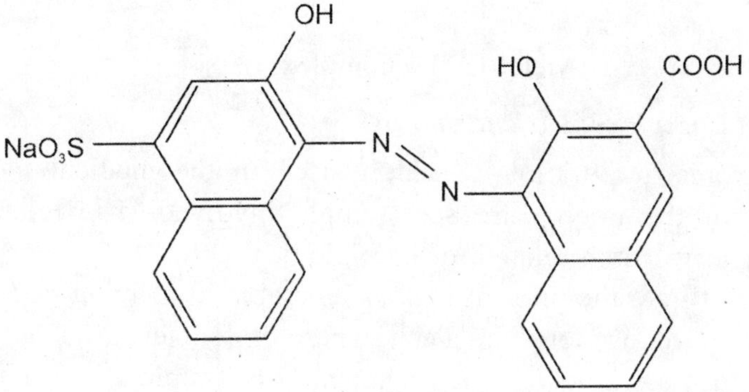

Calcone carboxylic acid

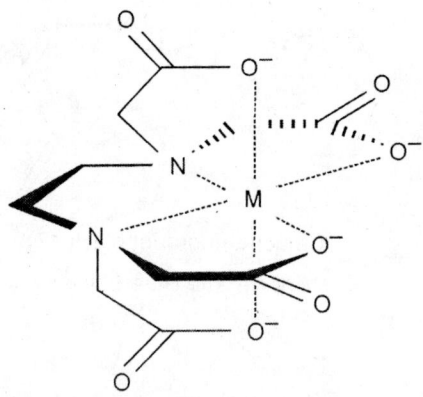

Catechol - violet

(Metal-EDTA complex

Applications of Complexometric titration:

- Complexometric titration is widely used in the medical industry because of the micro litre size sample involved. The method is efficient in research related to the biological cell.
- Ability to titrate the amount of ions available in a living cell.
- Ability to introduce ions into a cell in case of deficiencies. Complexometric titration involves the treatment of complex ions such as magnesium, calcium, copper, iron, nickel, lead and zinc with EDTA as the complexing agent.
- Complexometric titration is an efficient method for determining the level of hardness of water.

Types of Complexometric titration:

As mentioned earlier, EDTA is a versatile chelating titrant that has been used in innumerable complexometric determinations. The versatility of EDTA can be ascribed to the different ways in which the complexometric titration can be executed. Let us learn about different ways in which we can use EDTA titrations.

1. **Direct Titration:** It is the simplest and the most convenient method in which the standard solution of EDTA is slowly added to the metal ion solution till the end point is achieved. It is similar to simple acid-base titrations. For this method to be useful the formation constant must be large and the indicator must provide a very distinct colour change as mentioned earlier. Further we need standardized solution of EDTA and sometimes auxiliary complexing agents may be required. Some important elements which could be determined directly by the complexometric titration are Cu, Mn, Ca, Ba, Br, Zn, Cd, Hg, Al, Sn, Pb, Bi, Cr, Mo, Fe, Co, Ni, and Pd, etc. However, the presence of other ions may cause interference and need to be suitably handled.

2. **Back Titration:** In this method, an excess of a standard solution of EDTA is added to the metal solution being determined so as to complex all the metal ions present in the solution. The excess of EDTA left after the complex formation with the metal is back titrated with a standard solution of a second metal ion. This method becomes necessary if the analyte precipitates in the absence of EDTA or reacts too slowly with EDTA, or it blocks the indicator. For example, determination of Mn is done by this method because a direct titration is not possible due to precipitation of $Mn(OH)_2$. The excess EDTA remaining after complexation, is back titrated with a standard Zn solution using Eriochrome black T as indicator. However, one has to ensure the standard metal ion should not displace the analyte ion from their EDTA complex.

3. **Replacement Titration:** When direct or back titrations do not give sharp endpoints or when there is no suitable indicator for the analyte the metal may be determined by this method. The metal to be analyzed is added to a metal-EDTA complex. The analyte ion (with higher K_f) displaces EDTA from the metal and the metal is subsequently titrated with standard EDTA. For example, in the determination of Mn an excess of Mg EDTA chelate is added to Mn solution. The Mn ions quantitatively displace Mg from Mg-

EDTA solution because Mn forms a more stable complex with EDTA. The freed Mg metal is then directly titrated with a standard solution of EDTA using Eriochrome black T indicator. Ca, Pb and Hg may also be determined by this method.

4. **Indirect Titration:** Certain anions that form precipitate with metal cations and do not react with EDTA can be analyzed indirectly. The anion is first precipitated with a metal cation and the precipitate is washed and boiled with an excess of disodium EDTA solution to form the metal complex. The protons from disodium EDTA are displaced by a heavy metal and titrated with sodium alkali. Therefore, this method is also called alkalimetric titration. For example, barbiturates can be determined by this method.

Redox titration:

Principle: Determination of strength of unknown reducing agent by titration with standard oxidizing agent or vice versa is known as redox titration.

A reaction in which one or more electrons are lost is known as *oxidation* and a reaction in which one or more electrons are gained is known as *reduction*. Accordingly, a substance which can accept one or more electrons is known as *oxidizing agent* and a substance which can donate one or more electrons is called reducing agent. Titrations of this type are called *redox titrations*. Thus, redox titrations are those involving transfer of electrons from the reducing agent to the oxidizing agent.

Potassium permanganate, potassium dichromate, ceric sulphate, etc., are the common oxidizing agents used in redox titrations. Oxalic acid, Mohr's salt, arsenious oxide, etc., are the reducing agents commonly used in redox titrations.

Types-Redox (Iodine) titrations are of two types viz iodometry and iodimetry.

Iodometry and iodimetry:

An example of a redox titration is treating a solution of iodine with a reducing agent and using starch as indicator. Iodine forms an intensely blue complex with starch. Iodine (I_2) can be reduced to iodide (I'') by e.g. thiosulphate ($S_2O_3^{2''}$), and when all iodine is spent the blue colour disappears. When iodine solution is directly used for the estimation of reducing agents, the titration is called iodimetric titration (iodimetry).

While in the other type Iodine is not directly used, but iodine is liberated, The titrations involving the iodine liberated in a chemical reaction is called *iodometric titration (iodometry)*. Iodine is a mild oxidizing agent. In the presence of a suitable reducing agent it gets reduced to iodine ion, I^-. In addition to this, all oxidizing agents having electrode potential greater than 0.54 V can oxidize I^- to I_2.

In iodimetric titrations, free iodine is used. Since it is difficult to prepare the solution of iodine (iodine sublimates and is less soluble in water) it is dissolved in KI solution.

$$KI + I_2 \rightarrow KI_3$$

This solution is first standardized before use. With the standard solution of I_2, substances such as sulfite, thiosulphate, arsenite are estimated.

In iodometric titrations, an oxidizing agent is allowed to react in neutral medium or in acidic medium with excess of KI to liberate free iodine.

$$KI + \text{oxidizing agent} \rightarrow I_2$$

Free iodine is titrated against a standard reducing agent usually with sodium thiiosulfate. Halogens, oxyhalogens, cupric ions, peroxides etc can be estimated by this method.

$$I_2 + Na_2S_2O_3 \rightarrow 2NaI + Na_2S_2O_4$$

$$2CuSO_4 + 4KI \rightarrow Cu_2I_2 + 2K_2SO_4 + I_2$$

$$K_2Cr_2O_7 + 6KI + 7H_2SO_4 \rightarrow Cr_2(SO4)_3 + 4K_2SO_4 + 7H_2O + 3I2$$

In both iodometric and iodimetric titrations, starch is used as an indicator. Starch solution gives a blue or violet color with free iodine. At the end point the blue or violet color disappears when iodine is completely changed to iodide.

Iodometric (oxidation of iodide) titrations comprise of two steps –

In the first step oxidizing agents such as $KMnO4$, $K_2Cr_2O_7$, $CuSO_4$, peroxides etc are treated with an excess of KI when iodine is liberated quickly and quantitatively. For eg.

$$2MnO4^- + 16\ H^+ + 10\ I \rightarrow 2Mn^{2+} + 5I_2 + 8H2O$$

$$Cr2O7\ 2^- + 14\ H^+ + 6I^- \rightarrow 2Cr3^+ + 3I_2 + 7H_2O$$

$$2Cu2^+ + 4I^- \rightarrow Cu_2I_2 + I_2$$

In the second step-

The liberated iodine is titrated against a standard solution of sodium thiosulfate using starch as an indicator. All such titrations in which iodine is liberated from potassium iodide with the help of an oxidizing reagent and is titrated against a standard solution of sodium thiosulfate are called iodometric titrations.

Reactions of some compounds with iodide are given as:

M nO$_4^-$

$$2MnO_4^- + 10I^- + 16H^+ \rightarrow Mn^{2+} + 5I_2 + 8H_2O$$

$Cr_2O_7^-$

$$Cr_2O_7^{2-} + 6I^- + 14H^+ \rightarrow 2Cr^{3+} + I_2 + 7H_2O$$

IO_3^-

$$IO_3^- + 5I^- + 6H^+ \rightarrow 3I_2 + 3H_2O$$

BrO_3^-

$$BrO_3^- + 6I^- + 6H^+ \rightarrow Br^- + 3I_2 + 3H_2O$$

$Cr4^+$

$$2Cr^{4+} + 2I^- \rightarrow 2Cr^{3+} + I_2$$

$Fe3^+$

$$2Fe^{3+} + 2I^- \rightarrow 2Fe^{2+} + I_2$$

H_2O_2

$$H_2O_2 + 2I^- + 2H^+ \rightarrow 2H_2O + I_2$$

Cu^{2+}

$$2Cu^{2+} + 2I^- \rightarrow 2Cu\ I + I_2$$

O_3

$$O_3 + 2I^- + 2H^+ \rightarrow O2 + H_2 + H_2O$$

Cl_2

$$Cl2 + 2I^- \rightarrow 2\ Cl^- + I_2$$

In an Iodimetric titrations (reduction of iodine) the direct use of iodine as an oxidizing agent in neutral or slightly acidic medium using starch as an indicator is made. The various reducing agents used in these titrations are thiosulfates, sulfites, arsenites or antimonites.

$$I_2 + S_2O_3^{2-} \rightarrow 2I^- + S_4O_6^{2-}$$
thiosulfate   to   tetra thionate

$$I_2 + SO_3^{2-} + H_2O \rightarrow 2I^- + SO_4^{2-} + 2H^+$$
sulfite   to   sulfate

$H_2S + I_2 \rightarrow S + 2I^- + 2H^+$

$Sn^{2+} + I_2 \rightarrow Sn^{4+} + 2I^-$

$N_2H_4 + 2I_2 \rightarrow N_2 + 4H^+ + 4I^-$

Problem-A mixture of $K_2Cr_2O_7$ and $KMnO_4$ was treated with excess of KI in an acidic medium. The iodine liberated required 100 cc of 0.15 N sodium thiosulfate solution for titration. The % amount of each can now be determined.

The redox changes that occur in the reaction mixture are -

$5e + Mn^{7+} \rightarrow Mn^{2+}$ (reduction)

$6e + Cr_2^{6+} \rightarrow 2Cr^{3+}$ (reduction)

$2I^{1-} \rightarrow I_2 + 2e$ (oxidation)

$2S_2O_3 \rightarrow S_4O_6^{2-} + 2e$ (oxidation)

We can now calculate the amount of dichromate and permanganate.

Let the amount of dichromate and permanganate be a and b gms

$$a + b = 0.5 \text{ g Equation 1}$$

milli eq of dichromate + milli eq of permanganate = milli eq of Iodine = milli eq of sodium thiosulfate

$a/294/6 \times 1000 + b/158/5 \times 1000 = 100 \times 0.15$ Equation 2

From eqns 1 and 2

$$a = 0.073 \text{ and } b = 0.427$$

Therefore % of dichromate is 14.6% and % of permanganate is 85.4%

Precipitation Titration:

A precipitation titration is one in which the titrant forms a precipitate with the analyte. Basic principle is that when product of ionic concentrations of ions becomes more than the solubility product of the electrolyte then precipitation occurs

For example, the compound AB is precipitated when

Conc.of $(A^+)(B^-) > K_{sp}(AB)$

Similarly precipitation of AgCl in the solution of chloride ions occurs by adding $AgNO_3$ solution, when

Conc.of $(Ag^+)(Cl^-) > K_{sp}(AgCl)$

Precipitation frequently proceeds slowly or starts after some time. Many precipitates show a tendency to adsorb and thereby coprecipitate the species being titrated or the titrant. The indicator may also be adsorbed on the precipitate formed during the titration and thereby be unable to function appropriately at the end point. If a precipitate is highly coloured, visual detection of colour change at the end point may be impossible, but even where a white precipitate is formed like AgCl; the milky solution may still make location of the end point difficult. Due to these difficulties, precipitation titrations are not so popular in present–day routine analysis. The major areas of application include the determination of silver or halides by the precipitation of the silver salts (argentometric titrations) and the determination of sulphate by precipitation as barium sulphate

A precipitation titration curve has the same general shape as that of a strong acid titrated with a strong base in the case where the precipitate has very low solubility. It is shaped like the curve for the titration of a weak acid with a strong base when a more soluble precipitate is formed. As an example of the former, consider the titration of

100 ml of 0.01 M KI with the 0.1000 M AgNO3 titrant. The reaction is

$$Ag^+ + I^- \rightarrow AgI(s)$$

and the AgI product has a relatively low solubility product,

$$Ksp = [Ag^+] [I^-] = 1.0 \times 10^{-16}$$

In 100.0 ml of 0.0100 M I^- there is initially

100 ml $\times$ 0.01000 mmol/ml = 1.000 mmol of I^-

This requires the addition of 1.000 mmol of Ag^+

to precipitate all the I^- corresponding to a total of 10.00 ml of Ag^+ to reach the equivalence point.

Major Regions of a Precipitation Titration Curve:

There are three major regions of the titration curve i) prior to the equivalence point, ii) at the equivalence point where exactly 10.00 ml of Ag^+ titrant have been added, and iii) beyond the equivalence point where Ag^+ is in excess. Initially at 0 ml added titrant, no Ag^+ has been added and it is not possible to calculate a meaningful value of [Ag^+]. The addition of 1.00 ml of Ag^+titrant correspond to (1.00 ml Ag^+)(0.1000 m mol/ml) = 0.1000 m mol added Ag^+

According to above reaction ($Ag^+ + I^- \rightarrow AgI(s)$) the precipitates 0.1000 mmol of I^-, leaving 0.900 mmol I^- in 100.0 + 1.0 = 101.0 ml of solution. The concentration of I^- is [I^-] = 0.900 mmol/101.0 ml = 8.91 $\times$ 10^{-3} M. Both the unreacted KI and the slightly soluble AgI contribute to the species concentration of iodide ion. Thus, the equilibrium concentration of I^- is larger than the analytical concentration of KI by an amount equal to the molar solubility of the precipitate.

$$[I^-] = 8.91 \times 10^{-3} + [Ag^+]$$

$$[I^-] = 8.91 \times 10^{-3} + Ksp/[I^-]$$

Since, $[Ag^+] = Ksp/[I^-]$

The contribution of the AgI to the equilibrium iodide concentration is equal to $[Ag^+]$ because one silver ion is formed for each iodide ion from this source. Unless the concentration of KI is very small, this term can be neglected The values of $[Ag^+]$ and log Ag^+ are then calculated as follows:

$$[Ag+] = Ksp/[I^-] = 1.00 \times 10^{-16}/8.91 \times 10^{-3}$$

$$= 1.12 \times 10^{-14}M$$

$$\log [Ag^+] = \log 1.12 \times 10^{-14} = -13.95, + Ag\ p = 13.95$$

prior to the equivalence point and after it are calculated in an identical manner.

Plot of a Precipitation Titration Curve

The titration curve for the titration of 100 ml of 0.0100 M KI with 0.1000 M AgNO$_3$ plotted from the data is shown in Fig. The equivalence point volume corresponds to the point half way up on the titration curve break. A vertical line drawn from this point to the volume axis would intersect it at

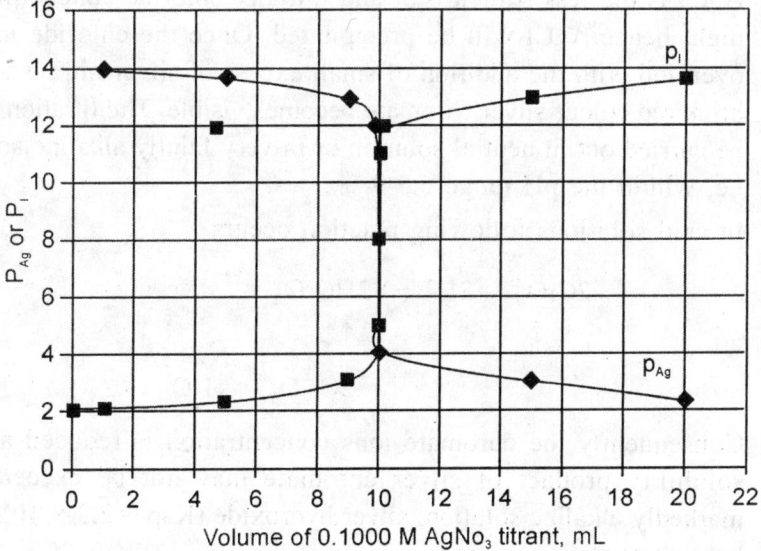

Fig.1.5: Curve for the titration of 100.0 ml of 0.0100 M KI with 0.1000 M AgNO$_3$

the equivalence volume of exactly 10.00 ml. This point could be determined graphically by the method similar to the titration of an acid with a base. Note that the break in this titration curve is extremely steep and the equivalence point could be readily found. Furthermore, if the general shape of the titration curve is known, only three points, commonly those at 50%, 100% and 150% titrated (5, 10 and 15 ml in Fig.) are enough to produce a reasonable sketch of the titration curve.

Another example. The most important precipitation process in titrimetric analysis utilizes silver nitrate as the reagent (Argentimetric process).

$$Ag^+_{(aq)} + Cl^-_{(aq)} \rightleftharpoons AgCl_{(s)}$$

Many methods are utilized in determining end points of these reactions, but the most important method, the formation of a coloured precipitate will be considered here.

1. In the titration of a neutral solution of chloride ions with silver nitrate, a small quantity of potassium chromate solution is added to serve as the indicator. At the end point the chromate ions combine with silver ions to form the sparingly soluble brick-red silver chromate. This is a case of fractional precipitation, the two sparingly soluble salts being AgCl (Ksp = 1.2×10^{-10}) and Ag_2CrO_4 (Ksp = 1.7×10^{-12}).

    AgCl is the less soluble salt and initially chloride concentration is high, hence AgCl will be precipitated. Once the chloride ions are over and with the addition of small excess of silver nitrate solution brick red colour silver chromate becomes visible. The titration should be carried out in neutral solution or in very faintly alkaline solution. i.e. within the pH range 6.5-9.

    In acid solutions following reaction occurs.

    $$2CrO_4^{2-} + 2H^+ \rightleftharpoons 2HCrO_4^-$$
    $$\uparrow\downarrow$$
    $$2Cr_2O_7^{2-} + H_2O$$

    Consequently the chromate ions concentration is reduced and the solubility product of silver chromate may not be exceeded. In markedly alkaline solution, silver hydroxide (Ksp = $2.3 \times 10^{8)}$ might be precipitated.

2. The titration can be carried out with dichlorofluorescein as the indicator. Dichlorofluorescein is an example of an adsorption

indicator. Adsorption indicators have the interesting property of changing colour when they stick (adsorb) to the surface of a precipitate. During the titration the dichlorofluorescein molecules exist as negatively charged ions (anions) in solution. As the AgCl precipitate is forming, the excess Cl^- ions in the solution form a layer of negative charge on the precipitate surface. As the equivalence point is reached and passed, the excess Cl^- ions on the precipitate surface are replaced by excess Ag^+ ions, giving the surface a positive charge. The negatively charged indicator will be attracted to the positively charged precipitate surface where it absorbs and changes colour. The suspended precipitate will have a pink tinge because of some premature displacement of chloride ion by the dichlorofluorescein ion. When the pink colour starts to persist for slightly longer periods of time, the drip rate is lowered. The end point is reached when the entire solution turns pink. It is important that the AgCl precipitate be prevented from coagulation during the titration. For this reason a small amount of dextrin is added to the solution.

SOLVED PROBLEMS

Q.1. 0.2640 g of sodium oxalate is dissolved in a flask and requires 30.74 mL of potassium permanganate (from a burette) to titrate it and cause it to turn pink (the end point).

The equation for this reaction is:

$5Na_2C_2O_4(aq) + 2KMnO_4(aq) + 8H_2SO_4(aq) \rightarrow 2MnSO_4(aq) + K_2SO_4(aq) + 5Na_2SO_4(aq) + 10\ CO_2(g) + 8\ H_2O(l)$

(a) How many moles of sodium oxalate are present in the flask?

(b) How many moles of potassium permanganate have been titrated into the flask to reach the end point?

(c) What is the molarity of the potassium permanganate?

Ans.

Solution to (a):

0.2640 g/134.00 g/mol = 0.001970149 mol

to four sig figs, this would be 0.001970 mol

Solution to (b):

From the balanced equation, the oxalate-permanganate molar ratio is five to two.

0.001970149 mol oxalate times (2 mol permanganate/5 mol oxalate)
= 0.00078806 mol permanganate

to four sig figs, this is 0.0007881 mol

Solution to (c):

0.00078806 mol / 0.03074 L = 0.02564 M (to four sig figs)

Q.2: Potassium dichromate is used to titrate a sample containing an unknown percentage of iron. The sample is dissolved in H_3PO_4/ H_2SO_4 mixture to reduce all of the iron to Fe^{2+} ions. The solution is then titrated with 0.01625 M $K_2Cr_2O_7$, producing Fe^{3+} and Cr^{3+} ions in acidic solution. The titration requires 32.26 mL of $K_2Cr_2O_7$ for 1.2765 g of the sample.

(a) Balance the net ionic equation using the half-reaction method.

(b) Determine the percent iron in the sample.

(c) Is the sample ferrous iodate, ferrous phosphate, or ferrous acetate?

Ans.

Solution to (a):

$$6Fe^{2+} + Cr_2O_7^{2-} + 14H^+ \rightarrow 6\ Fe^{3+} + 2Cr^{3+} + 7H_2O$$

The mechanics of balancing is left to the reader.

The key point is the ferrous ion-dichromate molar ratio, which is six to one.

Solution to (b):

(1) Determine Fe(II) in solution:

(0.01625 mol/L) (0.03226 L) = 0.000524225 mol dichromate

0.000524225 mol times (6 mol Fe(II)/1 mol dichromate)

= 0.00314535 mol Fe(II)

0.00314535 mol Fe(II) times 55.845 g/mol = 0.175652 g

(2) Determine percent of iron in the sample:

0.175652 g / 1.2765 g = 13.76%

Solution to (c):

Which compound contains 13.76% iron? The only way to determine this is to calculate the percent composition of the three sbstances.

Ferrous iodate: $Fe(IO_3)_2$

% Fe: 55.845 g/mol divided by 405.67 g/mol = 13.77%

Here's the percent composition calculator I used to calculate the three percent compositions. Here are the other two substances in the question:

$$Fe_3(PO_4)_2 = 46.87\%$$
$$Fe(C_2H_3O_2)_2 = 32.11\ \%$$

Q.3: A solution contains both iron(II) and iron(III) ions. A 50.0 mL sample of the solution is titrated with 35.0 mL of 0.00280 M $KMnO_4$, which oxidizes Fe^{2+} to Fe^{3+}. The permangante ion is reduced to manganese(II) ion. Another 50.0 mL sample of solution is treated with zinc metal, which reduces all the Fe^{3+} to Fe^{2+}. The resulting solution is again titrated with 0.00280 M $KMnO_4$, this time 48.0 mL is required. What are the concentrations of Fe^{2+} and Fe^{3+} in the solution?

Solution:

1) The stoichiometric relationship of permangante to Fe(II):

$$5Fe^{2+} + 8H^+ + MnO_4^- \rightarrow 5Fe^{3+} + Mn^{2+} + 4H_2O$$

is five to one.

2) Calculate moles of Fe(II) reacted:

(0.00280 mol/L) (0.0350 L) = 0.000098 mol of MnO_4^-

(0.0000980 mol Mn) (5 mol Fe/1 mol Mn) = 0.000490 mol Fe(II)

3) Determine the TOTAL iron content:

(0.00280mol/L) (0.0480 L) = 0.0001344 mol of MnO_4^-

(0.0000980mol Mn) (5mol Fe/1mol Mn) = 0.000672 mol of total Fe

4) Determine Fe(III) in solution and its molarity:

0.000672 mol – 0.000490 mol = 0.000182 mol

0.000182 mol / 0.050 L = 0.00364 M

5) Determine molarity of Fe(II):

0.000490 mol/0.050 L = 0.0098 M

Q.4. How do you calculate Equivalent weight of Oxidising and Reducing Agents.

Ans. Equivalent weight of Oxidising and Reducing Agents

Equivalent weight of a substance (oxidant or reductant) is equal to molecular weight divided by number of electrons lost or gained by one molecule of the substance in a redox reaction.

Eq. wt. of

$$\text{Oxidising agent} = \frac{\text{Molecular weight}}{\text{No. of electrons gained by one molecule}}$$

$$= \frac{\text{Molecular weight}}{\text{Change in O.N. per molde}}$$

Eq. wt. of

$$\text{Reducing agent} = \frac{\text{Molecular weight}}{\text{No. of electrons lost by one molecule}}$$

$$= \frac{\text{Molecular weight}}{\text{Change in O.N. per molde}}$$

Table : Equivalent weight of few oxidising/reducing agents

Agents	O.N.	Product	O.N.	Change in O.N. per atom	Total Change in O.N. per mole	Eq. wt.
$Cr_2O_2^{2-}$	+ 6	Cr^{1+}	+ 3	3	$3 \times 2 = 6$	Mol. wt./6
$C_2O_4^{2-}$	+ 3	CO_2	+ 4	1	$1 \times 2 = 2$	Mol. wt./2
$S_2O_2^{2-}$	+ 2	$S_4O_1^{2-}$	+ 2.5	0.5	$0.5 \times 2 = 1$	Mol. wt./1
H_2O_2	– 1	H_2O	– 2	1	$1 \times 2 = 2$	Mol. wt./2
H_2O_2	– 1	O_2	0	1	$1 \times 2 = 2$	Mol. wt./2
MnO_4^- (Acidic medium)	+ 7	Mn^{2+}	+ 2	5	$5 \times 1 = 5$	Mol. wt./5
MnO_4^- (Neutral medium)	+ 7	MnO_2	+ 4	3	$3 \times 1 = 3$	Mol. wt./3
MnO_4^- (Alkaline medium)	+ 7	MnO_4^{2-}	+ 6	1	$1 \times 1 = 1$	Mol. wt./1

Q.5. A solution of sodium hydroxide contained 0.250 mol dm^{-3}. Using phenolphthalein indicator, titration of 25.0 cm^3 of this solution required 22.5 cm³ of a hydrochloric acid solution for complete neutralisation.

(a) write the equation for the titration reaction.

(b) what apparatus would you use to measure out (i) the sodium hydroxide solution? (ii) the hydrochloric acid solution?

(c) what would you rinse your apparatus out with before doing the titration ?

(d) what is the indicator colour change at the end-point?

(e) calculate the moles of sodium hydroxide neutralised.

(f) calculate the moles of hydrochloric acid neutralised.

(g) calculate the concentration of the hydrochloric acid in mol/dm³ (molarity).

Ans.

(a) $NaOH_{(aq)} + HCl_{(aq)} \rightarrow NaCl_{(aq)} + H_2O_{(l)}$

(b) (i) pipette (ii) burette

(c) everything with distilled water, then pipette with a little of the NaOH(aq) and the burette with a little of the HCl(aq)

(d) pink to colourless, the first drop of excess acid removes the pink alkaline colour of phenolphthalein

(e) moles sodium hydroxide neutralised: 0.250 x 25.0/1000 = 0.00625 mol NaOH

(remember: moles = molarity x volume in dm³ and its two rearrangements and 1 dm³ = 1000 cm³)

(f) moles HCl = moles NaOH (equation) = 0.00625 mol HCl (in 22.5 cm³)

(g) concentration hydrochloric acid = 0.00625 × 1000 ÷ 22.5 = 0.278 mol dm⁻³ (3sf)

(scaling up to 1 dm³ = 1000 cm³ to get the molarity)

Another way to work it out is 22.5 cm³ = 22.5 ÷ 1000 = 0.0225 dm³

Therefore molarity = 0.00625 ÷ 0.0225 = 0.278 mol dm⁻³

Q.6. A solution made from pure barium hydroxide contained 2.74 g in exactly 100 cm³ of water. Using phenolphthalein indicator, titration of 20.0 cm³ of this solution required 18.7 cm³ of a hydrochloric acid solution for complete neutralisation.

[atomic masses: Ba = 137, O = 16, H = 1)

(a) write the equation for the titration reaction.

(b) calculate the molarity of the barium hydroxide solution.

(c) calculate the moles of barium hydroxide neutralised.

(d) calculate the moles of hydrochloric acid neutralised.

(e) calculate the molarity of the hydrochloric acid.

Ans.

(a) $Ba(OH)_{2(aq)} + 2HCl_{(aq)} \rightarrow BaCl_{2(aq)} + 2H_2O_{(l)}$

(b) formula mass of $Ba(OH)_2$ = 171, moles = 2.74 ÷ 171 = 0.016 mol in 100 cm³, (scaling up × 10)

therefore 0.16 mol in 1000 cm³, so molarity of $Ba(OH)_2$ is 0.16 mol dm⁻³

(c) moles $Ba(OH)_2$ used in titration = 0.16 x 20/1000 = 0.0032 mol

(d) moles HCl titrated = 2 × moles of $Ba(OH)_2$ used (2 : 1 in equation) 2 × .0032

= 0.0064 mol HCl in 18.7 cm³ of the acid solution,

18.7 cm³ = 0.0187 dm³

(e) therefore molarity of $HCl_{(aq)}$ = 0.0064/0.0187 = 0.342 mol dm⁻³

Q.7. 4.90g of pure sulphuric acid was dissolved in water, the resulting total volume was 200 cm³. 20.7 cm³ of this solution was found on titration, to completely neutralise 10.0 cm³ of a sodium hydroxide solution.   [atomic masses: S = 32, O = 16, H = 1)

(a) write the equation for the titration reaction.

(b) calculate the molarity of the sulphuric acid solution.

(c) calculate the moles of sulphuric acid neutralised.

(d) calculate the moles of sodium hydroxide neutralised.

(e) calculate the concentration of the sodium hydroxide in mol dm⁻³ (molarity).

Ans.

(a) $2NaOH_{(aq)} + H_2SO_{4(aq)} \rightarrow Na_2SO_{4(aq)} + 2H_2O_{(l)}$

(b) moles H_2SO_4 = 4.90 ÷ 98 = 0.050 mol in 200cm³

scaling up to get molarity of the sulphuric acid solution, 0.050 × 1000 ÷ 200 = 0.25 mol dm⁻³

(c) moles of sulphuric acid neutralised = $0.250 \times 20.7/1000$
= 0.005175 mol

(d) moles of sodium hydroxide neutralised = $2 \times 0.005175 = 0.01035$ mol ($2 : 1$ in equation)

(e) concentration of the sodium hydroxide = $0.01035 \times 1000 \div 10$
= 1.035 mol dm^{-3} (molarity 1.04, 3sf)

Q.8. 100 cm^3 of a magnesium hydroxide solution required 4.5 cm^3 of sulphuric acid (of concentration 0.100 mol dm^{-3}) for complete neutralisation.   [atomic masses: Mg = 24.3, O = 16, H = 1)

(a) give the equation for the neutralisation reaction.

(b) calculate the moles of sulphuric acid neutralised.

(c) calculate the moles of magnesium hydroxide neutralised.

(d) calculate the concentration of the magnesium hydroxide in mol dm^{-3} (molarity).

(e) calculate the concentration of the magnesium hydroxide in g cm^{-3}.

Ans.

(a) $Mg(OH)_{2(aq)} + H_2SO_{4(aq)} \rightarrow MgSO_{4(aq)} + 2H_2O_{(l)}$

(b) moles of sulphuric acid neutralised = $0.100 \times 4.5/1000 = 0.00045$ mol

(c) moles of magnesium hydroxide neutralised also = 0.00045 (1:1 in equation) in 100 cm^3

(d) concentration of the magnesium hydroxide in mol dm^{-3} = 0.00045 $\times 1000 \div 100 = 0.0045$

                                (scaling up to 1000cm^3 = 1dm^3, to get molarity)

(e) molar mass of Mg(OH)$_2$ = 58.3

so concentration of the magnesium hydroxide = 0.0045×58.3
= 0.26 g dm^{-3} (= g per 1000 cm^3),

so concentration = $0.26 \div 1000 = 0.00026$ g cm^{-3}

Q.9. Magnesium oxide is not very soluble in water, and is difficult to titrate directly.

Its purity can be determined by use of a 'back titration' method. 4.06 g of impure magnesium oxide was completely dissolved in 100 cm^3 of hydrochloric acid, of concentration 2.00 mol dm^{-3} (in excess).

The excess acid required $19.7 cm^3$ of sodium hydroxide (0.200 mol dm^{-3}) for neutralisation.

This 2nd titration is called a 'back-titration', and is used to determine the unreacted acid.

[atomic masses: Mg = 24.3, O = 16]

(a) write equations for the two neutralisation reactions.

(b) calculate the moles of hydrochloric acid added to the magnesium oxide.

(c) calculate the moles of excess hydrochloric acid titrated.

(d) calculate the moles of hydrochloric acid reacting with the magnesium oxide.

(e) calculate the moles and mass of magnesium oxide that reacted with the initial hydrochloric acid.

(f) hence the % purity of the magnesium oxide.

(g) what compounds could be present in the magnesium oxide that could lead to a false value of its purity ? explain.

Ans.

(a) (i) $M gO_{(s)} + 2HCl_{(aq)} \rightarrow MgCl_{2(aq)} + H_2O_{(l)}$

(a) (ii) $NaOH_{(aq)} + HCl_{(aq)} \rightarrow NaCl_{(aq)} + H_2O_{(l)}$

(b) moles of hydrochloric acid added to the magnesium oxide = 2 × 100/1000 = 0.20 mol HCl

(c) moles of excess hydrochloric acid titrated = 19.7 ÷ 1000 × 0.200 = 0.00394 mol HCl

{mole ratio NaOH:HCl is 1:1 from equation (ii)}

(d) moles of hydrochloric acid reacting with the magnesium oxide = 0.20 − 0.00394 = 0.196 mol HCl

(e) mole MgO reacted = 0.196 ÷ 2 = 0.098 {1: 2 in equation (i)} the formula mass of MgO = 40.3 therefore mass of MgO reacting with acid = 0.098 x 40.3 = 3.95 g

(f) % purity = 3.95 ÷ 4.06 × 100 = 97.3% MgO

(g) $Mg(OH)_2$ from MgO + H_2O, $MgCO_3$ from the original mineral source, both of these compounds react with acid and would lead to a false titration value.

Q.10. $2.00 dm^3$ of concentrated hydrochloric acid (10.0 M) was spilt onto a laboratory floor. It can be neutralised with limestone powder.

[atomic masses: Ca = 40, C = 12, O = 16)

(a) give the equation for the reaction between limestone and hydrochloric acid.

(b) how many moles of hydrochloric acid was spilt?

(c) how many moles of calcium carbonate will neutralise the acid?

(d) what minimum mass of limestone powder is needed to neutralise the acid?

(e) If 1000 dm^3 of sulphuric acid, of concentration 2.00 mol dm^{-3}, leaked from a tank, calculate the minimum mass of magnesium oxide required to neutralise it.

Ans.

(a) $CaCO_{3(s)} + 2HCl_{(aq)} \rightarrow CaCl_{2(aq)} + H_2O_{(l)} + CO_{2(g)}$

(b) moles of hydrochloric acid was spilt = 2.00 x 10.0 = 20 mol HCl

(c) moles of calcium carbonate to neutralise the acid = 20 ÷ 2 = 10.0 mol $CaCO_3$ (1:2 in equation)

(d) formula mass of $CaCO_3$ = 100,

so mass of limestone powder needed to neutralise the acid = 100 × 10 = 1000g $CaCO_3$

(e) the neutralisation reaction is $MgO + H_2SO_4 \rightarrow MgSO_4 + H_2O$, moles H_2SO_4 = 1000 × 2 = 2000 mol acid, 2000 mol MgO needed (1:1 in equation), mass MgO needed = 2000 x 40.3 = 80600 g or 80.6 kg

Q.11. A 50.0 cm^3 sample of sulphuric acid was diluted to 1.00 dm^3. A sample of the diluted sulphuric acid was analysed by titrating with aqueous sodium hydroxide. In the titration, 25.0 cm^3 of 1.00 mol dm^{-3} aqueous sodium hydroxide required 20.0 cm^3 of the diluted sulphuric acid for neutralisation.

(a) give the equation for the full neutralisation of sulphuric acid by sodium hydroxide.

(b) calculate how many moles of sodium hydroxide were used in the titration?

(c) calculate the concentration of the diluted acid.

(d) calculate the concentration of the original concentrated sulphuric acid solution.

Ans.

(a) $2NaOH_{(aq)} + H_2SO_{4(aq)} \rightarrow Na_2SO_{4(aq)} + 2H_2O_{(l)}$

(b) moles of sodium hydroxide used in the titration = 25.0 x 1/1000
= 0.025 mol NaOH

(c) mol H_2SO_4 = mol NaOH ÷ 2 = 0.0125 mol in 20.0 cm^3,

so scaling up to 1000 cm^3 to get molarity of diluted acid = 0.0125 × 1000 ÷ 20 = 0.625 mol dm^{-3}

(or molarity = 0.0125 mol/0.02 dm^3 = 0.625 mol dm^{-3})

(d) scaling up from 50 to 1000 cm^3, gives the concentration of the original concentrated sulphuric acid solution,

= 0.625 × 1000 ÷ 50 = 12.5 mol dm^{-3}

Q.12. 25.0 cm^3 of seawater was diluted to 250 cm^3 in a graduated volumetric flask.

A 25.0 cm^3 aliquot of the diluted seawater was pipetted into a conical flask and a few drops of potassium chromate(VI) indicator solution was added.

On titration with 0.100 mol dm^{-3} silver nitrate solution, 13.8 cm^3 was required to precipitate all the chloride ion.

[Atomic masses: Na = 23, Cl = 35.5]

(a) Give the ionic equation for the reaction of silver nitrate and chloride ion.

(b) Calculate the moles of chloride ion in the titrated 25.0 cm^3 aliquot.

(c) Calculate the molarity of chloride ion in the diluted seawater.

(d) Calculate the molarity of chloride ion in the original seawater.

(e) Assuming that for every chloride ion there is a sodium ion, what is the theoretical concentration of sodium chloride salt in g dm^{-3} in seawater?

Ans.

(a) $Ag^+_{(aq)} + Cl^-_{(aq)} \rightarrow AgCl_{(s)}$ (sodium ions and nitrate ions etc. are spectator ions)

(b) from equation: moles silver nitrate ($AgNO_3$) = moles chloride ion (Cl^-)

moles = molarity $AgNO_3$ × volume of $AgNO_3$ in dm^3

= 0.100 × 13.8/1000 = 1.38 × 10^{-3} mol Cl$^-$ (in 25.0 cm^3 aliquot)

(c) moles in 1 dm^3 of diluted seawater = $1.38 \times 10^{-3} \times 1000/25$ = 0.0552 (scaling up to 1000 cm^3)

So molarity of chloride in diluted seawater is 0.0552 mol dm^{-3}

(d) Now in the titration 25.0 cm^3 of the 250 cm^3 was used,

so the molarity of chloride ion in the original seawater must be scaled up accordingly.

molarity of chloride ion in seawater = $0.0552 \times 250/25.0 = 0.552$ mol dm^{-3}

(e) $M_r(NaCl) = 23 + 35.5 = 58.5$

concentration of NaCl in g dm^{-3} = molarity × formula mass = $0.552 \times 58.5 = 32.3$ g dm^{-3}

Q.13. 0.12 g of rock salt was dissolved in water and titrated with 0.100 mol dm^{-3} silver nitrate until the first permanent brown precipitate of silver chromate is seen.

19.7 cm^3 was required to titrate all the chloride ion.

[Atomic masses: Na = 23, Cl = 35.5]

(a) How many moles of chloride ion was titrated?

(b) What mass of sodium chloride was titrated?

(c) What was the % purity of the rock salt in terms of sodium chloride?

Ans.

(a) moles = molarity $AgNO_3$ × volume in dm^3 = $0.100 \times 19.7/1000$
= 1.97×10^{-3} mol Cl^- ion

[$AgNO_3$:NaCl or Ag^+:Cl^- is 1:1, see Q10(a)/(b)] f. mass NaCl = 23 + 35.5 = 58.5

(b) mass = mol × formula mass = $1.97 \times 10^{-3} \times 58.5$

= 0.1152 g NaCl

(c) % purity = $0.1152 \times 100/0.12 = 96.0$ % in terms of NaCl (3sf)

Q.14. How to determine the water of crystallisation in hydrated sodium carbonate crystals ('washing soda') by titration with standard hydrochloric acid solution.

If 0.352g of hydrated sodium carbonate crystals, $Na_2CO_3 \times H_2O$, was titrated with 0.100 mol dm^{-3} (0.100M) standard hydrochloric solution. If the titration value was 24.65 cm^3, calculate the moles of

Na_2CO_3 titrated and hence deduce x, the number of molecules of water of crystallisation in washing soda crystals.

Ans. $Na_2CO_3 + 2HCl \rightarrow 2NaCl + H_2O + CO_2$, 1 mol hydrochloric acid relates to 0.5 moles of sodium carbonate mol HCl used = 0.100 × 24.65/1000 = 0.002465, mol Na_2CO_3 titrated = 0.002465/2 = 0.0012325 $M_r(Na_2CO_3)$ = 106, so mass Na_2CO_3'titrated = 106 x 0.0012325 = 0.130645

Therefore mass of H_2O in sample= 0.352 - 0.130645 = 0.221355 g mole ratio $Na_2CO_3 : H_2O$ is therefore 0.0012325 : 0.221355/18, giving 0.0012325 : 0.0122975 diving through by 0.0012325 gives a ratio of 1 : 9.98 (only a 0.2% error if x = 10)

Therefore the value of x can be reliably deduced as 10, since it would be expected to be an integer.

i.e. the formula of hydrated sodium carbonate crystals ('washing soda') is $Na_2CO_3.10H_2O$

Q.15. Calculate the equivalent weight of $KMnO_4$ in acidic and basic medium.

Ans. $KMnO_4$ has a Molar mass of 158.04 g/mol

There are two possibillities:

1. $KMnO_4$ as an oxidizer in acidic media:

    $M nO_4^- + 8 H^+ + 5e^- \rightarrow Mn^{2+} + 4H_2O$ (gained 5 electrons from reductant)

    i.e. Eq. wt. of $KMnO_4$ = 158.04/5 = 31.61 grams/equivalent

2. $KMnO_4$ as an oxidizer in basic media:

    $MnO_4^- + 2H_2O + 3e^- \rightarrow MnO_{2(s)} + 4OH^-$ (gained 3 electrons)

    In which case, Eq. wt. of $KMnO_4$ = 158.04/3 = 52.68 grams/equivalent.

THEORETICAL QUESTIONS FOR EXAMINATION

Q.1. Define Normality, molarity & molality of a solution.

Q.2. Explain the principle of Volumetric analysis.

Q.3. Explain Acid –base titration with example.

Q.4. Explain the principle of acid-alaklimetry and explain the titration curves for strong acid and weak base.

Q.5. Explain redox titration with example.

Q.6. Explain complexometric titration by giving the example of hardness of water.

Q.7. Explain precipitation titration for chloride ion determination in the water.

Q.8. Differentiate between iodimetry and iodometry titration with exaplme.

Q.9. Write molecular formula for 2 strong acid, 2 strong base,weak acid weak base and calculate their molecular weight and equivalent weight.

Q.10. Write the names and reactions of 2 reducing agent and 2 oxidising agent with their equivalent weight.

Chapter 2
SPECTROSCOPIC METHODS
OF ANALYSIS

➢ **Laws of Spectroscopy**
➢ **UV-Visible**
➢ **IR**
➢ **NMR and Mass Spectroscopy**
➢ **Numerical Problems**

Spectroscopy was originally the study of the interaction between radiation and matter as a function of wavelength (λ). In fact, historically, spectroscopy referred to the use of visible light dispersed according to its wavelength, e.g. by a prism. Later the concept was expanded greatly to comprise any measurement of a quantity as function of either wavelength or frequency. Thus it also can refer to interactions with particle radiation or to a response to an alternating field or varying frequency (v). A further extension of the scope of the definition added energy (E) as a variable, once the very close relationship $E = hv$ for photons was realized. A plot of the response as a function of wavelength (λ) or more commonly frequency is referred to as a spectrum.

Spectrometry is the spectroscopic technique used to assess the concentration or amount of a given species. In those cases, the instrument that performs such measurements is a spectrometer or spectrograph.

Spectroscopy/spectrometry is often used in physical and analytical chemistry for the identification of substances through the spectrum emitted from or absorbed by them. Spectroscopy/spectrometry is also heavily used in astronomy and remote sensing. Most large telescopes have spectrometers, which are used either to measure the chemical composition and physical properties of astronomical objects or to measure their velocities from the Doppler shift of their spectral lines.

Classification of Methods

The type of spectroscopy depends on the physical quantity measured. Normally, the quantity that is measured is an intensity(I), either of energy(E) absorbed or produced.

- Electromagnetic spectroscopy involves interactions of matter with electromagnetic radiation, such as light.
- Electron spectroscopy involves interactions with electron beams. Auger spectroscopy involves inducing the Auger effect with an electron beam. In this case the measurement typically involves the kinetic energy of the electron as variable.
- Mass spectrometry involves the interaction of charged species with magnetic and/or electric fields, giving rise to a mass spectrum. The term "mass spectroscopy" is deprecated, for the technique is primarily a form of measurement, though it does produce a spectrum for observation. This spectrum has the mass m as variable, but the measurement is essentially one of the kinetic energy of the particle.
- Acoustic spectroscopy involves the frequency of sound.
- Dielectric spectroscopy involves the frequency of an external electrical field
- Mechanical spectroscopy involves the frequency of an external mechanical stress, e.g. a torsion applied to a piece of material.

Measurement Process

Most spectroscopic methods are differentiated as either atomic or molecular based on whether or not they apply to atoms or molecules. Along with that distinction, they can be classified on the nature of their interaction:

- Absorption spectroscopy uses the range of the electromagnetic spectra in which a substance absorbs. This includes atomic absorption spectroscopy and various molecular techniques, such as infrared spectroscopy in that region and nuclear magnetic resonance (NMR) spectroscopy in the radio region. Absorption spectroscopy is a technique in which the power of a beam of light measured before and after interaction with a sample is compared
- Emission spectroscopy uses the range of electromagnetic spectra in which a substance radiates (emits). The substance first must absorb energy. This energy can be from a variety of sources, which determines the name of the subsequent emission, like luminescence. Molecular luminescence techniques include spectrofluorimetry.
- Scattering spectroscopy measures the amount of light that a substance

scatters at certain wavelengths, incident angles, and polarization angles. The scattering process is much faster than the absorption/emission process. One of the most useful applications of light scattering spectroscopy is Raman spectroscopy.

Electromagnetic spectrum is shown here

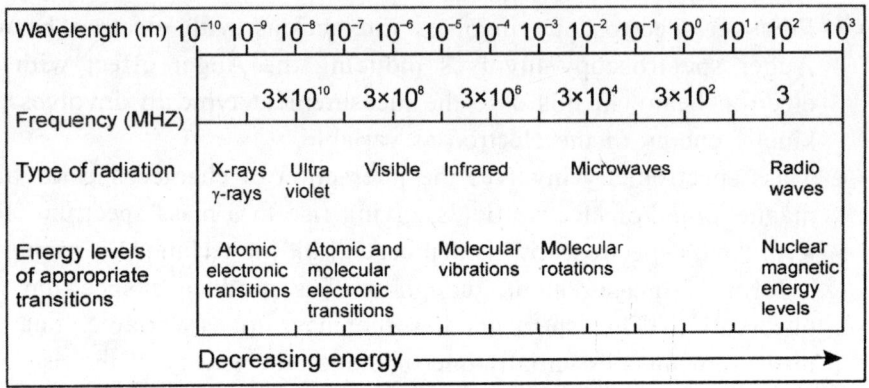

Fig. 2.1:

LAWS OF SPECTROSCOPY: BEER-LAMBERT LAW

The Beer-Lambert law states that the absorbance of a solution is directly proportional to the concentration(c) of solutions and pathlength (L) of the sample cell (cuvette). Thus UV/VIS spectroscopy can be used to determine the concentration of a solution. It is necessary to know how quickly the absorbance changes with concentration. This can be taken from references (tables of molar extinction coefficients), or more accurately, determined from a calibration curve.

The method is most often used in a quantitative way to determine concentrations of an absorbing species in solution, using the Beer-Lambert law:

$$A = \log_{10} (I/I_0) = \varepsilon \cdot c \cdot L$$

where A is the measured absorbance, I_0 is the intensity of the incident light at a given wavelength, I is the transmitted intensity, L the pathlength through the sample, and c the concentration of the absorbing species. For each species and wavelength, a is a constant known as the molar absorptivity or extinction coefficient. This constant is a fundamental molecular property in a given solvent, at a particular temperature and pressure, and has units of $1/M^* \; cm$ or often $AU/M^* \; cm$.

The absorbance and extinction *a* are sometimes defined in terms of the natural logarithm instead of the base-10 logarithm.

Visible and Ultraviolet Spectroscopy

Many atoms emit or absorb visible light. In order to obtain a fine line spectrum, the atoms must be in a gas phase. This means that the substance has to be vaporised. The spectrum is studied in absorption or emission. Visible absorption spectroscopy is often combined with UV absorption spectroscopy in UV/Vis spectroscopy. Although this form may be uncommon as the human eye is a similar indicator, it still proves useful when distinguishing colours.

All atoms absorb in the Ultraviolet (UV) region because these photons are energetic enough to excite outer electrons. If the frequency is high enough, photo ionisation takes place. UV spectroscopy is also used in quantifying protein and DNA concentration as well as the ratio of protein to DNA concentration in a solution..

Principle of Ultraviolet-visible spectroscopy (UV/ VIS)

Principle: It involves the spectroscopy of photons in the UV-visible region i.e from 10 nm to 800 nm broadly, UV range is 10 to 400 nm while 400 to 800 nm for Visisble. 200 to 400 nm is close to visible hence known as near UV and 10 to 200 nm is far UV. In this region of the electromagnetic spectrum, molecules undergo electronic transitions i.e these wavelengths have sufficient energy to cause electronic excitations or transitions.

Molecular electronic transitions occur when electrons in a molecule are excited from one energy level to a higher energy level. The energy change associated with this transition provides information on the structure of a molecule and determines many molecular properties such as color. Planck's law gives the relationship between the energy involved in the electronic transition and the frequency of radiation. In a molecule electrons may be of three types, π (pi electron in pi molecular orbital), σ (present in sigma bonded molecular orbital) and *n* electrons (non bonding).

Electronic transitions are of following four types :

1. sigma to sigma antibonding
2. pi to pi antibonding
3. n to sigma antibonding
4. n to pi antibonding

Diagram of Possible *electronic* transitions of π, σ, and *n* electrons is shown in Fig. 2.2.

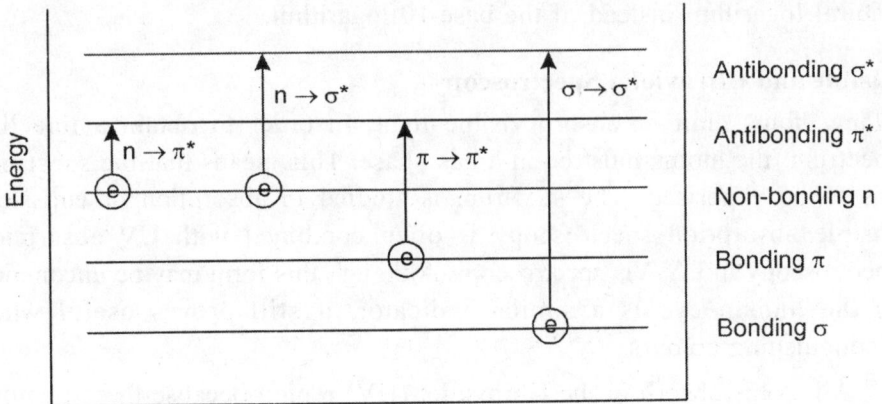

Fig. 2.2.

1. σ → σ* Transitions

An electron in a bonding s orbital is excited to the corresponding antibonding orbital. The energy required is large or wavelength is minimum than other transitions,. For example, methane (which has only C-H bonds, and can only undergo σ → σ* transitions) shows an absorbance maximum at 125 nm or less than. Absorption maxima due σ → σ* transitions are not seen in typical UV-Vis. spectra (200 – 700 nm)

2. *n* → σ* Transitions

Saturated compounds containing atoms with lone pairs (non-bonding electrons) are capable of *n* → σ* transitions. These transitions usually need less energy than σ → σ* transitions. They can be initiated by light whose wavelength is in the range 150 – 250 nm. The number of organic functional groups with *n* → σ* peaks in the UV region is small.

3. *n* → π* and

4. π → π* Transitions

Most absorption spectroscopy of organic compounds is based on transitions of *n* or π electrons to the π* excited state. This is because the absorption peaks for these transitions fall in an experimentally convenient region of the spectrum (200 – 700 nm). These transitions need an unsaturated group in the molecule to provide the p electrons.

Molar absorbtivities from *n* → π* transitions are relatively low, and range from 10 to100 L mol^{-1} cm^{-1}. π → π* transitions normally give molar absorbtivities between 1000 and 10,000 L mol^{-1} cm^{-1}.

The solvent in which the absorbing species is dissolved also has an effect on the spectrum of the species. Peaks resulting from $n \to \pi^*$ transitions are shifted to shorter wavelengths (*blue shift*) with increasing solvent polarity. This arises from increased solvation of the lone pair, which lowers the energy of the n orbital. Often (but *not* always), the reverse (i.e. *red shift*) is seen for $\pi \to \pi^*$ transitions. This is caused by attractive polarisation forces between the solvent and the absorber, which lower the energy levels of both the excited and unexcited states. This effect is greater for the excited state, and so the energy difference between the excited and unexcited states is slightly reduced - resulting in a small red shift. This effect also influences $n \to \pi^*$ transitions but is overshadowed by the blue shift resulting from solvation of lone pairs.

UV/Visible is spectroscopy is routinely used in the quantitative determination of solutions of transition metal ions and highly conjugated organic compounds.

Instrumentation

Instrumentation-The basic parts of a spectrophotometer are a light source (often an incandescent bulb for the visible wavelengths, or a deuterium arc lamp in the ultraviolet), a holder for the sample, a diffraction grating or monochromator to separate the different wavelengths of light, and a detector. The cells in the spectrometer must be made of pure silica for ultraviolet spectra because soda glass absorbs below 365 nm, and pyrex glass below 320 nm.Detection of the radiation passing through the sample or reference

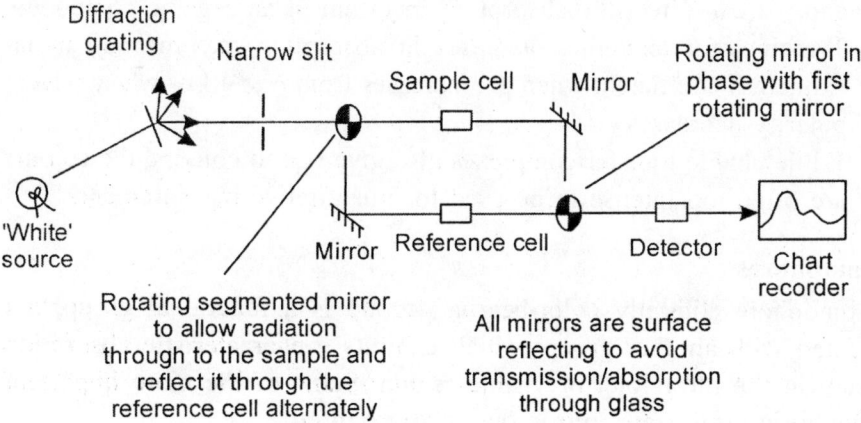

Fig. 2.3

cell can be achieved by either a photomultiplier or a photodiode. The spectrum is produced by comparing the currents generated by the sample and the reference beams.Modern instruments are self-calibrating, though the accuracy of the calibration can be checked if necessary. Wavelength checks are made by passing the sample beam through glass samples (containing holmium oxide) that have precise absorption peaks, and the absorption is calibrated by passing the sample beam through either a series of filters, each with a specific and known absorption, or a series of standard solutions.

Some points to be noted

- Solutions of transition metal ions can be coloured (i.e., absorb visible light) because d electrons within the metal atoms can be excited from one electronic state to another. The colour of metal ion solutions is strongly affected by the presence of other species, such as certain anions or ligands. For instance, the colour of a dilute solution of copper sulfate is a very light blue; adding ammonia intensifies the colour and changes the wavelength of maximum absorption (λ_{max}).

- Organic compounds, especially those with a high degree of conjugation, also absorb light in the UV or visible regions of the electromagnetic spectrum. The solvents for these determinations are often water for water soluble compounds, or ethanol for organic-soluble compounds. (Organic solvents may have significant UV absorption; not all solvents are suitable for use in UV spectroscopy. Ethanol absorbs very weakly at most wavelengths.) Solvent polarity and pH can effect the absorption spectrum of an organic compound. Tyrosine, for example, increases in absorption maxima and molar extinction coefficient when pH increases from 6 to 13 or when solvent polarity decreases.

- While charge transfer complexes also give rise to colours, the colours are often too intense to be used for quantitative measurement.

Chromophores

A chromophore (literally color-bearing) group is a functional group, not conjugated with another group, which exhibits a characteristic absorption spectrum in the ultraviolet or visible region. Some of the more important chromophoric groups are: nitrogroup, azo group etc.

If any of the simple chromophores is conjugated with another (of the same type or different type) a multiple chromophore is formed having a new absorption band which is more intense and at a longer wavelength that the strong bands of the simple.

Auxochromes

The color of a molecule may be intensified by groups called auxochromes which generally do not absorb significantly in the 200-800nm region, but will affect the spectrum of the chromophore to which it is attached. The most important auxochromic groups are OH, NH_2, CH_3 and OCH_3 and their properties are acidic (phenolic) or basic. The actual effect of an auxochrome on a chromophore depends on the polarity of the auxochrome, e.g. groups like CH_3^-, $CH_3CH_2^-$, and Cl.

Effect of modification on the wavelength (λ_{max}) or absorbance

Bathochromic shift: This displacement of an absorption maximum (λ_{max}) towards a longer wavelength (i.e. from blue to red) is termed a bathochromic shift. This is obtained by auxochrome.

Hypsochromic shift: When some modification is done in the organic compound and (λ_{max}) absorption maximum is shifted towards lower side i.e. from the red to ultraviolet is termed a hypsochromic shift.

Hyperchromic and Hypochromic effect: When on certain modification in the compound, λ_{max} is not changed but peak of absoption or absorbance is increased up side, that is known as Hyperchromic effect while absorption peak is shifted down ward then this shift is hypochromic shift and effect is hypochromic effect.

Theoretical calculation of (λ_{max}): Woodward–Fieser rules

Woodward's rules, named after Robert Burns Woodward and also known as Woodward–Fieser rules (for Louis Fieser) are several sets of empirically derived rules which attempt to predict the wavelength of the absorption maximum (λ_{max}) in an ultraviolet–visible spectrum of a given compound. Inputs used in the calculation are the type of chromophores present, the substituents on the chromophores, and shifts due to the solvent compounds, conjugated dienes, and polyenes.

Application in Conjugated diene compound

Open chain diene compound

For open chain conjugated diene, basic value of diene is 217nm. 5nm is to be added for each alky substituent present on the double bonded carbon.

30 nm is to added for extra double bond for extending conjugation. Other increments are given in the table

Cyclic diene compound

One set of Woodward–Fieser rules for dienes is outlined in table 2.1. A cyclic diene is either **homoannular** with both double bonds contained in one ring or **heteroannular** with two double bonds distributed between two rings.

Table 2.1

Structural	λ_{max} effect (nm)
Base value for open chain diene	217
Base value for heteroannular diene	214
Base value for homoannular diene	253
Increments	
Double bond extending conjugation	+30
Alkyl substituent or ring residue	+5
Exocyclic double bond	+5
acetate group	+0
Ether group	+6
Thioether group	+30
bromine, chlorine	+5
secondary amine group	+60

With the aid of these rules the UV absorption maximum can be predicted, for example in these two compounds:

Absorption maximum : 214 + 20 + 5 = 239 nm

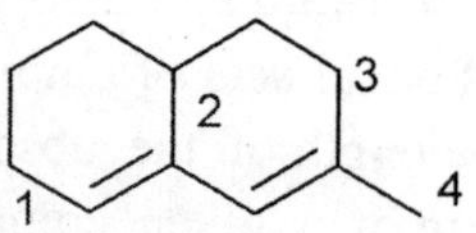

heteroannular diene : 214
alkyl and ring residue
substitutents 4 × 5 = 20
exocyclic double bond : 5

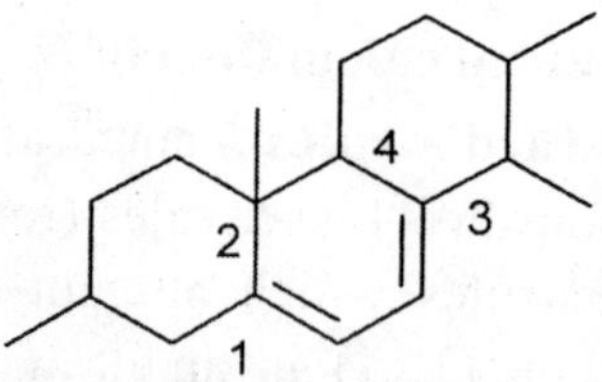

heteroannular diene : 253
alkyl substitutents 4 × 5
exocyclic double bond : 2 × 5
Absorption maximum : 253 + 20 + 10 = 283 nm

In the compound on the left, the base value is 214 nm (a heteroannular diene). This diene group has 4 alkyl substituents (labeled 1, 2, 3, 4) and the double bond in one ring is exocyclic to the other (adding 5 nm for an exocyclic double bond). In the compound on the right, the diene is homoannular with 4 alkyl substituents. Both double bonds in the central B ring are exocyclic with respect to rings A and C.

Example

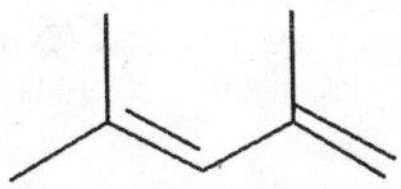

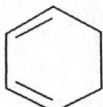

Open chain conjugated diene = 217 nm
Alkyl groups or ring residues: 3 × 5 = 15 nm
Calculated: 232 nm
Observed: 234 nm

Example

Cisoid: base value (homoanular) =   253 nm
Alkyl groups or ring residues: 2 × 5 = 10 nm
Calculated: 263 nm
Observed: 256 nm

Example

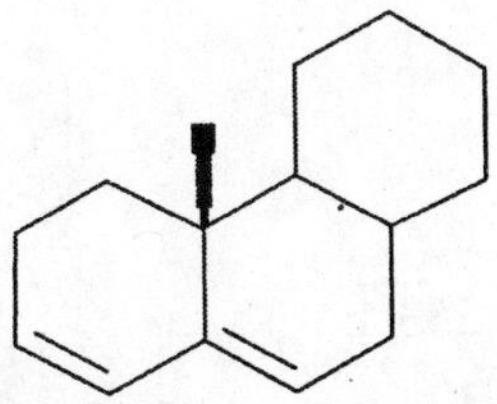

Base value:(hetero anular diene) =   214 nm
Alkyl groups or ring residues: 3 × 5 = 15 nm
Exocyclic double bond: 5 nm
Calculated: 234 nm
Observed: 235 nm

Example

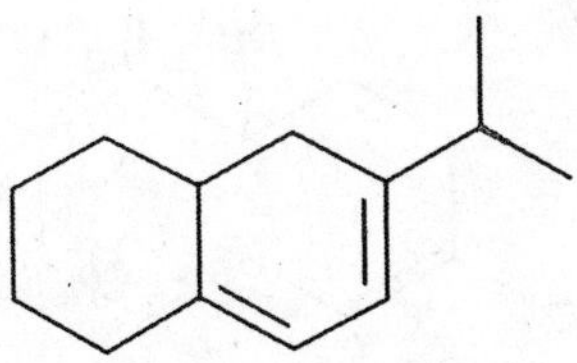

Cisoid: (homo anular diene) =   253 nm
Alkyl groups or ring residues: 4 × 5 = 20 nm
Exocyclic double bond: 5 nm
Calculated: 278 nm
Observed: 275 nm

Example

Exocyclic Double Bond

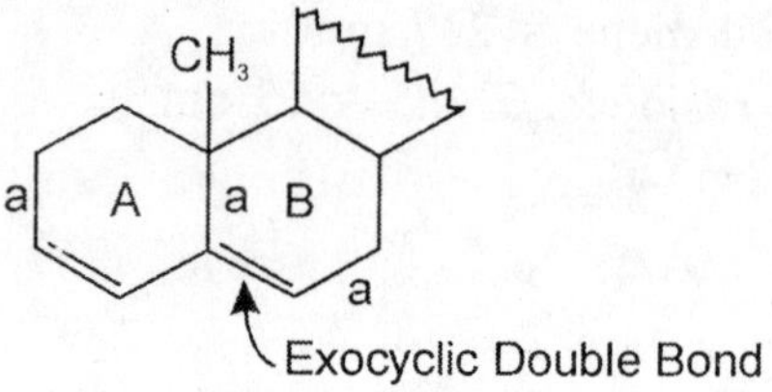

transoid :   214 mm
ring residues: 3 × 5 =   15
exocyclic double bond: 15
exocyclic double bond: 5
                               234 nm
observed: 235 nm

Example

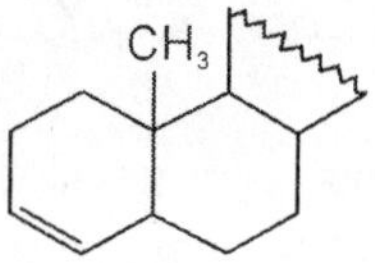

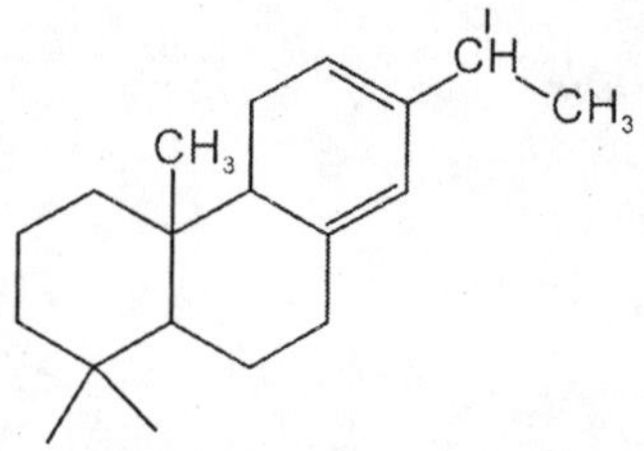

cisoid: 253 nm
ring residues: 3 × 5 =   15
exocyclic double bond: 5
                               273 nm   278 nm
observed: 255 nm   observed: 275 nm

Example

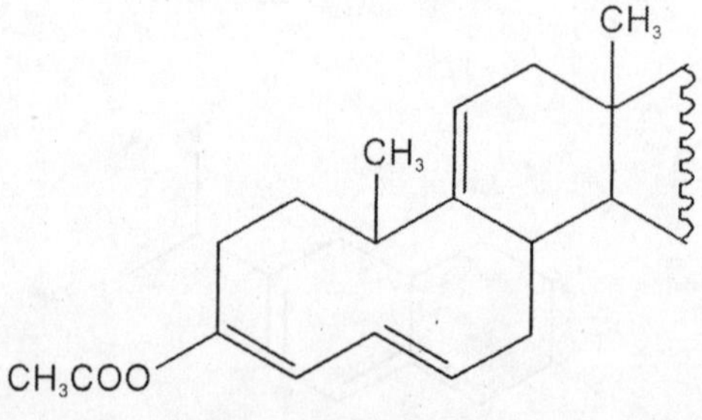

cisoid:	253 nm
ring residues: 5 × 5 =	25
double bond extending	
conjugation: 2 × 30 =	60
exocyclic double bonds: 3 × 5 = 15	
CH_3COO- :	0
	353 nm
observed:	355 nm

Woodward's Rules for Conjugated Carbonyl Compounds

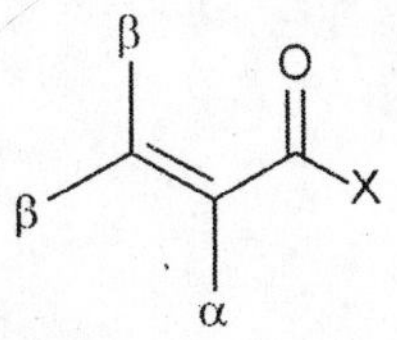

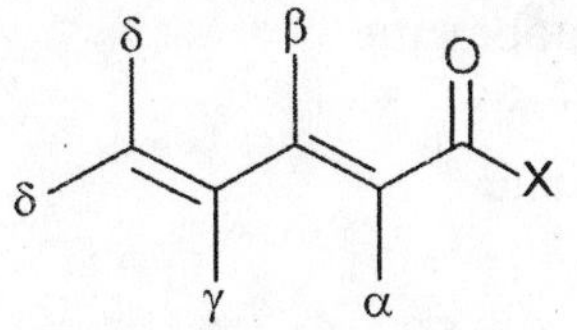

Base values:

  X = R

Six-membered ring or acyclic parent enone	$\lambda = 215$ nm
Five-membered ring parent enone	$\lambda = 202$ nm
X = H	$\lambda = 208$ nm
X = OH, OR	$\lambda = 195$ nm

Increments for:

Double bond extending conjugation		30
Exocyclic double bond		5
Endocyclic double bond in a 5- or 7-membered ring for		
X = OH, OR		5
Homocyclic diene component		39
Alkyl substituent or ring residue	α	10
	β	12
	γ or higher	18

Polar groupings:

–OH	α	35
	β	30
	δ	50
–OC(O)CH₃	α,β,γ,δ	6
–OCH₃	α	35
	β	30
	γ	17

	δ	31
–Cl	α	15
	β,γ,δ	12
–Br	α	30
	α,γ,δ	25
$-NR_2$	β	95

*Solvent shifts for various solvents: (if required)

Solvent	λ_{max} shift (nm)
water	+ 8
chloroform	− 1
ether	− 7
cyclohexane	− 11
dioxane	− 5
hexane	− 11

Example 1:

Acyclic enone:		215 nm
α-Alkyl groups or ring residues:		10 nm
β-Alkyl groups or ring residues:	$2 \times 12 =$	<u>24 nm</u>
Calculated:		249 nm
Observed:		249 nm

Example 2:

Five-membered ring parent enone:		202 nm
β-Alkyl groups or ring residues:	$2 \times 12 =$	24 nm
Exocyclic double bond:		<u>5 nm</u>
Calculated:		231 nm
Observed:		226 nm

Example 3:

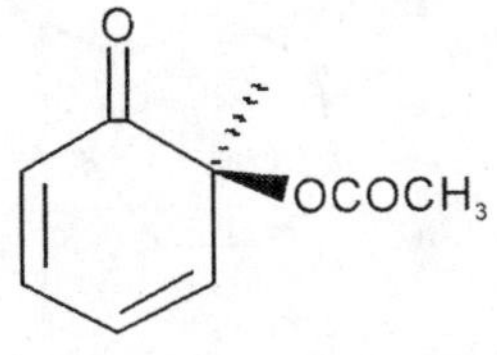

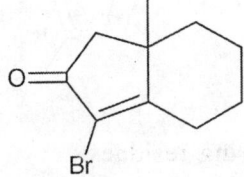

Six-membered ring or	
alicyclic parent enone:	215 nm
Extended conjugation:	30 nm
Homocyclic diene component:	39 nm
δ-Alkyl groups or ring residues:	<u>18 nm</u>
Calculated:	302 nm
Observed:	300 nm

Example 4:

Five-membered ring parent enone:	202 nm
α-Br:	25 nm
β-Alkyl groups or ring residues: 2 × 12 =	24 nm
Exocyclic double bond:	<u>5 nm</u>
Calculated:	256 nm
Observed:	251 nm

Example 5:

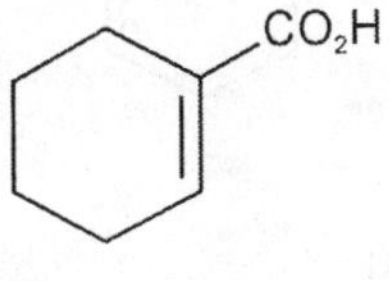

Carboxylic acid:	195 nm
α-Alkyl groups or ring residues:	10 nm
β-Alkyl groups or ring residues:	<u>12 nm</u>
Calculated:	217 nm
Observed:	217 nm

Example 6:

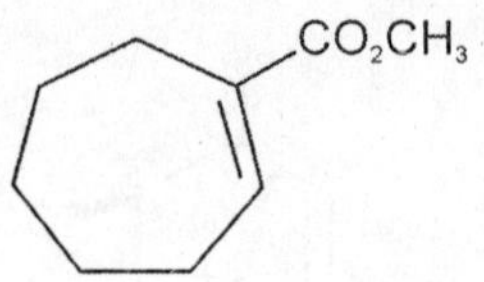

Ester:	195 nm
α-Alkyl groups or ring residues:	10 nm
β-Alkyl groups or ring residues:	12 nm
Endocyclic double bond in 7-membered ring:	5 nm
Calculated:	222 nm

Example 7:

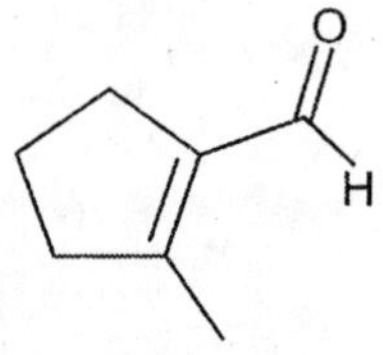

Aldehyde:		208 nm
α-Alkyl groups or ring residues:		10 nm
β-Alkyl groups or ring residues:	2 x 12 =	24 nm
Calculated:		242 nm
Observed:		242 nm

Example 8:

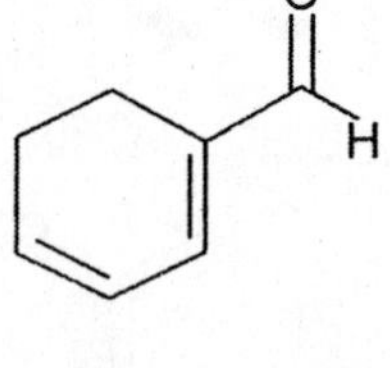

Aldehyde:	208 nm
Extended conjugation:	30 nm
Homodiene component:	39 nm
α-Alkyl groups or ring residues:	10 nm
δ-Alkyl groups or ring residues:	18 nm
Calculated:	304 nm
Observed:	302 nm

acyclic enone:	215 mm
α —CH$_3$:	10
β —CH$_3$:	24
	249 nm
observed:	249 nm

6-membered enone:	215 nm
double bond extending	
conjugation:	30
homocyclic diene	39
	302 nm
observed:	300 nm

5-membered enone:	202 mm
β-ring residue: 2 × 12 =	24
exocyclic double bond:	5
	231 nm
observed:	249 nm

5-membered enone:	202 nm
α-Br.	25
β-ring residue: 2 × 12 =	24
exocyclic double bond:	5
	256 nm
observed:	251 nm

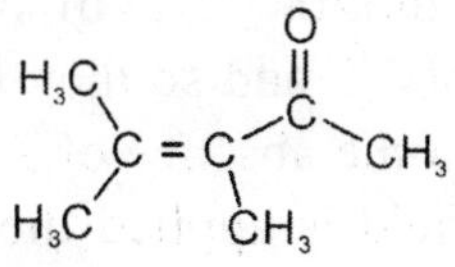

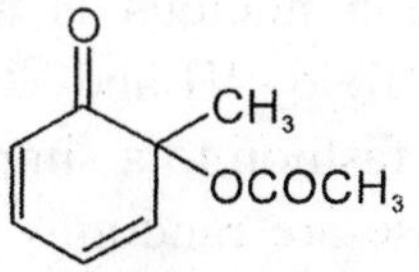

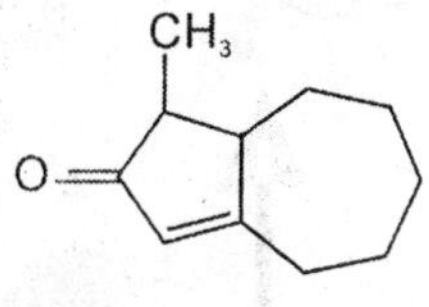

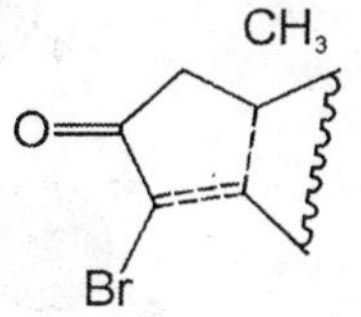

NMR SPECTROSCOPY

Nuclear magnetic resonance spectroscopy is the use of the NMR phenomenon to study physical, chemical, and biological properties of matter. As a consequence, NMR spectroscopy finds applications in several areas of science. NMR spectroscopy is routinely used by chemists to study chemical structure using simple one-dimensional techniques. Two-dimensional techniques are used to determine the structure of more complicated molecules. Nuclear magnetic resonance was first described and measured in molecular beams by *Isidor Rabi* in 1938.

Basics

Nuclei with an odd mass or odd atomic number have "nuclear spin" (in a similar fashion to the spin of electrons). This includes ^{1}H and ^{13}C (but **not** ^{12}C). The spins of nuclei are sufficiently different that NMR experiments can be sensitive for only one particular isotope of one particular element.

Since a nucleus is a charged particle in motion, it will develop a magnetic field. ^1H and ^{13}C have nuclear spins of 1/2 and so they behave in a similar fashion to a simple, tiny bar magnet. In the absence of a magnetic field, these are randomly oriented but when a field is applied they line up parallel to the applied field, either spin aligned or spin opposed. The more highly populated state is the lower energy spin state spin aligned situation. Two schematic representations of these arrangements are shown below:

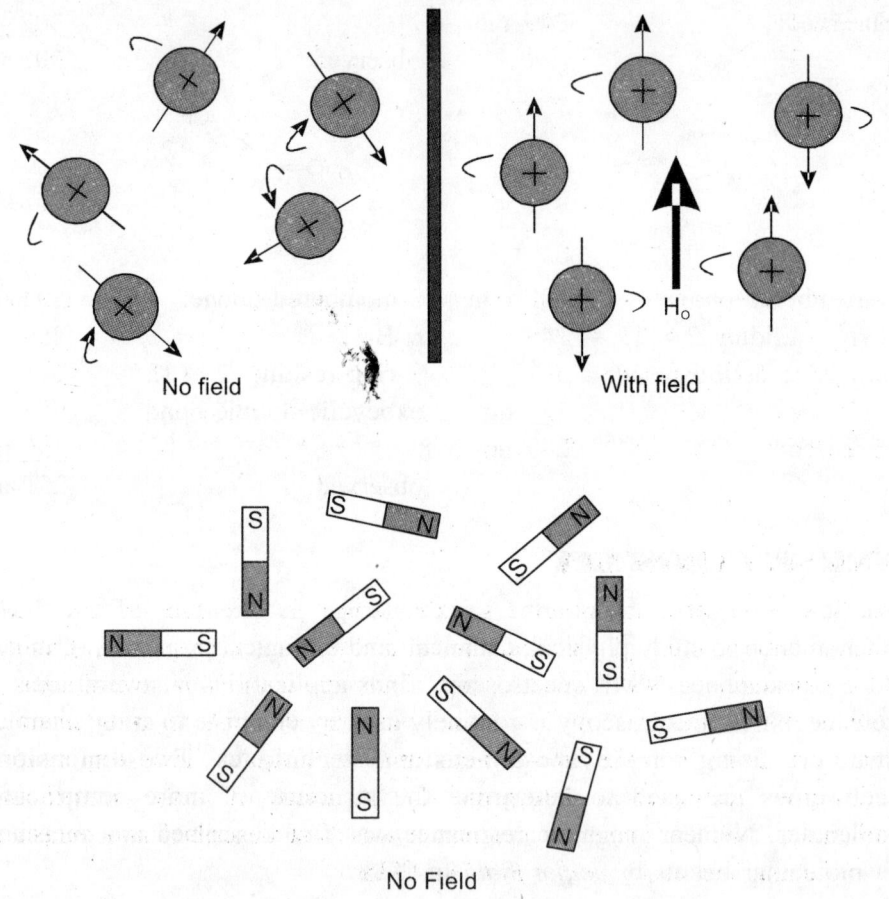

No field   With field H_o

No Field

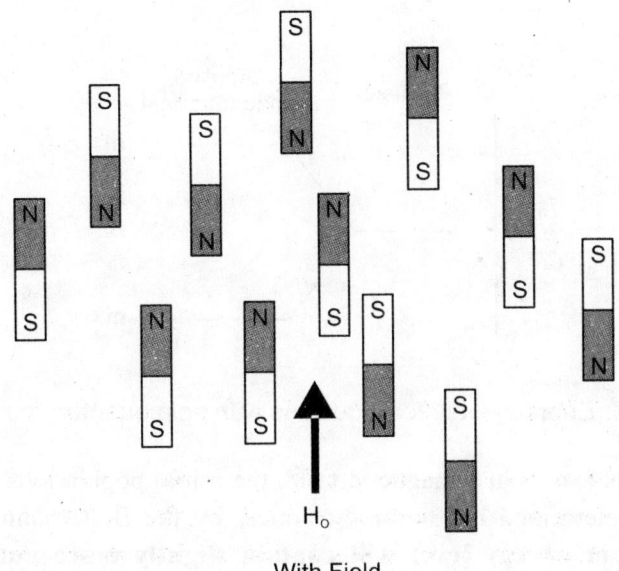

With Field

All nucleons, that is neutrons and protons, composing any atomic nucleus, have the intrinsic quantum property of spin. The overall spin of the nucleus is determined by the spin quantum number S. If the number of both the protons and neutrons in a given nuclide are even then $S = 0$, i.e. there is no overall spin; just as electrons pair up in atomic orbitals, so do even numbers of protons or even numbers of neutrons (which are also spin-$^1D_2$ particles and hence fermions) pair up giving zero overall spin. A non-zero spin is thus always associated with a non-zero magnetic moment.

The rules for determining the net spin of a nucleus are as follows;

1. If the number of neutrons **and** the number of protons are both even, then the nucleus has **NO** spin.

2. If the number of neutrons **plus** the number of protons is odd, then the nucleus has a half-integer spin (i.e. 1/2, 3/2, 5/2)

3. If the number of neutrons **and** the number of protons are both odd, then the nucleus has an integer spin (i.e. 1, 2, 3))

The overall spin, I, is important. Quantum mechanics tells us that a nucleus of spin I will have $2I + 1$ possible orientations. A nucleus with spin 1/2 will have 2 possible orientations. In the absence of an external magnetic field, these orientations are of equal energy. If a magnetic field is applied,

then the energy levels split. Each level is given a *magnetic quantum number,*
m.

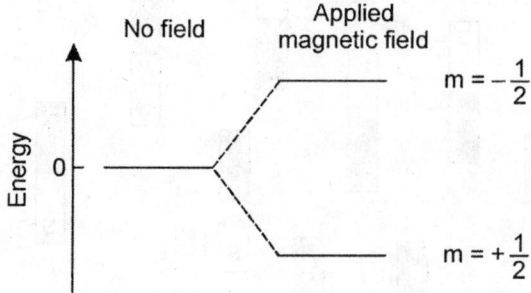

Fig. 2.4: Energy levels for a nucleus with spin quantum number 1/2

When the nucleus is in a magnetic field, the initial populations of the energy
levels are determined by thermodynamics(by the Boltzmann distribution)
that **the lower energy level will contain slightly more nuclei than the
higher level**. It is possible to excite these nuclei into the higher level with
electromagnetic radiation. The frequency of radiation needed is determined
by the difference in energy (ΔE) between the energy levels. If this energy is
supplied by external source in the form of radio frequency, then the nucleus
attains the state of resonance and a signal is obtained, knwon as NMR
signal.

Calculating transition energy

The nucleus has a positive charge and is spinning. This generates a small
magnetic field. The nucleus therefore possesses a magnetic moment, μ, which
is proportional to its spin, *I*.

$$\mu = \frac{\gamma I h}{2\pi}$$

The constant, γ, is called the *magnetogyric ratio* and is a fundamental
nuclear constant which has a different value for every nucleus. *h* is Plancks
constant.

The energy of a particular energy level is given by;

$$E = \frac{\gamma h}{2\pi} = m\,B$$

Where *B* is the strength of the magnetic field **at the nucleus**.

The difference in energy between levels (the transition energy) can be found from

$$\Delta E = \frac{\gamma h B}{2\pi}$$

This means that if the magnetic field, B, is increased, so is ΔE. It also means that if a nucleus has a relatively large magnetogyric ratio, then DE is correspondingly large.

Instrumentation: Diagram of NMR Spectrometer is shown in the Fig. 2.5. The instrument consists of 2 strong magnets,between them sample is placed in the sample tube. Radiofrequency oscillator (RFO) is used to match the frequency, when nucleus is in resonance then NMR signal is obtained. Generally RFO is set between 40 to 100MHz frequency.

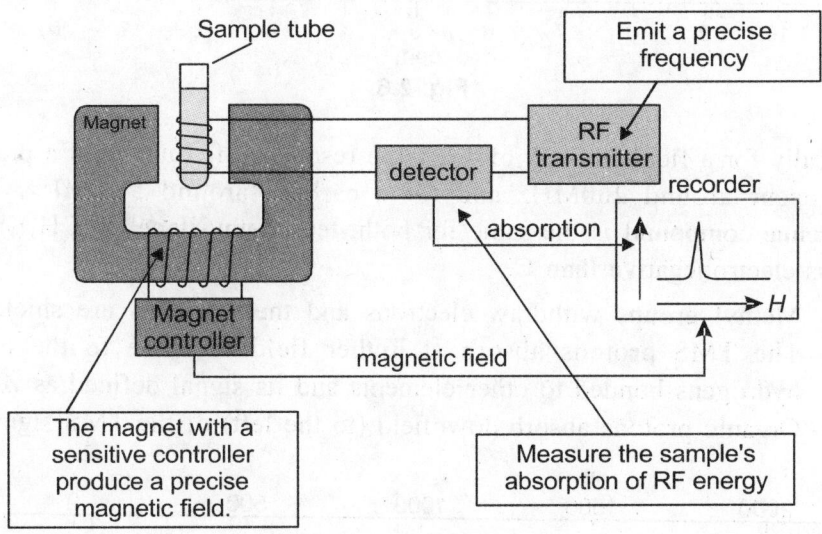

Fig. 2.5: NMR Spectrometer

Chemical Shift: It is a measure of how far the signal of the proton (sample) is from the reference signal.

The chemical shift in absolute terms is defined by the frequency of the resonance expressed with reference to a standard compound which is *defined* to be at 0 ppm. The scale is made more manageable by expressing it in parts per million (ppm) and is independent of the spectrometer frequency.

- An NMR spectrum is a plot of the *radio frequency applied* against *absorption*.

- A signal in the spectrum is referred to as a *resonance*.
- The frequency of a signal is known as its *chemical shift*, δ.
  Chemical shift,

$$\delta = \frac{\text{frequency of signal} - \text{frequency of reference}}{\text{spectrometer frequency}} \times 10^6$$

It is often convienient to describe the relative positions of the resonances in an NMR spectrum. For example, a peak at a chemical shift, δ, of 10 ppm is said to be *downfield* or *deshielded* with respect to a peak at 5 ppm,. The terms shielded and deshielded will be explained later.

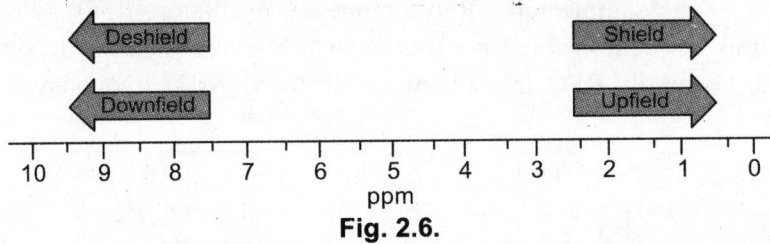

Fig. 2.6.

Typically for a field strength of 4.7 T the resonance frequency of a proton will occur around 200MHz and for a carbon, around 50.4MHz. The **reference** compound is the same for both, tetramethysilane ($Si(CH_3)_4$). Si is less electronegative than C.

- Methyl groups withdraw electrons and their protons are shielded. The TMS protons absorb at higher field compare to the most hydrogens bonded to other elements and its signal defined as zero.
- Organic protons absorb downfield (to the left) of the TMS signal.

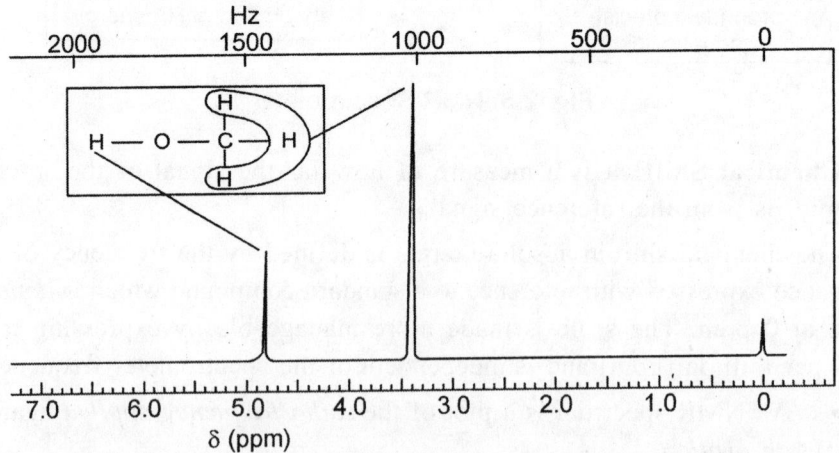

Fig. 2.7

TMS is used as a standard or reference compound in NMR because TMS has very low boiling point i.e volatie in nature at room temperature, it is unreactive, it cab be obtained in the pure form, it gives single NMR peak with out splitting, when analysis is over, it can be separated easily.

H-NMR Chemical Shifts

- The <u>chemical shift</u> is the position on the δ scale (in ppm) where the peak occurs.
- Typical ppm values for protons in different chemical environments are shown in the Fig. 2.8 and 2.9 below.
- There are two major factors that influence chemical shifts
  - (a) deshielding due to reduced electron density (due electronegative atoms). More electronegative substituent deshield more and give larger chemical shifts. Effect of an electronegative group on the chemical shift depends on its distance from the protons.

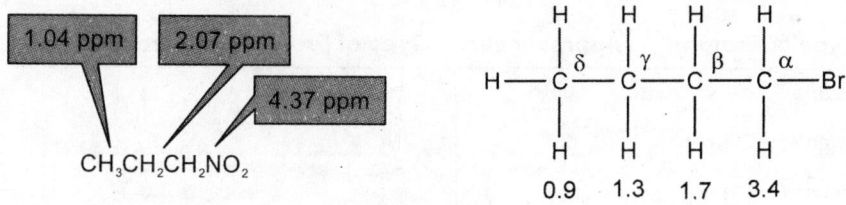

Fig. 2.8.

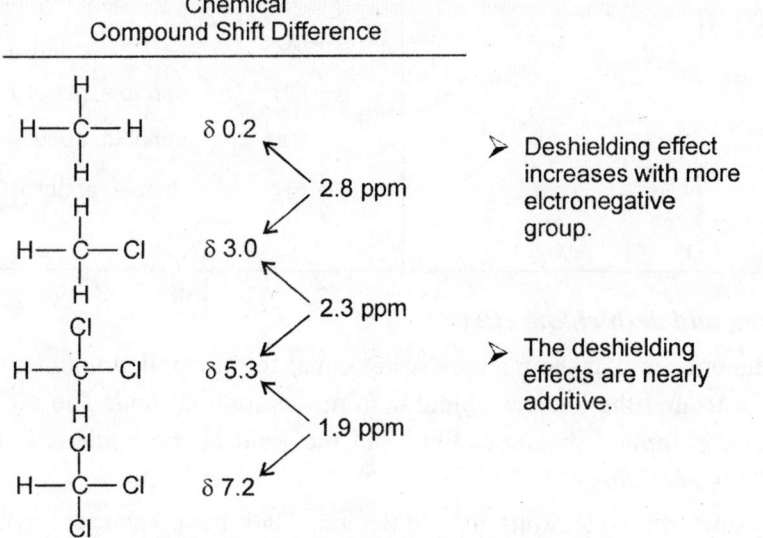

Fig. 2.9.

The effect decreases with increasing distance. The effects can be negligible if the protons are separated from the electronegative group by four or more bonds.

(b) anisotropy (due to magnetic fields generated by À bonds).

Some values of chemical shift for different type of H atom attached to C are given Fig. 2.10:

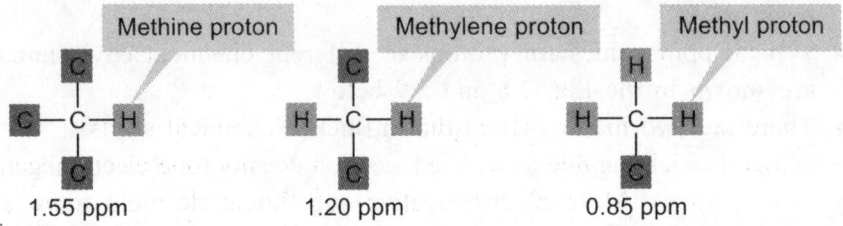

Some chraracteristics values of chemical shifts are given Fig. 2.10:

Type of Proton	Approximate δ	Type of Proton	Approximate δ
alkane (—CH₃)	0.9	$>C=C<_{CH_3}$	1.7
alkane (—CH₂—)	1.3	Ph—H	7.2
alkane ($-\underset{\mid}{C}H-$)	1.4	Ph—CH₃	2.3
		R—CHO	9 – 10
$-\overset{O}{\underset{\parallel}{C}}-CH_3$	2.1	R—COOh	10 – 12
—C≡C—H	2.5	R—OH	variable, about 2–5
R—CH₂—X	3 – 4	Ar—OH	variable, about 4–7
(X = halogen, O)		R—NH₂	variable, about 1.5–4
$>C=C<_H$	5 – 6		

Shielding and deshielding effect

The magnetic field at the nucleus is **not** equal to the applied magnetic field; electrons around the nucleus shield it from the applied field. The difference between the applied magnetic field and the field at the nucleus is termed the *nuclear shielding*.

Consider the s-electrons in a molecule. They have spherical symmetry and circulate in the applied field, producing a magnetic field which opposes the applied field. This means that the applied field strength must be increased for the nucleus to absorb at its transition frequency. This *upfield shift* is also termed *diamagnetic shift.*, while the electrons which create external magnetic field and that field (secondary magnetic field) is along the external magnetic, in this state proton or nucleus is said to deshielded and deshielded proton requires less energy to flip or resonance.Deshielding effect given down field signal. Electrons in p-orbitals have **no** spherical symmetry. They produce comparatively large magnetic fields at the nucleus, which give a *low field shift*. This "deshielding" is also termed *paramagnetic shift.*

In proton (^{1}H) NMR, p-orbitals play no part, which is why only a small range of chemical shift (10 ppm) is observed. We can easily see the effect of s-electrons on the chemical shift by looking at substituted methanes, CH_3X. As X becomes increasingly electronegative, so the electron density around the protons decreases, and they resonate at lower field strengths (increasing d_H values).

Depending on their chemical environment, protons in a molecule are shielded by different amounts. Hydrogen bonding in concentrated solutions deshield the protons, so signal is around δ–3.5 for N-H and δ–4.5 for O-H. The presence of electronegative atom will withdraw electron from the proton, hence it is deshielded.

Hydrogen bonding and oxygen atom strongly deshield the carboxylic acid proton in acid.

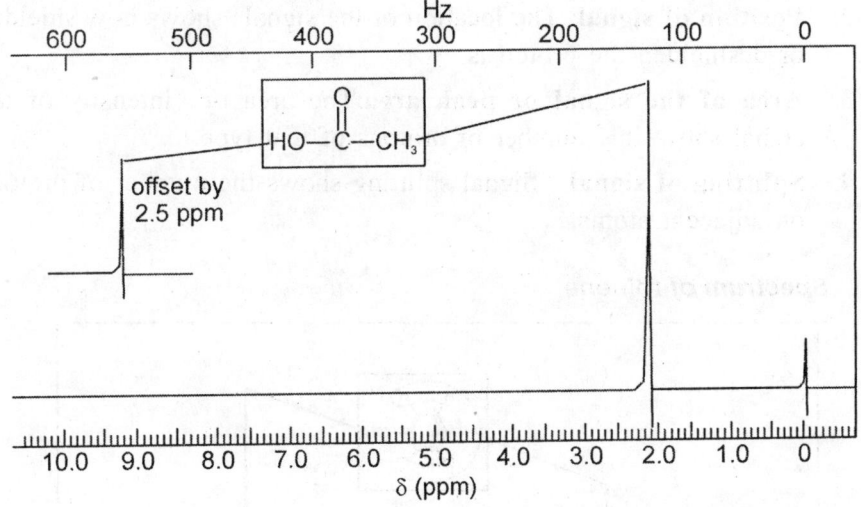

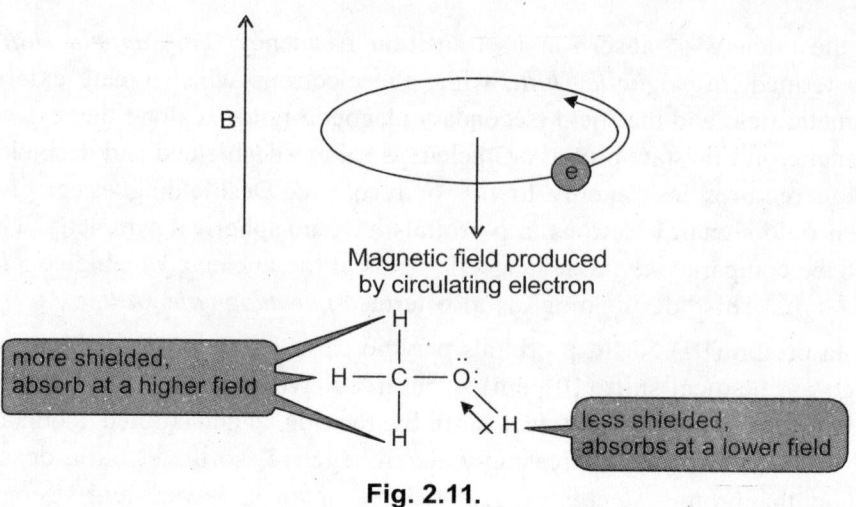

Magnetic field produced
by circulating electron

more shielded,
absorb at a higher field

less shielded,
absorbs at a lower field

Fig. 2.11.

In toluene, it is the protons attached directly to the aromatic ring that will be the most deshielded.

Study of NMR spectrum: NMR Signals

NMR spectrum consists of NMR signals and study of NMR signal is mainly dependent on following four points:-

1. **Number of singal/peaks:** The number of signals shows how many different kinds of protons are present.

2. **Position of signal**: The location of the signals shows how shielded or deshielded the proton is.

3. **Area of the signal or peak area:** The area or intensity of the signal shows the number of protons of that type.

4. **Splitting of signal**: Signal splitting shows the number of protons on adjacent atoms.

Spectrum of toluene

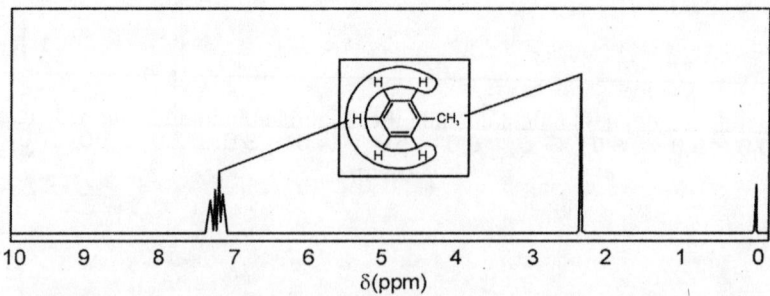

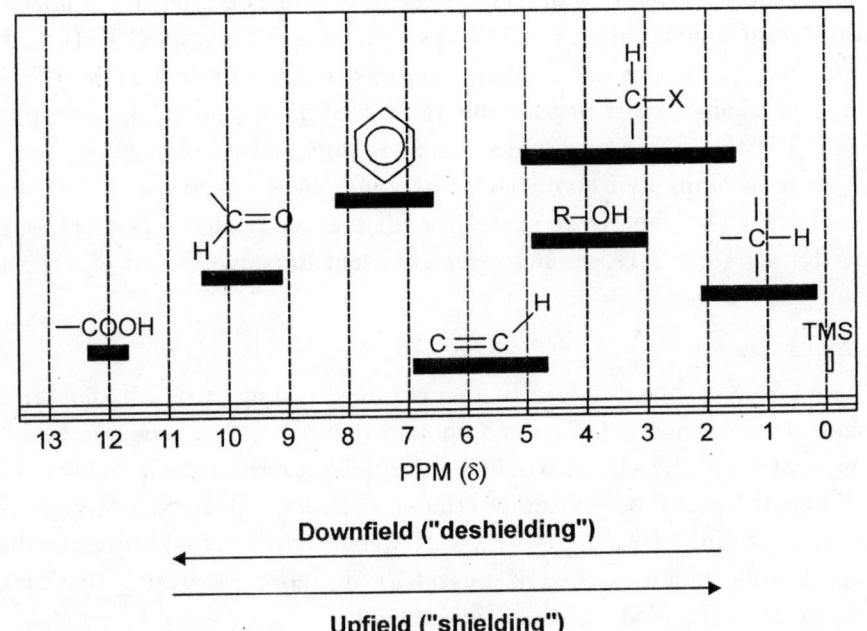

Fig. 2.12.

1. Number of signals/peaks

Number of peaks or signal in aspectrum of acompound are proportional to the different kinds of proton present in that molecule.

A hydrogen atom is "different" to another hydrogen atom if it is not in an identical environment to the other hydrogen. This could mean it's attached to a different type of atom (e.g. CH vs OH, or sp3 CH vs sp2 CH) or due to the number of adjacent H (e.g. CH_3– vs –CH_2–) or just at a different point in a chain (e.g. compare the H in the methylene (CH_2) groups in $CH_3CH_2CH_2OH$

Counting different types of Hydrogen

There are variuos methods that can be used to count the number of kinds of H (each achieve the same result).

Substitution method (simplest but slowest)

The idea is that we replace each H in the molecule in turn with a "dummy" atom (for example a –Cl) to see if you get a different product (*i.e.* one that will require a different name). Each new product, indicates a different type of H. This idea is related to the radical chlorination of alkanes where some of each possible product is usually obtained.

A hydrogen atom is "different" to another hydrogen atom if it is not in an identical environment to the other hydrogen. This could mean it's attached to a different type of atom (e.g. CH vs OH, or sp3 CH vs sp2 CH) or due to the number of adjacent H (e.g. CH_3- vs $-CH_2-$) or just at a different point in a chain (e.g. compare the H in the methylene (CH_2) groups in $CH3CH_2CH_2OH$. Only one NMR signal is obtained corresponding to all equivalent protons in a compound like, one NMR signal for all the four H atoms of CH_4, one NMR signal for all the six H atoms of C_2H_6 but 2 signal for C_2H_5Cl(3 H are equivalent, present on same C and other 2 are like attached to second C).

Position of signal

Position of NMR signal is largely affected by shielding or deshielding effect present in the compound.If an acompound more than one type of H atoms are present then one signal would be deshielded most (down fielded) and other signal would be upfielded (most shielded).Electronegativity and hydrogen bonding affect the position of signal. NMR signal corresponding to the H atom which is closely present to the more electronegative atom, would more deshielded or down field signal.

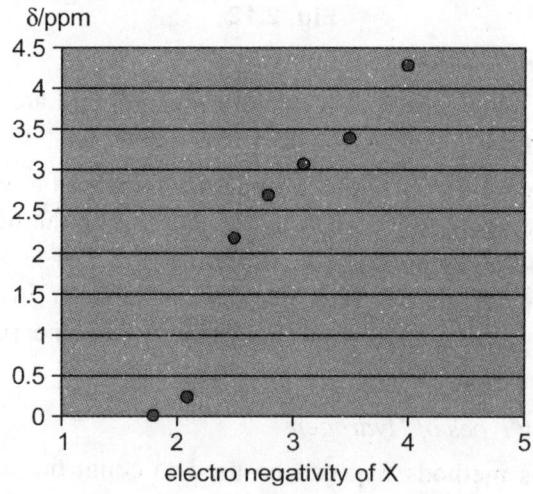

Fig. 2.13.

Since the field experienced by the proton defines the energy difference between the two spin states, the frequency and hence the chemical shift, δ/ppm, will change depending on the electron density around the proton. Electronegative groups attached to the C—H system decrease the electron density around the protons, and there is less shielding (*i.e.* deshielding) so the chemical shift increases. This is reflected by the plot shown in the graph to the left which is based on the data shown below:

Compound, CH_3X	CH_3F	CH_3OH	CH_3Cl	CH_3Br	CH_3I	CH_4	$(CH_3)_4Si$
X	F	O	Cl	Br	I	H	Si
Electronegativity of X	4.0	3.5	3.1	2.8	2.5	2.1	1.8
Chemical shift, δ/ppm	4.26	3.4	3.05	2.68	2.16	0.23	0

These effects are cumulative, so the presence of more electronegative groups produce more deshielding and therefore, larger chemical shifts.

Compound	CH_4	CH_3Cl	CH_2Cl_2	$CHCl_3$
δ/ppm	0.23	3.05	5.30	7.27

These **inductive effects** are not just felt by the immediately adjacent protons as the disruption of electron density has an influence further down the chain. However, the effect does fade rapidly as you move away from the electronegative group. As an example, look at the chemical shifts for part of a primary bromide

H signal	$-CH_2-CH_2-CH_2Br$		
δ / ppm	1.25	1.69	3.30

3. Area of signal or relative intensity of signal (Integration)

Area of a particular signal is directly proportional to the number of corresponding H atoms present in that signal. It gives the idea about the number of H atoms present in different NMR signal of a compound, with the help of calculation of relative area we can find out total and individual H atoms present in various signals. It is important to remember that integration only provides ratios of protons, not the absolute number. For convenience in calculating the relative signal strengths, the smallest

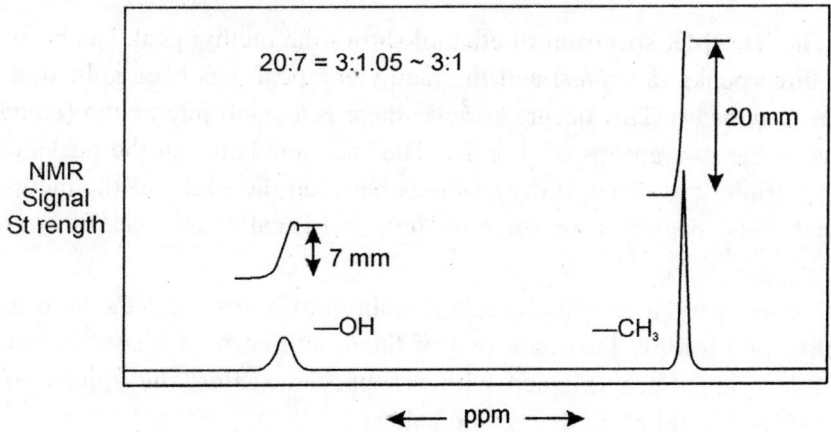

integration is set to 1 and the other values are converted accordingly. Like in ethanol, CH_3CH_2OH, 3 NMR signal areas are in the ratio of 3:2:1.

Integrals appear as lines on the spectra above the signals, in which their heights correspond to the integration ratios. In this spectra, the area corresponding to –OH H is correctly determined to be in a 3:1 ratio with the 3 CH_3 H's.

4. Splitting of signal (Spin - spin coupling)

NMR signals are not usually single triangles, but a complex pattern of split triangles labeled as doublets (2peaks), triplets (3 peaks), quartets (4 peaks), etc. The distance between the split peaks are called coupling constants, denoted by J. The interaction between nearby protons produce different spin flip energies (E) as they can orient themselves in a pattern of parallel or antiparallel to the applied magnetic force. This phenomenon, where the spin of the nucleus of one proton is close enough to affect the spin of another, is called spin-spin coupling. Splitting is always reciprocated between the protons—if Ha splits Hb, then Hb must split Ha—and provides information on the neighbors of a proton within the molecule.

N + 1 Rule: For a proton with n neighbours, its signal will be split into n + 1 lines

Consider the structure of ethanol;

Methylene
↓
CH_3—CH_2—OH
↑
Methyl

The ^1H NMR spectrum of ethanol shows the methyl peak has been split into three peaks (a *triplet*) and the methylene peak has been split into four peaks (a *quartet*). This occurs because there is a small interaction (*coupling*) between the two groups of protons. The spacings between the peaks of the methyl triplet are equal to the spacings between the peaks of the methylene quartet. This spacing is measured in Hertz and is called the *coupling constant, J.*

To see why the methyl peak is split into a triplet, let's look at the **methylene** protons. There are two of them, and each can have one of two possible orientations (aligned with or opposed against the applied field). This gives a total of four possible states;

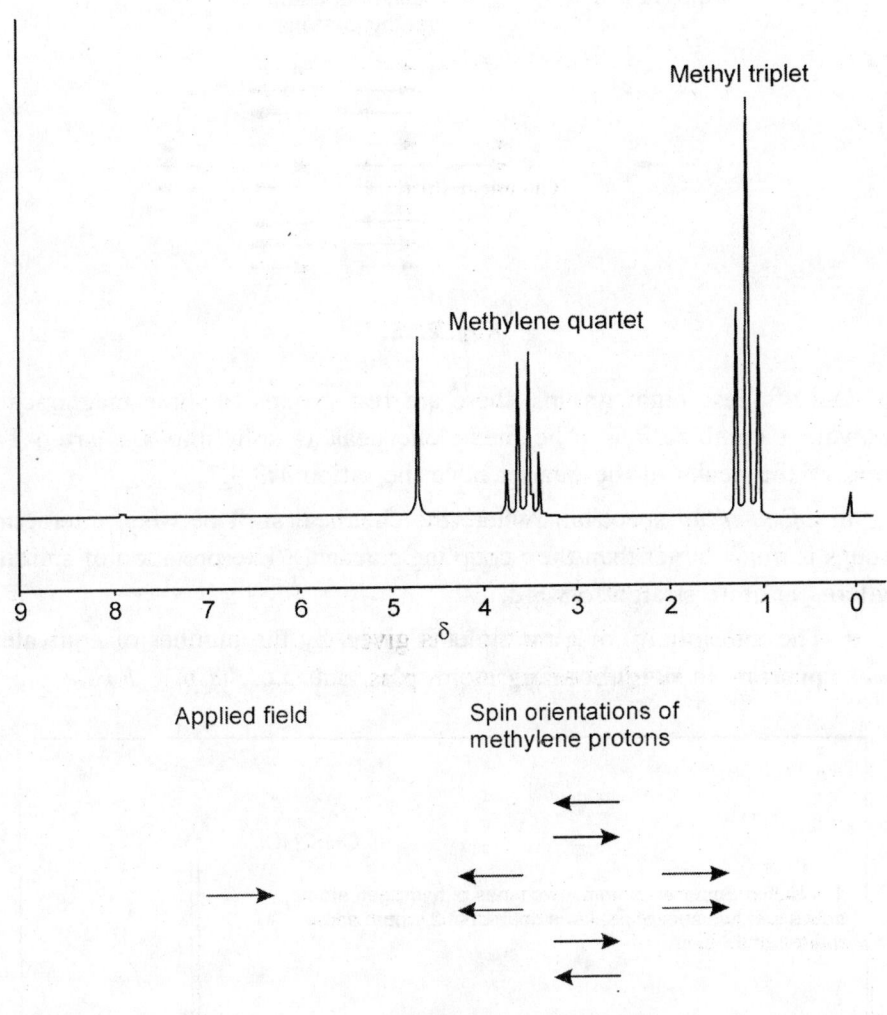

Fig. 2.14.

In the first possible combination, spins are paired and opposed to the field. This has the effect of reducing the field experienced by the **methyl** protons; therefore a slightly higher field is needed to bring them to resonance, resulting in an upfield shift. Neither combination of spins opposed to each other has an effect on the methyl peak. The spins paired in the direction of the field produce a downfield shift. Hence, the methyl peak is split into three, with the ratio of areas 1:2:1. Similarly, the effect of the methyl protons on the methylene protons is such that here are eight possible spin combinations for the three methyl protons;

Applied field   Spin orientations of
                                       methyl protons

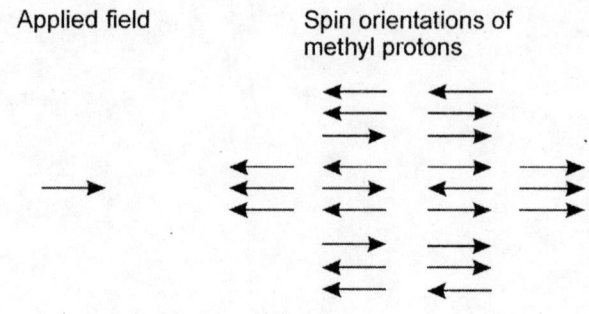

Fig. 2.15.

Out of these eight groups, there are two groups of three magnetically equivalent combinations. The methylene peak is split into a quartet. The areas of the peaks in the quartet have the ration 1:3:3:1.

In a *first-order* spectrum (where the chemical shift between interacting groups is much larger than their coupling constant), interpretation of splitting patterns is quite straightforward;

- The multiplicity of a multiplet is given by the number of equivalent **protons** in **neighbouring** atoms plus one, i.e. *the n + 1 rule*.

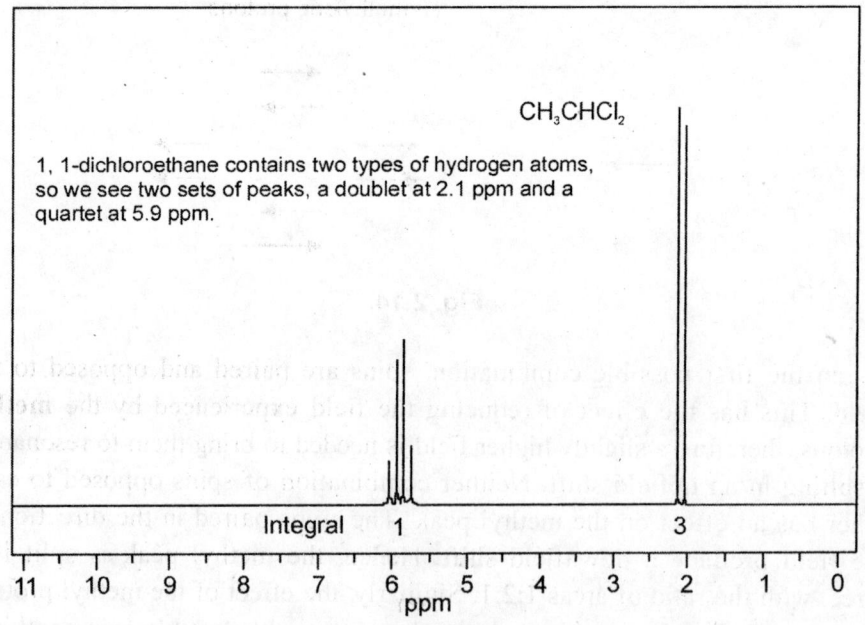

CH_3CHCl_2

1, 1-dichloroethane contains two types of hydrogen atoms, so we see two sets of peaks, a doublet at 2.1 ppm and a quartet at 5.9 ppm.

Integral   1   3

11   10   9   8   7   6   5   4   3   2   1   0
                          ppm

Fig. 2.16.

- Equivalent nuclei do not interact with each other. The three methyl protons in ethanol cause splitting of the neighbouring methylene protons; they do not cause splitting among themselves.
- The coupling constant is not dependant on the applied field. Multiplets can be easily distinguished from closely spaced chemical shift peaks.

For another example, see the spectra of 1, 1-dichloroethane shown Fig. 2.16:

Before we look at the coupling, lets review the assignment of the peaks first:

- δ = 5.9 ppm, integration = 1H deshielded: agrees with the —$CHCl_2$ unit
- δ = 2.1 ppm, integration = 3H : agrees with —CH_3 unit

Now, what about the coupling patterns?

Coupling arises because the magnetic field of vicinal (adjacent) protons influences the field that the proton experiences.

- The proximity of "n" equivalent H on neighbouring carbon atoms, causes the signals to be split into "n + 1" lines.
- This is known as the *multiplicity* or *splitting* or *coupling pattern* of each signal.
- Equivalent protons (or those with the same chemical shift) **do not couple** to each other.
- If the neighbours are not all equivalent, more complex patterns arise.
- To a first approximation, protons on adjacent sp^3 C tend to behave as if they are equivalent.

Now we can do more a complete analysis, including the application of the "n + 1" rule to 1,1-dichloroethane:

- δ = 5.9 ppm, quartet, integration = 1H, deshielded : agrees with the —$CHCl_2$ unit next to a –CH_3 unit (n = 3, so n + 1 = 4 lines)
- δ = 2.1 ppm, doublet, integration = 3H : agrees with —CH_3 unit, next to a —CH— (n = 1, so n + 1 = 2 lines)

Coupling Constant, J

The coupling constant, J (usually in frequency units, Hz) is a measure of the interaction between a pair of protons.

In a vicinal system of the general type, H_a—C—C—H_b then the coupling of H_a with H_b, J_{ab},

Must be Equal to the coupling of H_b with H_a, J_{ba}, therefore $J_{ab} = J_{ba}$.

The implications are that the spacing between the lines in the coupling patterns are the same as can be seen in the coupling patterns from the H-NMR spectra of 1,1-dichloroethane (see left).

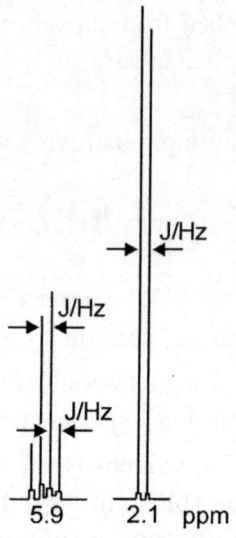

Fig. 2.17.

Pascal's Triangle

The relative intensitites of the lines in a coupling pattern is given by a binomial expansion or more conviently by Pascal's triangle.

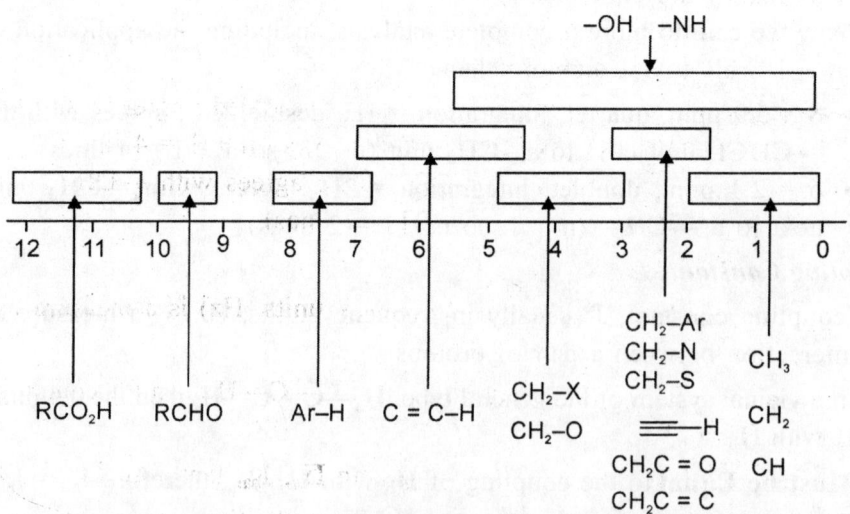

Fig. 2.18.

To derive Pascal's triangle, start at the apex, and generate each lower row by creating each number by adding the two numbers above and to either side in the row above together. The first six rows are shown to the Fig. 2.18.

So for H-NMR a proton with zero neighbours, n = 0, appears as a single line, a proton with one neighbours, n = 1 as two lines of equal intensity, a proton with two neighbours, n = 2, as three lines of intensities 1 : 2 : 1, etc.

Note that the figure shows the typical chemical shifts for protons being influenced by a *single group*.

Some H-NMR Spectra of -ethyl bromide, propy bromide and isopropyl alcohol are shown here in the given Fig. (2.19, 2.20 and 2.21).

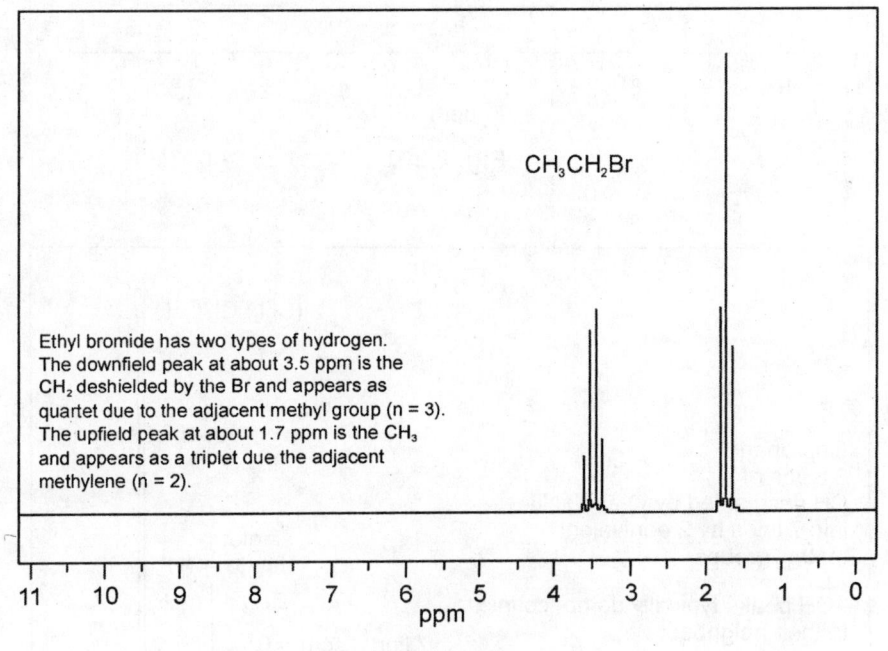

CH_3CH_2Br

Ethyl bromide has two types of hydrogen. The downfield peak at about 3.5 ppm is the CH_2 deshielded by the Br and appears as quartet due to the adjacent methyl group (n = 3). The upfield peak at about 1.7 ppm is the CH_3 and appears as a triplet due the adjacent methylene (n = 2).

ppm

Fig. 2.19.

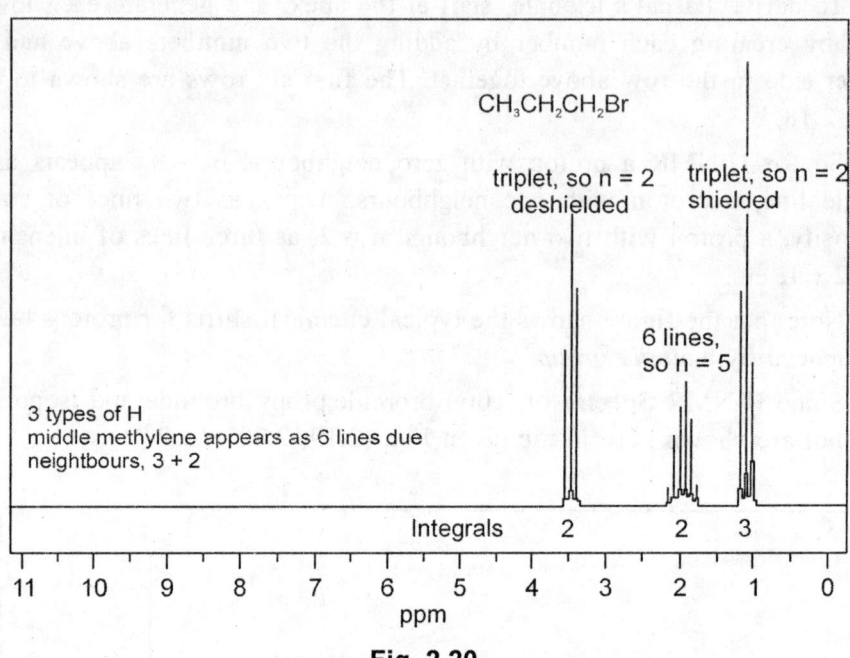

Fig. 2.20.

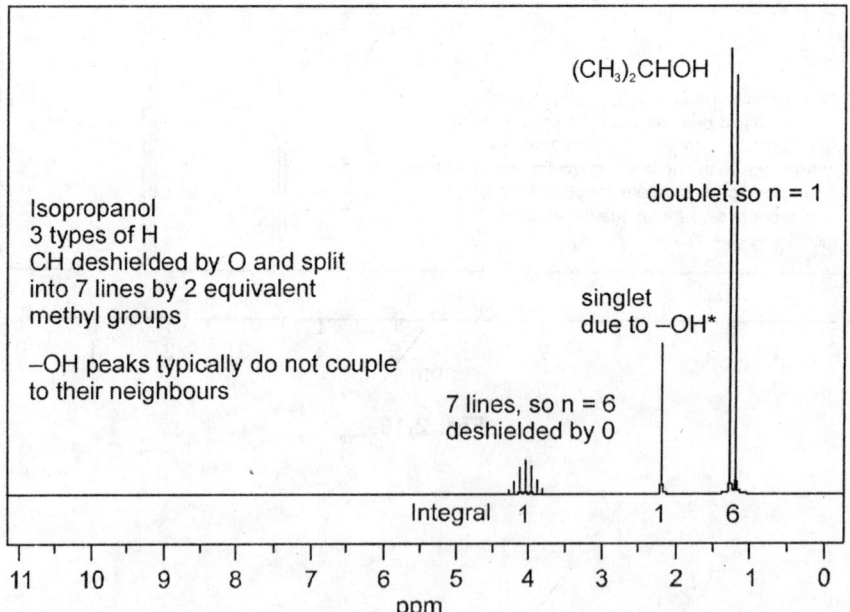

Fig. 2.21.

Interpretting ¹H-NMR Spectra

Let's summarise what can be obtained from a ¹H NMR spectrum:

How many types of H?

Indicated by how many groups of signals there are in the spectra

What types of H?

Indicated by the chemical shift of each group

How many H of each type are there?

Indicated by the integration (relative area) of the signal for each group.

What is the connectivity?

Look at the coupling patterns. This tells you what is next to each group

An example of an H NMR is shown below:

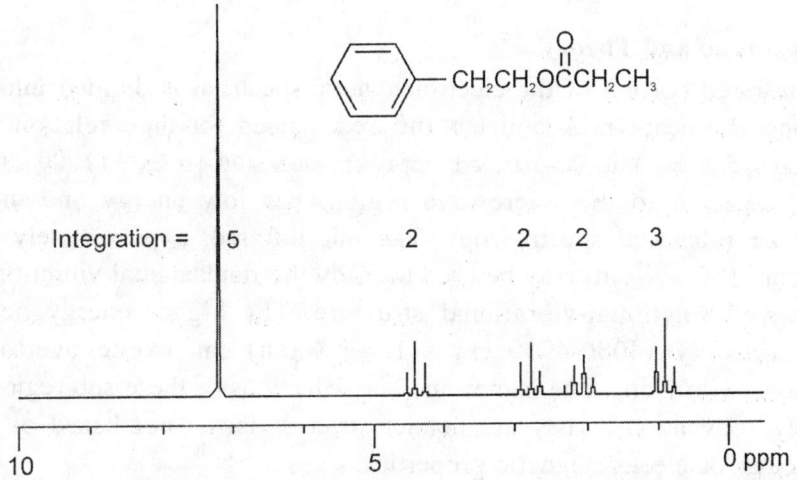

Based on the outline given above the four sets of information we get are:

5 basic types of H present in the ratio of 5 : 2 : 2 : 2 : 3.

These are seen as a 5H "singlet" (ArH), two 2H triplets, a 2H quartet and a 3H triplet. Each triplet tells us that there are 2H in the adjacent position, and a quartet tells us that there are 3H adjacent.

(Think of it as the lines you see, L = n + 1, where n = number of equivalent adjacent H)

This tells us we that the peaks at 4.4 and 2.8 ppm must be connected as a CH_2CH_2 unit.

The peaks at 2.1 and 0.9 ppm as a CH_2CH_3 unit. Using the chemical shift charts, the H can be assigned to the peaks as below:

7.2ppm (5H) = Ar**H**

4.4ppm (2H) = **CH**$_2$O

2.8ppm (2H) = Ar-**CH**$_2$

2.1ppm (2H) = O=C**CH**$_2$CH$_3$ and

0.9ppm (3H) = CH$_2$**CH**$_3$

INFRARED SPECTROSCOPY

Infrared spectroscopy offers the possibility to measure different types of inter atomic bond vibrations at different frequencies. Especially in organic chemistry the analysis of IR absorption spectra shows what type of bonds are present in the sample.

Background and Theory

The infrared portion of the electromagnetic spectrum is divided into three regions; the near-, mid- and far- infrared, named for their relation to the visible spectrum . The far–infrared, approximately 400–10 cm^{-1} (1000–30 μm), lying adjacent to the microwave region, has low energy and may be used for rotational spectroscopy. The mid-infrared, approximately 4000-400 cm^{-1} (30–1.4 μm) may be used to study the fundamental vibrations and associated rotational-vibrational structure. The higher energy near-IR, approximately 14000-4000 cm^{-1} (1.4–0.8 μm) can excite overtone or harmonic vibrations. The names and classifications of these sub regions are merely conventions. They are neither strict divisions nor based on exact molecular or electromagnetic properties.

Infrared spectroscopy exploits the fact that molecules have specific frequencies at which they rotate or vibrate corresponding to discrete energy levels (vibrational modes). These resonant frequencies are determined by the shape of the molecular potential energy surfaces, the masses of the atoms and, by the associated vibronic coupling. In order for a vibrational mode in a molecule to be IR active, it must be associated with changes in the permanent dipole.

In particular, in the Born-Oppenheimer and harmonic approximations, i.e. when the molecular Hamiltonian corresponding to the electronic ground state can be approximated by a harmonic oscillator in the neighborhood of the equilibrium molecular geometry, the resonant frequencies are determined by the normal modes corresponding to the molecular electronic ground state

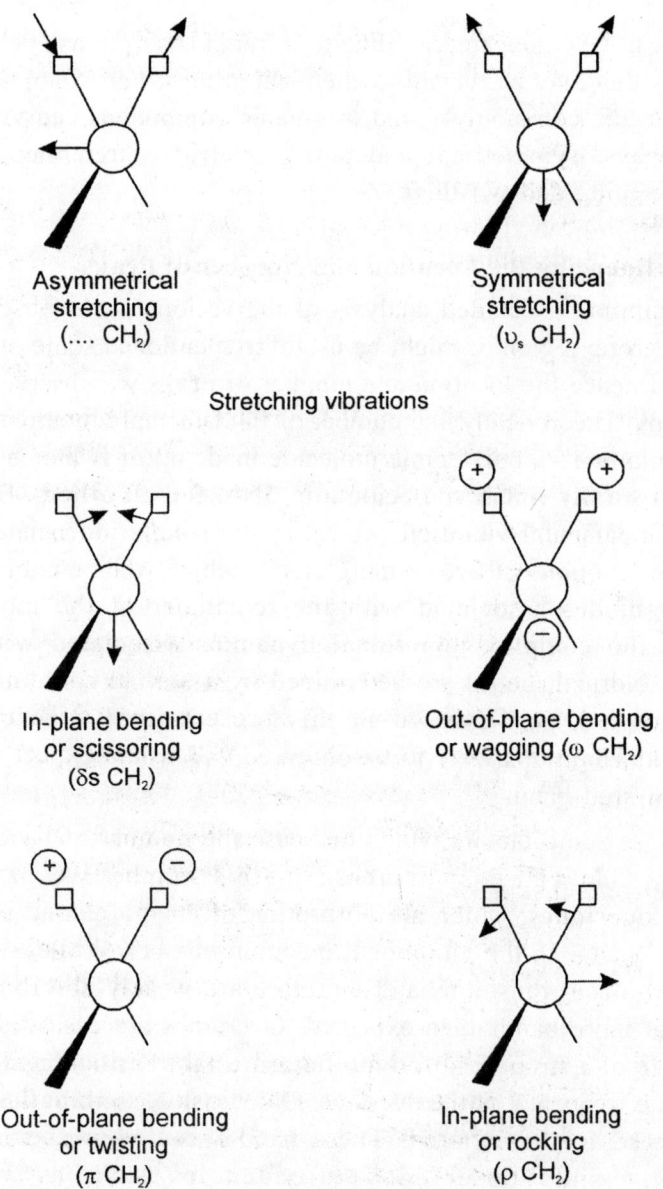

Asymmetrical stretching (.... CH_2)

Symmetrical stretching (υ_s CH_2)

Stretching vibrations

In-plane bending or scissoring (δs CH_2)

Out-of-plane bending or wagging (ω CH_2)

Out-of-plane bending or twisting (π CH_2)

In-plane bending or rocking (ρ CH_2)

Fig. 2.22: Bending Vibrations

potential energy surface. Nevertheless, the resonant frequencies can be in a first approach related to the strength of the bond, and the mass of the atoms at either end of it. Thus, the frequency of the vibrations can be associated with a particular bond type. Simple diatomic molecules have only one bond, which may stretch. More complex molecules have many bonds, and vibrations can be conjugated, leading to infrared absorptions at characteristic frequencies that may be related to chemical groups. For example, the atoms in a CH_2 group, commonly found in organic compounds can vibrate in six different ways: symmetrical and antisymmetrical stretching, scissoring, rocking, wagging and twisting:

Factors Influencing the Location and Number of Peaks

Before beginning a detailed analysis of the various peaks observed in the functional group region, it might be useful to mentioned some of the factors that can influence the location and number of peaks we observe in infrared spectroscopy. Theoretically, the number of fundamental vibrations or **normal modes** available to a polyatomic molecule made up of N atoms is given by **3N-5 for a totally linear molecule and 3N-6 for all others.** By a normal mode or fundamental vibration, we mean the simple independent bending or stretching motions of two or more atoms, which when combined with all of normal modes associated with the remainder of the molecule will reproduce the complex vibrational dynamics associated with the real molecules. Normal modes are determined by a normal coordinate analysis (which will not be discussed in this presentation). If each of these fundamental vibrations were to be observed, we would expect either 3N-5 or 3N-6 infrared bands.

There are some factors which decrease the number of bands observed and others that cause an increase in this number. We have already mentioned **overtones**, which are absorption of energy caused by a change of 2 rather than 1 in the vibrational quantum number. While overtones are usually forbidden transitions and therefore are weakly absorbing, they do give rise to more bands than expected. Overtones are easily identified by the presence of a strongly absorbing fundamental transition at slightly more than half the frequency of the overtone. On occasion, **combination bands** are also observed in the infrared. These bands, as their name implies, are absorption bands observed at frequencies such as $_1 + _2$ or $_1 - _2$, where $_1$ and $_2$ refer to fundamental frequencies. Other combinations of frequencies are possible. The symmetry properties of the fundamentals play a role in determining which combinations are observed. Fortunately, combination bands are seldom observed in the functional group region of most polyatomic molecules and the presence of these bands seldom cause a problem in identification. Another cause of splitting of bands in infrared is due to a phenomena called **Fermi Resonance**. While a discussion of Fermi Resonance is beyond the scope of this presentation, this splitting can be observed whenever two fundamental motions or a fundamental and combination band have nearly the same energy (*i.e.* $_1$ and 2_2 or $_1$ and $_2 + _3$). In this case, the two levels split each other. One level increases while the other decreases in energy. In order to observe Fermi Resonance, in addition to the requirement that a near coincidence of energy levels occurs, other symmetry properties of these vibrations must also be satisfied. As a consequence, Fermi Resonance bands are not frequently encountered.

There are also several factors which decrease the number of infrared bands observed. Symmetry is one of the factors that can significantly reduce the number of bands observed in the infrared. If stretching a bond does not cause a change in the dipole moment, the vibration will not be able to interact with the infrared radiation and the vibration will be infrared inactive. Other factors include the near coincidence of peaks that are not resolved by the spectrometer and the fact that only a portion of the infrared spectrum is usually accessed by most commercial infrared spectrometers.

The infrared spectrum of a sample is collected by passing a beam of infrared light through the sample. Examination of the transmitted light reveals how much energy was absorbed at each wavelength. This can be done with a monochromatic beam, which changes in wavelength over time, or by using a Fourier transform instrument to measure all wavelengths at once. From this, a transmittance or absorbance spectrum can be produced, showing at which IR wavelengths the sample absorbs. Analysis of these absorption characteristics reveals details about the molecular structure of the sample.

This technique works almost exclusively on samples with covalent bonds. Simple spectra are obtained from samples with few IR active bonds and high levels of purity. More complex molecular structures lead to more absorption bands and more complex spectra. The technique has been used for the characterization of very complex mixtures.

Sample preparation

Gaseous samples require little preparation beyond purification, but a sample cell with a long pathlength (typically 5-10 cm) is normally needed, as gases show relatively weak absorbances.

Liquid samples can be sandwiched between two plates of a high purity salt (commonly sodium chloride, or common salt, although a number of other salts such as potassium bromide or calcium fluoride are also used). The plates are transparent to the infrared light and will not introduce any lines onto the spectra. Some salt plates are highly soluble in water, so the sample and washing reagents must be anhydrous (without water).

Solid samples can be prepared in four major ways. The first is to crush the sample with a mulling agent (usually nujol) in a marble or agate mortar, with a pestle. A thin film of the mull is applied onto salt plates and measured.

The second method is to grind a quantity of the sample with a specially purified salt (usually potassium bromide) finely (to remove scattering effects from large crystals). This powder mixture is then crushed in a mechanical die press to form a translucent pellet through which the beam of the spectrometer can pass.

The third technique is the Cast Film technique, which is used mainly for polymeric materials. The sample is first dissolved in a suitable, non hygroscopic solvent. A drop of this solution is deposited on surface of KBr or NaCl cell. The solution is then evaporated to dryness and the film formed on the cell is analysed directly. Care is important to ensure that the film is not too thick otherwise light cannot pass through. This technique is suitable for qualitative analysis.

The final method is to use microtomy to cut a thin (20-100 micrometre) film from a solid sample. This is one of the most important ways of analysing failed plastic products for example because the integrity of the solid is preserved.

It is important to note that spectra obtained from different sample preparation methods will look slightly different from each other due to differences in the samples' physical states

Instrumentation: An infrared spectrophotometer is composed of an IR light source, a sample container, a prism to separate light by wavelength, a detector, and a recorder (which produces the infrared spectrum). A schematic for a typical infrared spectrophotometer is shown in Fig. 2.23.

A beam of infrared light is produced and split into two separate beams. One is passed through the sample, the other passed through a reference which is often the substance the sample is dissolved in. The beams are both reflected back towards a detector, however first they pass through a splitter which quickly alternates which of the two beams enters the detector. The two signals are then compared and a printout is obtained.

A reference is used for two reasons:

- This prevents fluctuations in the output of the source affecting the data
- This allows the effects of the solvent to be cancelled out (the reference is usually a pure form of the solvent the sample is in)

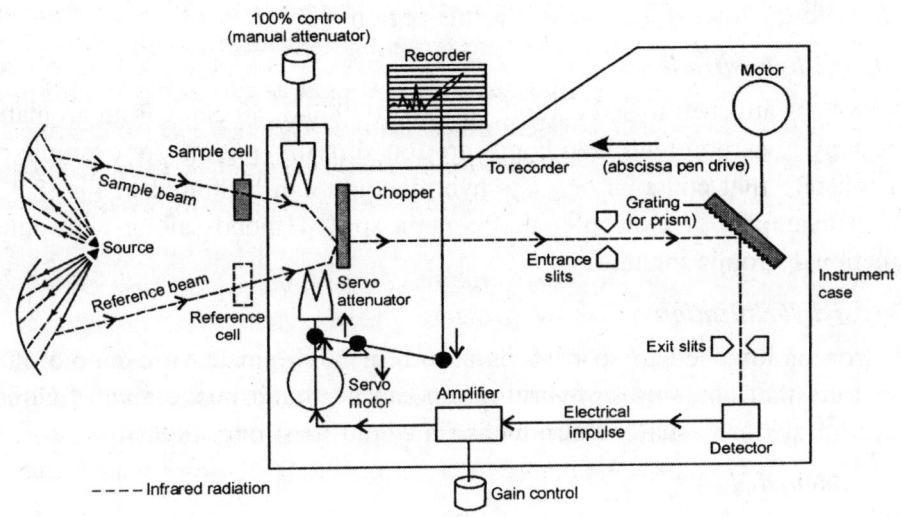

Fig. 2.23

Summary of absorptions of bonds in organic molecule:(Frequency)

C-H sp3 hybridization

Methyl groups, methylene groups and methine hydrogens on sp3 carbon atoms all absorb between 2850 and 3000 cm-1. While it is sometimes possible to differentiate between these types of hydrogen, the beginning student should probably avoid this type of interpretation. It should be pointed out however, that molecules that have local symmetry, will usually show symmetric and asymmetric stretching frequencies. Take, for example, a CH2 group. It is not possible to isolate an individual frequency for each hydrogen. These two hydrogens will couple and will show two stretching frequencies, a symmetric stretching frequency in which stretching and compression of both hydrogens occurs simultaneously, and an asymmetric stretching frequency in which stretching of one hydrogen is accompanied by compression of the other. While these two motions will occur at different frequencies, both will be found between the 2850-3000 cm-1 envelope. Similarly for a CH$_3$ group, symmetric and asymmetric vibrations are observed. This behavior is found whenever this type of local symmetry is present. We will find other similar examples in the functional groups we will be discussing. Some examples of spectra containing only sp3 hybridization can be found in Figs. 2.31-2.32, and located at the end of this discussion. These peaks are usually sharp and of medium intensity.

Considerable overlap of several of these bands usually results in absorption that is fairly intense and broad in this region.

C-H sp2 hybridization

Hydrogens attached to sp2 carbons absorb at 3000-3250 cm^{-1}. Both aromatic and vinylic carbon hydrogen bonds are found in this region. An example of a molecule that contains only sp^2 hybridization can be found in Fig. 2.32. Other examples of molecules that contain sp^2 C-H bonds along with other functional groups include.

C-H sp hybridization

Hydrogens attached to sp carbons absorb at 3300 cm^{-1}. An example of a spectrum that contains sp hybridization can be found in the given figures. These peaks are usually sharp and of medium to strong intensity.

C-H aldehydes

Before concluding the discussion of the carbon hydrogen bond, one additional type of C-H stretch can be distinguished, the C-H bond of an aldehyde. The C-H stretching frequency appears as a doublet, at 2750 and 2850 cm^{-1}. You may (should) question why the stretching of a single C-H bond in an aldehyde leads to the two bands just described. The splitting of C-H stretching frequency into a doublet in aldehydes is due to the phenomema we called "Fermi Resonance". It is believed that the aldehyde C-H stretch is in Fermi resonance with the first overtone of the C-H bending motion of the aldehyde. The normal frequency of the C-H bending motion of an aldehyde is at 1390 cm^{-1}. As a result of this interaction, one energy level drops to *ca.* 2750 and the other increases to *ca.* 2850 cm^{-1}. Only one C-H stretch is observed for aldehydes that have the C-H bending motion of an aldehyde significantly shifted from 1390 cm^{-1}.

C-H exceptions

In summary, it is possible to identify the type of hydrogen based on hybridization by examining the infrared spectra in the 3300 to 2750 cm^{-1} region. Before concluding, we should also mention some exceptions to the rules we just outlined. Cyclopropyl hydrogens which are formally classified as sp3 hybridized actually have more s character than 25%. Carbon-hydrogen frequencies greater than 3000 cm^{-1} are observed for these stretching vibrations. Halogen substitution can also affect the C-H stretching frequency. The C-H stretching frequencies of hydrogens attached to a carbon also bearing halogen substitution can also be shifted above 3000 cm^{-1}.

Nitrogen Hydrogen Stretching Frequencies

Much of what we have discussed regarding C-H stretching frequencies is also applicable here. There are three major differences between the C-H and N-H stretching frequencies. First, the force constant for N-H stretching is stronger, there is a larger dipole moment associated with the N-H bond, and finally, the N-H bond is usually involved in hydrogen bonding. The stronger force constant leads to a higher frequency for absorption. The N-H stretching frequency is usually observed from 3500-3200 cm^{-1}. The larger dipole moment leads to a stronger absorption and the presence of hydrogen bonding has a definite influence on the band shape and frequency position. The presence of hydrogen bonding has two major influences on spectra. First, its presence causes a shift toward lower frequency of all functional groups that are involved in hydrogen bonding and second, the peaks are generally broadened. Keep these two factors in mind as you examine the following spectra, regardless of what atoms and functional groups are involved in the hydrogen bonding.

The N-H stretching frequency is most frequently encountered in amines and amides. The following examples will illustrate the behavior of this functional group in a variety of circumstances.

Primary amines and amides derived from ammonia

The N-H stretching frequency in primary amines and in amides derived from ammonia have the same local symmetry as observed in CH2. Two bands, a symmetric and an asymmetric stretch are observed. It is not possible to assign the symmetric and asymmetric stretches by inspection but their presence at approximately 3300 and 3340 cm-1 are suggestive of a primary amine or amide. These bands are generally broad and a third peak at frequencies lower than 3300 cm^{-1}, presumably due to hydrogen bonding, is also observed.

Secondary amines and amides

Secondary amines and amides show only one peak in the infrared. This peak is generally in the vicinity of 3300 cm^{-1}.

Tertiary amines and amides

Tertiary amines and amides from secondary amines have no observable N-H stretching band.

N-H bending motions

You may recall that we will be ignoring most bending motions because these occur in the fingerprint region of the spectrum. One exception is the N-H bend which occurs at about 1600 cm^{-1}. This band is generally very broad and relatively weak. Since many other important bands occur in this region it is important to note the occurrence of this absorption lest it be mistakenly interpreted as another functional group.

Hydroxyl Stretch

The hydroxyl stretch is similar to the N-H stretch in that it hydrogen bonds but does so more strongly. As a result it is often broader than the N-H group. In those rare instances when it is not possible to hydrogen bond, the stretch is found as a relative weak to moderate absorption at 3600-3650 cm^{-1}. In tri-t-butylmethanol where steric hindrance prevents hydrogen bonding, a peak at 3600 cm^{-1} is observed. Similarly for hexanol, phenol, and hexanoic acid, gas phase and liquid phase spectra illustrate the effect of hydrogen bonding on both the O-H stretch and on the rest of the spectrum. In should be pointed out that, in general, while gas phase spectra are usually very similar, frequencies are generally shifted to slightly higher values in comparison to condensed phase spectra. Gas phase spectra that differ significantly from condensed phase spectra are usually taken as evidence for the presence of some sort of molecular association in the condensed phase.

The hydroxyl group in phenols and alcohols usually is found as a broad peak centered at about 3300 cm^{-1} in the condensed phase as noted above and in the additional examples of Figs. 2.31 and 2.32. The O-H of a carboxylic acid, so strongly associated that the O-H absorption in these materials, is often extended to approximately 2500 cm^{-1}. This extended absorption is clearly observed in Figs. 2.29, 2.30 and 2.31 and serves to differentiate the O-H stretch of a carboxylic acid from that of an alcohol or phenol. In fact, carboxylic acids associate to form intermolecular hydrogen bonded dimers both in the solid and liquid phases.

The nitrile group

The nitrile group is another reliable functional group that generally is easy to identify. There is a significant dipole moment associated with the CN bond which leads to a significant change when it interacts with infrared radiation usually leading to an intense sharp peak at 2200-2280 cm^{-1}. Very few other groups absorb at this region with this intensity. The spectrum illustrates the typical behavior of this functional group. If another electronegative atom such as a halogen is attached to the same carbon as the nitrile group, the intensity of this is markedly reduced.

The carbon-carbon triple bond

The CC bond is not considered to be a very reliable functional group. This stems in part by considering that the reduced mass is likely to vary. However it is characterized by a strong force constant and because this stretching frequency falls in a region where very little else absorbs, 2100-2260 cm^{-1}, it can provide useful information. The terminal carbon triple bond (CC-H) is the most reliable and easiest to identify. We have previously discussed the C-H stretching frequency; coupled with a band at 3300 cm^{-1}, the presence of a band at approximately 2100 cm^{-1} is a strong indication of the -CC-H group.

An internal -CC- is more difficult to identify and is often missed. Unless an electronegative atom such as nitrogen or oxygen is directly attached to the sp hybridized carbon, the dipole moment associated with this bond is small; stretching this bond also leads to a very small change. In cases where symmetry is involved, such as in diethyl acetylenedicarboxylate, Fig. 2.32, there is no change in dipole moment and this absorption peak is completely absent. In cases where this peak is observed, it is often weak and difficult to identify with a high degree of certainty.

The carbonyl group

The carbonyl group is probably the most ubiquitous group in organic chemistry. It comes in various disguises. The carbonyl is a polar functional group that frequently is the most intense peak in the spectrum. We will begin by discussing some of the typical acyclic aliphatic molecules that contain a carbonyl group. We will then consider the effect of including a carbonyl as part of a ring and finally we will make some comments of the effect of conjugation on the carbonyl frequency.

Acyclic aliphatic carbonyl groups

Esters, aldehydes, and ketones

Esters, aldehydes, and ketones are frequently encountered examples of molecules exhibiting a C = O stretching frequency. The frequencies, 1735, 1725, 1715 cm^{-1} respectively, are too close to allow a clear distinction between them. However, aldehydes can be distinguished by examining both the presence of the C-H of an aldehyde (2750, 2850 cm^{-1}) and the presence of a carbonyl group. Examples of an aliphatic aldehyde, ester, and ketone are given in Fig. 2.32.

Carboxylic acids, amides and carboxylic acid anhydrides

Carboxylic acids, amides and carboxylic acid anhydrides round out the remaining carbonyl groups frequently found in aliphatic molecules. The carbonyl frequencies of these molecules, 1700-1730 (carboxylic acid), 1640-1670 (amide) and 1800-1830, 1740-1775 cm^{-1} (anhydride), allow for an easy differentiation when the following factors are also taken into consideration.

A carboxylic acid can easily be distinguished from all the carbonyl containing functional groups by noting that the carbonyl at 1700-1730cm^{-1} is strongly hydrogen bonded and broadened as a result. In addition it contains an O-H stretch which shows similar hydrogen bonding as noted above.

Amides are distinguished by their characteristic frequency which is the lowest carbonyl frequency observed for an uncharged molecule, 1640-1670 cm^{-1} (Amide I). In addition, amides from ammonia and primary amines exhibit a weaker second band (Amide II) at 1620-1650 cm^{-1} and 1550 cm^{-1} respectively, when the spectra are run on the solids. Amides from secondary amines do not have a hydrogen attached at nitrogen and do not show an Amide II band. The Amide I band is mainly attributed to the carbonyl stretch. The Amide II involves several atoms including the N-H bond. We will return to the frequency of the amide carbonyl when we discuss the importance of conjugation and the effect of resonance on carbonyl frequencies.

Anhydrides can be distinguished from other simple carbonyl containing compounds in that they contain and exhibit two carbonyl frequencies. However, these frequencies are not characteristic of each carbonyl. Rather they are another example of the effects of local symmetry similar to what we have seen for the CH2 and NH2 groups. The motions involved here encompass the entire anhydride (–(C = O)–O–(O = C–) in a symmetric and asymmetric stretching motion of the two carbonyls. The two carbonyl frequencies often differ in intensity. It is not possible to assign the peaks to the symmetric or asymmetric stretching motion by inspection nor to predict the more intense peak. However, the presence of two carbonyl frequencies and the magnitude of the higher frequency (1800 cm^{-1}) are a good indication of an anhydride.

Cyclic aliphatic carbonyl containing compounds

The effect on the carbonyl frequency as a result of including a carbonyl group as part of a ring is usually attributed to ring strain. Generally ring strain is believed to be relieved in large rings because of the variety of conformations available. However as the size of the ring gets smaller, this option is not available and a noticeable effect is observed. The effect of increasing ring stain is to increase the carbonyl frequency, independent of whether the carbonyl is a ketone, part of a lactone(cyclic ester), anhydride or lactam (cyclic amide).

Like the CC bond, the C = C bond stretch is not a very reliable functional group. However, it is also characterized by a strong force constant and because of this and because the effects of conjugation which we will see can enhance the intensity of this stretching frequency, this absorption can provide useful and reliable information.

Terminal C = CH2

In simple systems, the terminal carbon carbon double bond (C = CH2) is the most reliable and easiest to identify since the absorption is of moderate intensity at 1600-1675 cm^{-1}. We have previously discussed the C-H stretching frequency of an sp2 hybridized C-H. In addition the terminal C = CH2 is also characterized by a strong band at approximately 900 cm^{-1}. Since this band falls in the fingerprint region, some caution should be exercised in its identification.

Internal C = C

An internal non-conjugated C=C is difficult to identify and can be missed. The dipole moment associated with this bond is small; stretching this bond also leads to a very small change. In cases where symmetry is involved, such as in 4-octene, Figure 10, there is no change in dipole moment and this absorption peak is completely absent. In cases where this peak is observed, it is often weak. In 2,5-dihydrofuran, it is difficult to assign the C=C stretch because of the presence of other weak peaks in the vicinity. The band at approximately 1670 cm^{-1} may be the C=C stretch. In 2,5-dimethoxy-2,5-dihydrofuran, the assignment at 1630 cm^{-1} is easier but the band is weak.

There is one circumstance that can have a significant effect on the intensity of both internal and terminal olefins and acetylenes. Substitution of a heteroatom directly on the unsaturated carbon to produce, for example, a vinyl or acetylenic ether, or amine leads to a significant change in the polarity of the C=C or CC bond and a substantial increase in intensity is observed. The C=C in 2,3-dihydrofuran is observed at 1617.5 cm^{-1} and is one of the most intense bands in the spectrum

Aromatic ring breathing motions

Benzene rings are encountered frequently in organic chemistry. Although we may write benzene as a six membered ring with three double bonds, most are aware that this is not a good representation of the structure of the molecule. The vibrational motions of a benzene ring are not isolated but involve the entire molecule. To describe one of the fundamental motions of benzene, consider imaginary lines passing through the center of the molecule and extending out through each carbon atom and beyond. A symmetric stretching and compression of all the carbon atoms of benzene along each line is one example of what we might describe as a ring breathing motion. Simultaneous expansions and compressions of these six carbon atoms lead to other ring breathing motions. These vibrations are usually observed between 1450 and 1600 cm^{-1} and often lead to four observable absorptions of variable intensity.

Effect of resonance and conjugation on infrared frequencies

Let's continue our discussion of the importance of resonance but shift from the nitro group to the carboxylate anion. The carboxylate anion is represented as a resonance hybrid by the following figure:

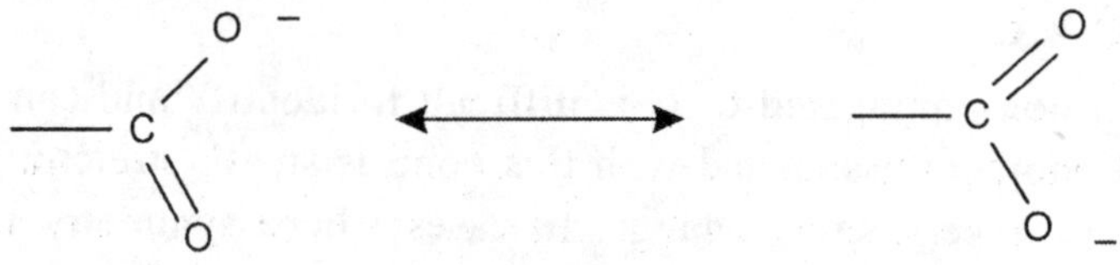

Fig. 2.24.

Unlike the nitro group which contained functional groups we will not be discussing, the carboxyl group is made up of a resonance hybrid between a carbon oxygen single bond and a carbon oxygen double bond. According to resonance, we would expect the C-O bond to be an average between a single and double bond or approximately equal to a bond and a half. We can use the carbonyl frequency of an ester of 1735 cm^{-1} to describe the force constant of the double bond. We have not discussed the stretching frequency of a C-O single bond for the simple reason that it is quite variable and because it falls in the fingerprint region. However the band is known to vary from 1000 to 1400 cm^{-1}. For purposes of this discussion, we will use an average value of 1200 cm^{-1}. The carbonyl frequency for a bond and a half would be expected to fall halfway between 1735 and 1200 or at approximately 1465 cm^{-1}. The carboxyl group has the same symmetry as the nitro and CH2 groups. Both a symmetric and asymmetric stretch should be observed. An asymmetric and symmetric stretch at 1410 and 1560 cm^{-1} is observed that averages to 1480 cm-1, in good agreement with the average frequency predicted for a carbon oxygen bond with a bond order of 1.5. While this is a qualitative argument, it is important to realize that the carboxylate anion does not show the normal carbonyl and normal C-O single bond stretches (at approximately 1700 and 1200 cm^{-1}) suggested by each of the static structures above.

In the cases of the nitro group and the carboxylate anion, both resonance forms contribute equally to describing the ground state of the molecule. We will now look at instances where two or more resonance forms contribute unequally to describing the ground state and how these resonance forms can effect the various stretching frequencies.

Carbonyl frequencies

Most carbonyl stretching frequencies are found at approximately 1700 cm^{-1}. A notable exception is the amide carbonyl which is observed at approximately 1600 cm^{-1}. This suggests that the following resonance form makes a significant contribution to describing the ground state of amides:

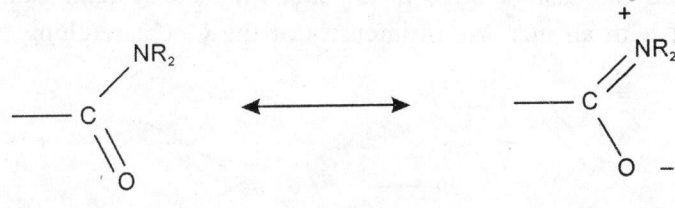

Fig. 2.25

You may recall that resonance forms that lead to charge separation are not considered to be very important. However the following information support the importance of resonance in amides. X-ray crystal structures of amides show that in the solid state the amide functional group is planar. This suggests sp2 hybridization at nitrogen rather than sp3. In addition the barrier to rotation about the carbon nitrogen bond has been measured. Unlike the barrier of rotation of most aliphatic C-N bonds which are of the order of a few kcal/mol, the barrier to rotation about the carbon nitrogen bond in dimethyl formamide is approximately 18 kcal/mol. This suggests an important contribution of the dipolar structure to the ground state of the molecule and the observed frequency of 1600 cm^{-1}, according to the arguments given above for the carboxylate anion, is consistent with more C-O single bond character than would be expected otherwise.

Conjugation of a carbonyl with a C=C bond is thought to lead to an increase in resonance interaction. Again the resonance forms lead to charge separation which clearly de-emphasizes their importance.

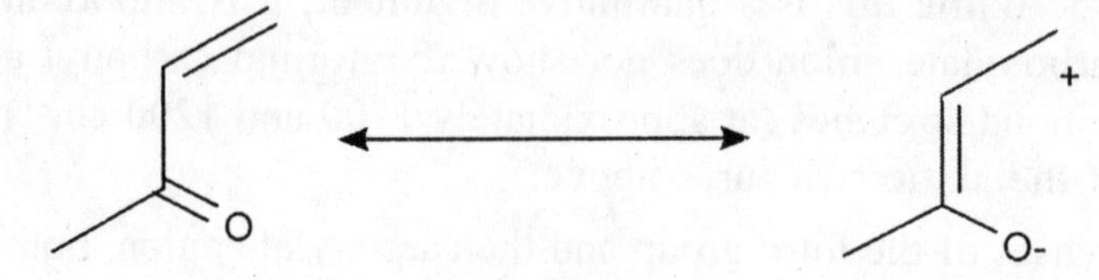

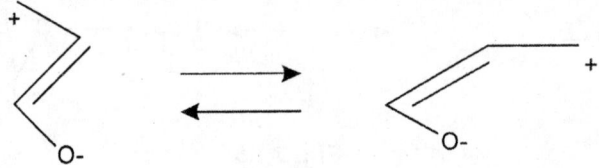

Fig. 2.26.

However this conjugative interaction is useful in interpreting several features of the spectrum. First it predicts the small but consistent shift of approximately 10 cm⁻¹ to lower frequency, observed when carbonyls are conjugated to double bonds or aromatic rings. This feature is summarized in Table 4 for a variety of carbonyl groups. Next, the dipolar resonance form suggests a more polar C=C than that predicted for an unconjugated C=C. In terms of the change in dipole moment, contributions from this structure suggest that the intensity of infrared absorption of a C=C double bond would increase relative to an unconjugated system. Conjugation is associated with an increase in intensity of the C=C stretching frequency.

Fig. 2.27

If the resonance interaction in these two forms differ, the effect of resonance on the carbonyl will differ leading to similar but different frequencies. The presence of multiple carbonyl frequencies is a good indication of a conjugated carbonyl. In some conjugated systems such as

Table 2.1: The effect of conjugation on carbonyl frequencies

Non-conjugated Compound	Frequency cm⁻¹	Conjugated Compound	Frequency cm⁻¹		Frequency cm⁻¹
butanal	1725	2-butenal	1691	benzaldehyde	1702
2-butanone	1717	methyl vinyl ketone	1700, 1681	acetophenone	1685
propanoic acid	1715	propenoic acid	1702	benzoic acid	1688
ethyl propionate	1740	ethyl acrylate	1727	ethyl benzoate	1718
butanoic	1819,	2-butenoic	1782,	benzoic	1786,
anhydride	1750	anhydride	1722	anhydride	1726
cis-cyclohexane-		1-cyclohexene-			
1,2-	1857,	1,2-	1844,	phthalic	1852,
dicarboxylic	1786	dicarboxylic	1767	anhydride	1762
anhydride		anhydride			

benzaldehyde and benzyl 4-hydroxyphenylketone, only one conformation by symmetry is possible and conjugation does not lead to any additional carbonyl frequencies. It should also be noted that in many of the examples given above, *cis-trans* isomerization about the carbon-carbon double bond is also possible. Some of the observed bands may also be due to the presence of these additonal isomers. Since the intensity of the peak is determined by the change in dipole moment, the presence of a small amount of geometric isomer can still lead to a detectable peak.

Interpretation of Infrared Spectra

We have just concluded a discussion of a large number of frequencies and the functional groups that are generally associated with these frequencies. At this point you may be asking yourself how to begin to interpret these frequencies with regards to obtaining information of molecular structure. There are a number of different approaches that can be used and often the best approach to use depends on the nature of the information you would like to obtain from your infrared spectrum. For example, if you are repeating a synthesis in the laboratory and you wish to determine whether you have successfully isolated the material you intended to prepare, you may be able to compare your spectrum to an infrared spectrum of an authentic sample. In this case, you are using infrared analysis for establishing the identity of your sample. Assuming that your spectrum has been run under the same conditions, as your reference, i.e. neat sample, KBr pellet, etc., you should be able to reproduce the spectrum of the reference material, peak for peak. The presence of some additional peaks in your spectrum may indicate a contamination with solvent, starting material or an impurity that has not been removed. The presence of fewer peaks than your reference is of more concern. This generally indicates a failure to obtain the desired material.

If the structure of the material of interest is unknown, then a more systematic analysis of your spectrum will be necessary. You should be aware that it is not usually possible to determine molecular structure from the infrared spectrum alone. Usually, some supplemental spectroscopic and/or structural information (such as molecular formula) is also necessary. For the unknowns in this course, you will generally be using infrared spectroscopy to differentiate between a few possible compounds. Frequently, this can be achieved by an analysis of the functional groups in your spectrum. The discussion which follows, uses a more generalized approach to analyze spectra. This approach should be applicable in a variety of different circumstances. If a portion of the discussion is not relevant to you, simply skip it and continue until it does become relevant.

The Degree of Unsaturation

Once the molecular formula of an unknown is known, it is a simple matter to determine the degree of unsaturation. The degree of unsaturation is simply the sum of the number of carbon-carbon double bonds and rings. Each reduces the number of hydrogens or any other element with a valance of one by two. Although there is a general formula that can be memorized and used, a much simpler procedure is to note the number of carbon atoms and any other elements in your molecular formula and simply draw a molecule that contains the requisite number of carbons atoms and any other elements that are present. Make sure there are no rings or carbon-carbon double bonds in your structure. Each carbon, nitrogen, sulfur and oxygen should have four, three, two and two single bonds, respectively. Use as many hydrogens as you need to make up the appropriate number of bonds for each element. Be sure to include all halogens and any other elements in your structure as well. Count the number of hydrogens in your structure and subtract this number from the number in your original molecular formula. The difference, divided by two equals the degree of unsaturation, the sum of the number of rings and double bonds.

Consider C_6Cl_6 as an example: CH_2Cl-$CHCl$-$CHCl$-$CHCl$-$CHCl$-CH_2Cl. The number of hydrogens in my sample molecule is 8; there are none in the original molecular formula. The difference, divided by two is four. The degree of unsaturation is four. An unsaturation factor of four is quite common and characteristic of benzene and its derivatives.

Application of the degree of unsaturation to the interpretation of an infrared spectrum is quite straightforward. Clearly some functional groups can be eliminated by composition. Amines, amides, nitriles and nitro groups can be eliminated if the molecule does not contain any nitrogen. Alternatively everything but amines can be eliminated if the molecular formula contains nitrogen and no degrees of unsaturation. The following steps should serve as a general protocol to follow and should prove useful regardless of the structure of your unknown or whether the degree of unsaturation is known.

1. Examine the C-H stretching frequencies at 3000 cm^{-1}. Absorption bands bands at frequencies slightly larger than 3000 cm^{-1} are indicative of vinyl or/and aromatic hydrogens. The presence of these peaks should be consistent with the degree of unsaturation of your molecule. The absence of absorption above 3000 cm^{-1} but the

presence of some unsaturation in the molecular formula are consistent with a cyclic compound.

If your degree of unsaturation is 4 or greater, look for 2 to 4 absorption peaks between 1600-1450 cm^{-1} and weak peaks at 2000-1667 cm^{-1}. These are characteristic of aromatic compounds.

2. Next look for a doublet at 2750 and 2850 cm-1 characteristic of an aldehyde. The presence of these two bands should also be accompanied by a strong absorption at approximately 1700 cm^{-1}. Most spectra display strong absorption in the 1800-1700 cm^{-1} region. If your spectrum does, check to see if the carbonyl is a closely spaced doublet or multiplet. Closely spaced multiplicity in the carbonyl region accompanied by C-H absorption at 3000-3100 cm^{-1} is frequently characteristic of an α, β- unsaturated carbonyl compounds. Check to make sure that the carbonyl frequency is consistent with conjugation.

3. If you unknown contains broad absorption from 3600-3000, your molecule could have an O-H or N-H stretch. Your molecular formula may allow you to differentiate. Check the multiplicity of this peak. A doublet is characteristic of a primary amine or and amide derived from ammonia. Check the carbonyl region at around 1650-1600 cm^{-1}. Two bands in this region are consistent of an amide from ammonia or a primary amine. Remember a broad and relatively weak band at about 1600 cm^{-1} is characteristic of N-H bending. Usually you will only see this band in amines, since that carbonyl group of the amide will interfere. Be sure to look for the effect of hydrogen bonding which usually results in a general broadening of the groups involved.

4. If the broad band starting at 3600 expands to nearly 2400 cm^{-1}, look for the presence of a broad carbonyl at approximately 1700 cm^{-1}. This extremely broad OH band is only observed in carboxylic acids and enols from b-diketones. The presence of a relatively intense but broad band at approximately 1700 cm^{-1} is good evidence for a carboxylic acid.

5. Don't try to over-interpret your spectrum. Often, it is not possible to arrive at a unique structure based on infrared analysis alone. You should use your infrared analysis much like you would use other classification tests. You can learn a great deal about your unknown from your spectrum but be sure to use other important

physical data such as melting point, boiling point and solubility characteristics of your unknown to assist you in narrowing down the different structural possibilities.

Summary of some functional groups and bonds: IR in table 2.2.

Functional Group	Type		Frequencies cm^{-1}	Peak Intensity
C-H	sp3 hybridized	R3C-H	2850-3000	M(sh)
	sp2 hybridized	=CR-H	3000-3250	M(sh)
	sp hybridized	C-H	3300	M-S(sh)
	aldehyde C-H	H-(C=O)R	2750, 2850	M(sh)
N-H	primary amine,	RN-H2, RCON-H2	3300, 3340	S, S(br)
	amide secondary amine, amide	RNR-H, RCON-HR	3300-3500	S(br)
	tertiary amine, amide	RN(R3), RCONR2	none	
O-H	alcohols, phenols	free O-H	3620-3580	W(sh)
		hydrogen bonded	3600-3650	S(br)
	carboxylic acids	R(C=O)O-H	3500-2400	S(br)
CN	nitriles	RCN	2280-2200	S(sh)
CC	acetylenes	R-CC-R	2260-2180	W(sh)
		R-CC-H	2160-2100	M(sh)
C=O	aldehydes	R(C=O)H	1740-1720	S(sh)
	ketones	R(C=O)R	1730-1710	S(sh)
	esters	R(CO2)R	1750-1735	S(sh)
	anhydrides	R(CO2CO)R	1820, 1750	S, S(sh)
	carboxylates	R(CO2)H	1600, 1400	S,S(sh)
C=C	olefins	R2C=CR2	1680-1640	W(sh)
		R2C=CH2	1600-1675	M(sh)
		R2C=C(OR)R	1600-1630	S(sh)
-NO2	nitro groups	RNO2	1550, 1370	S,S(sh)

Uses and applications

Infrared spectroscopy is widely used in both research and industry as a simple and reliable technique for measurement, quality control and dynamic measurement. It is of especial use in forensic analysis in both criminal and civil cases, enabling identification of polymer degradation for example. It is perhaps the most widely used method of applied spectroscopy.

The instruments are now small, and can be transported, even for use in field trials. With increasing technology in computer filtering and manipulation of the results, samples in solution can now be measured accurately (water produces a broad absorbance across the range of interest, and thus renders the spectra unreadable without this computer treatment). Some machines will also automatically tell you what substance is being measured from a store of thousands of reference spectra held in storage.

By measuring at a specific frequency over time, changes in the character or quantity of a particular bond can be measured. This is especially useful in measuring the degree of polymerization in polymer manufacture. Modern research machines can take infrared measurements across the whole range of interest as frequently as 32 times a second. This can be done whilst simultaneous measurements are made using other techniques. This makes the observations of chemical reactions and processes quicker and more accurate.

Techniques have been developed to assess the quality of tea-leaves using infrared spectroscopy. This will mean that highly trained experts (also called 'noses') can be used more sparingly, at a significant cost saving.

Infrared spectroscopy has been highly successful for applications in both organic and inorganic chemistry. Infrared spectroscopy has also been successfully utilized in the field of semiconductor microelectronics for example, infrared spectroscopy can be applied to semiconductors like silicon, gallium arsenide, gallium nitride, zinc selenide, amorphous silicon, silicon nitride, etc.

Isotope effects

The different isotopes in a particular species may give fine detail in infrared spectroscopy. For example, the O-O stretching frequency of oxyhemocyanin is experimentally determined to be 832 and 788 cm^{-1} for $v(^{16}O^{-16}O)$ and v $(^{18}O^{-18}O)$ respectively.

By considering the O-O as a spring, the wavelength of absorbance, v can be calculated:

$$v = \frac{1}{2\pi}\sqrt{\frac{k}{\mu}}$$

where k is the spring constant for the bond, and μ is the reduced mass of the A–B system:

$$\mu = \frac{m_A m_B}{m_A + m_B}$$

(m_i is the mass of atom i).

The reduced masses for ^{16}O-^{16}O and ^{18}O-^{18}O can be approximated as 8 and 9 respectively. Thus

$$\frac{v^{16}O}{v^{18}Q} = \sqrt{\frac{9}{8}} \approx \frac{832}{788}$$

For diatomic molecules, the absorption can be calculated.

$$v = \frac{1}{2Pc}\sqrt{\frac{k(m1+m2)}{m1*m2}}$$

$m1$, $m2$ = masses of vibrating atoms, g

c = velocity of light, 3×10^{10} cm/sec

v = wave number, cm^{-1}

k = force constant (bond strength), dynes/cm

P = 3.1416 (pi)

Bond Strength

For a single bond $k = 5 \times 10^5$ dynes/cm

double bond $k = 10 \times 10^5$ dynes/cm

triple bond $k = 15 \times 10^5$ dynes/cm

Example: Calculate the fundamental frequency expected in the infrared absorption spectrum for the C-0 stretching frequency.

$$v = \frac{\sqrt{\dfrac{(5\times10)(12+16)(6.023\times10)*}{(12)\times(16)}}}{2(3.1416)(3\times10)}$$

$$= 1110 \text{ cm}^{-1}$$

*Avogadro's number = 6.023×10^{23} atoms/mole

Fourier transform infrared spectroscopy

Fourier transform infrared (FTIR) spectroscopy is a measurement technique for collecting infrared spectra. Instead of recording the amount of energy absorbed when the frequency of the infra-red light is varied (monochromator), the IR light is guided through an *interferometer*. After passing the sample the measured signal is the interferogram. Performing a mathematical *Fourier transform* on this signal results in a spectrum identical to that from conventional (dispersive) infrared spectroscopy.

FTIR spectrometers are cheaper than conventional spectrometers because building of interferometers is easier than the fabrication of a monochromator. In addition, measurement of a single spectrum is faster for the FTIR technique because the information at all frequencies is collected simultaneously. This allows multiple samples to be collected and averaged together resulting in an improvement in sensitivity. Because of its various advantages, virtually all modern infrared spectrometers are FTIR instruments.

IR spectroscopy- IR Absorption of Selected Functional Groups (cm-1)

C — C (alkane) 800 - 1300

C == C (alkene) 1640 – 1680 *(med)*

C ≈ C (aromatic) 1600 and 1500 *(strong)*

C — H (alkane) 2850 – 2960 *(med – strong)*

C — H (alkene) 3020 – 3100 *(med)*

C — H (aromatic) 3030 *(med)*

C — Cl (alkane) 600 - 800 *(strong)*

C — N (amine) 1030, 1230 *(med)*

C — O (alcohol) 1050 – 1150 *(strong)*

C == O (acid) 1710 – 1780 *(strong)*

C == O (esters) 1735 – 1750 *(strong)*

C == O (amide) 1630 – 1690 *(strong)*

C ≡ ≡ N (nitriles) 2210 – 2260 *(med)*

O — H (acid) 2500 – 3100 *(broad, strong)*

O — H (alcohol) 3400 – 3650 *(broad, strong)*

O — H (phenol) 3200 – 3550

N — H (amine) 3300 – 3500 *(sharp, me*

IR Absorption of Selected Functional Groups (cm^{-1})

C — C (alkane) 800 – 1300

C == C (alkene) 1640 – 1680 *(med)*

C ≈ ≈ C (aromatic) 1600 and 1500 *(strong)*

C — H (alkane) 2850 – 2960 *(med – strong)*

C — H (alkene) 3020 – 3100 *(med)*

C — H (aromatic) 3030 *(med)*

C — Cl (alkane) 600 - 800 *(strong)*

C — N (amine) 1030, 1230 *(med)*

C — O (alcohol) 1050 – 1150 *(strong)*

C == O (acid) 1710 – 1780 *(strong)*

C == O (esters) 1735 – 1750 *(strong)*

C == O (amide) 1630 – 1690 *(strong)*

C ≡ ≡ N (nitriles) 2210 – 2260 *(med)*

O — H (acid) 2500 – 3100 *(broad, strong)*

O — H (alcohol) 3400 – 3650 *(broad, strong)*

O — H (phenol) 3200 – 3550

N — H (amine) 3300 – 3500 *(sharp, me)*

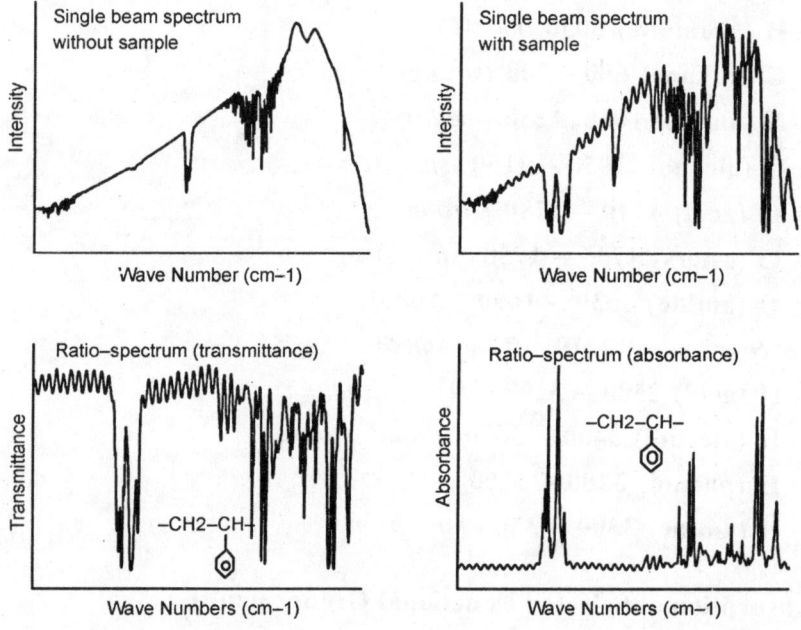

Fig. 2.28.

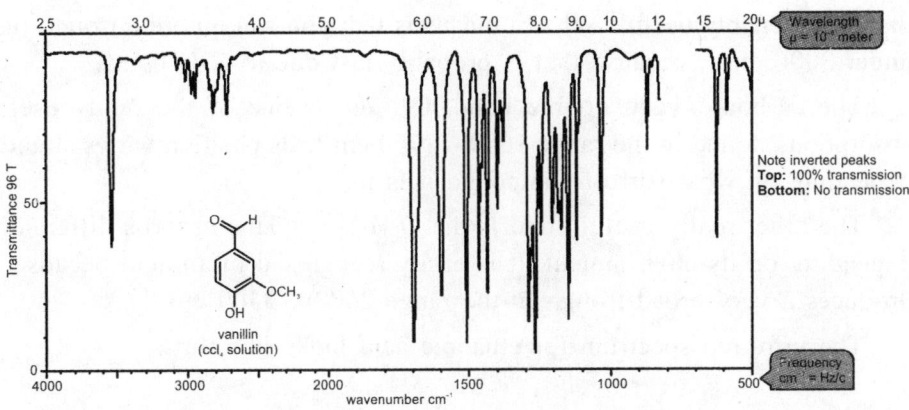

The infra-red spectrum for a simple carboxylic acid (Ethanoic acid)

Ethanoic acid has the structure:

$$CH_3-C\underset{O-H}{\overset{O}{\diagup\kern-0.5em\diagdown}}$$

we see that it contains the following bonds:

carbon-oxygen double, C=O

carbon-oxygen single, C-O

oxygen-hydrogen, O-H

carbon-hydrogen, C-H

carbon-carbon single, C-C

The carbon-carbon bond has absorptions which occur over a wide range of wavenumbers in the fingerprint region - that makes it very difficult to pick out on an infra-red spectrum.

The carbon-oxygen single bond also has an absorbtion in the fingerprint region, varying between 1000 and 1300 cm^{-1} depending on the molecule it is in. You have to be very wary about picking out a particular trough as being due to a C-O bond.

The other bonds in ethanoic acid have easily recognised absorptions outside the fingerprint region.

The C-H bond (where the hydrogen is attached to a carbon which is singly-bonded to everything else) absorbs somewhere in the range from

2853 – 2962 cm^{-1}. Because that bond is present in most organic compounds, that's not terribly useful! What it means is that you can ignore a trough just under 3000 cm^{-1}, because that is probably just due to C-H bonds.

The carbon-oxygen double bond, C = O, is one of the really useful absorptions, found in the range 1680 – 1750 cm^{-1}. Its position varies slightly depending on what sort of compound it is in.

The other really useful bond is the O-H bond. This absorbs differently depending on its environment. It is easily recognised in an acid because it produces a very broad trough in the range 2500 – 3300 cm^{-1}.

The infra-red spectrum for ethanoic acid looks like this:

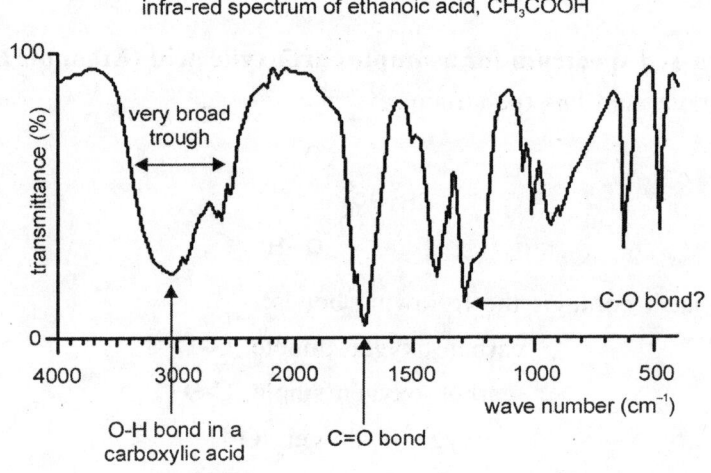

Fig. 2.29.

- The infra-red spectrum for an alcohol
- Ethanol

The O-H bond in an alcohol absorbs at a higher wavenumber than it does in an acid - somewhere between 3230 – 3550 cm^{-1}. In fact this absorption would be at a higher number still if the alcohol isn't hydrogen bonded - for example, in the gas state. All the infra-red spectra on this page are from liquids.

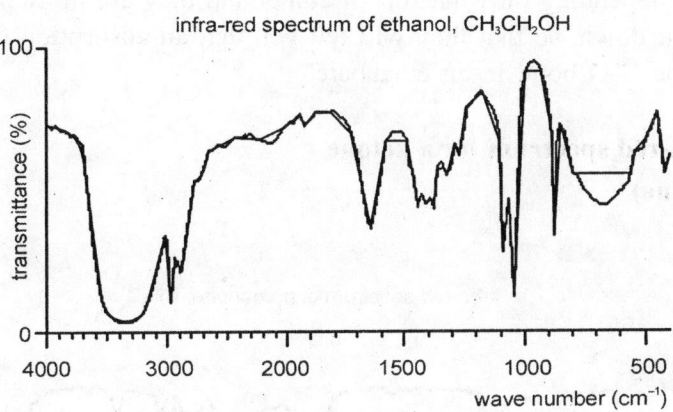

Fig. 2.30

The infra-red spectrum for an ester
Ethyl ethanoate

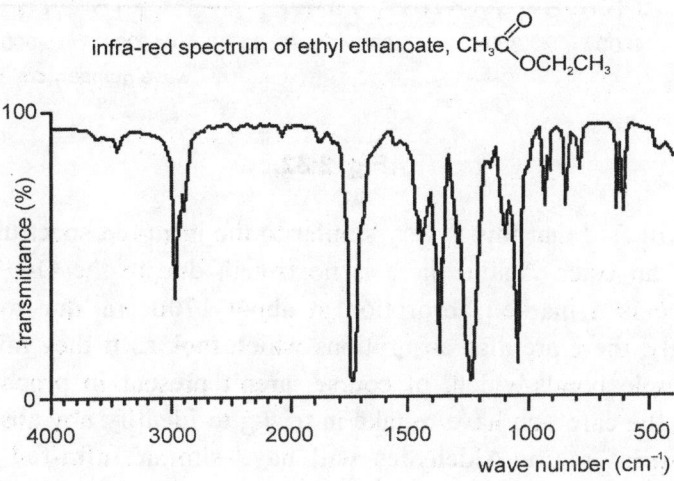

Fig. 2.31.

This time the O-H absorption is missing completely. Don't confuse it with the C-H trough fractionally less than 3000 cm^{-1}. The presence of the C = O double bond is seen at about 1740 cm^{-1}. The C-O single bond is the absorption at about 1240 cm^{-1}. Whether or not you could pick that out would depend on the detail given by the table of data which you get in your exam, because C-O single bonds vary anywhere between 1000 and 1300 cm^{-1}depending on what sort of compound they are in. Some tables of data fine it down, so that they will tell you that an absorption from 1230 - 1250 is the C-O bond in an ethanoate.

The infra-red spectrum for a ketone
(Propanone)

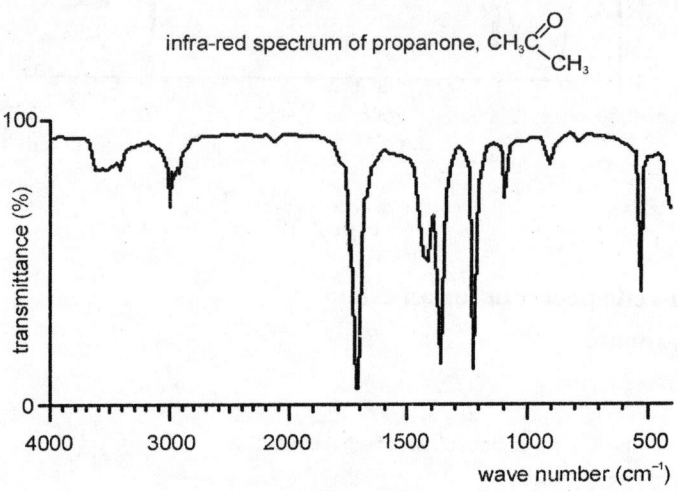

Fig. 2.32.

You will find that this is very similar to the infra-red spectrum for ethyl ethanoate, an ester. Again, there is no trough due to the O-H bond, and again there is a marked absorption at about 1700 cm^{-1}due to the C=O. Confusingly, there are also absorptions which look as if they might be due to C-O single bonds-which, of course, aren't present in propanone. This reinforces the care you have to take in trying to identify any absorptions in the fingerprint region.Aldehydes will have similar infra-red spectra to ketones.

Mass Spectroscopy (MS)

Basics - Mass spectrometry is the spectroscopic technique which is used for mass i.e molecular formula or Mwt determination of the compound. Mass spectrometry is based on slightly different principles to the other spectroscopic methods.

Terminology used

Molecular ion	The ion obtained by the loss of an electron from the molecule
Base peak	The most intense peak in the MS, assigned 100% intensity
M^+	Symbol often given to the molecular ion
Radical cation	+ve charged species with an odd number of electrons
Fragment ions	Lighter cations formed by the decomposition of the molecular ion. These often correspond to stable carbcations.

The principle behind mass spectrometry is that a charged particle passing through a magnetic field is deflected along a circular path on a radius that is proportional to the mass to charge ratio, m/e.

Working:

MS instruments consist of three modules:

- An ion source, which can convert gas phase sample molecules into ions (or, in the case of electrospray ionization, move ions that exist in solution into the gas phase)
- A mass analyzer, which sorts the ions by their masses by applying electromagnetic fields
- A detector, which measures the value of an indicator quantity and thus provides data for calculating the abundances of each ion present

In an electron impact mass spectrometer, sample of the compound is injected and then it is vaporised.A high energy beam of electrons (from electron gun) is bombarded to displace an electron from the organic molecules to form a radical cation known as the molecular ion, then this is passed through a magnetic field, from where ions are deflected and more becomes unstable then they can fragment to give other smaller ions. The collection, of ions is then focused into a beam and accelerated into the magnetic field and deflected along circular paths according to the masses of the ions or m/ ratio. By adjusting the magnetic field, the ions can be focused on the detector and recorded.The set of ions is analyzed in such a way that a signal is obtained for each value of m/e, the intensity of each signal reflects the relative abundance of the ion producing the signal. The largest peak is called as base peak, its intensity is taken as 100,intensities of other signal are expressed relative to base peak. In this way, a spectrum is obtained known as mass spectrum, which is characteristic of a particular compound. Some specta are shown in the Fig. 2.35 and 2.36..

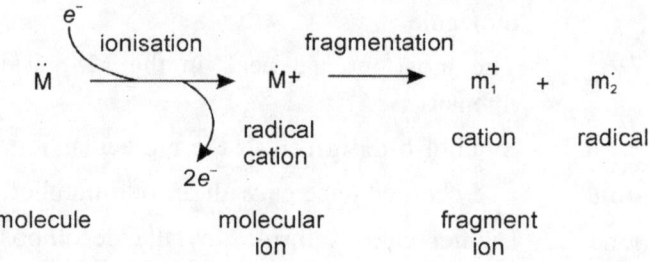

Fig. 2.33 : Schematic diagram for Mass spectrometer

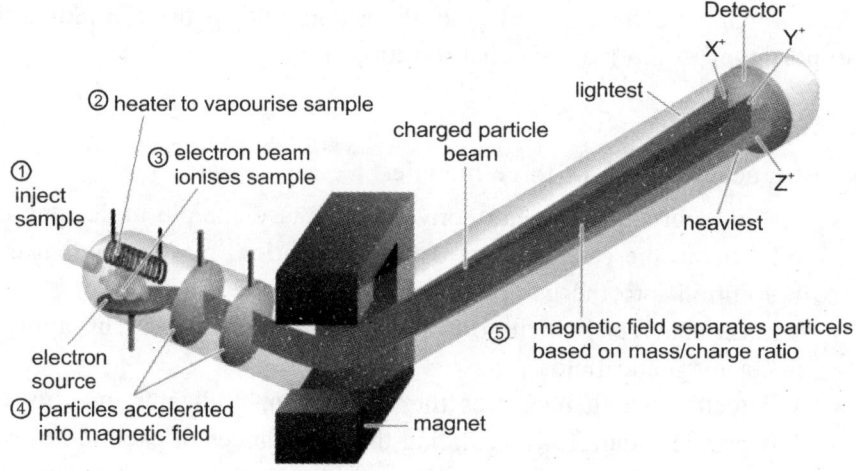

Fig. 2.34.

The MS of a typical hydrocarbon, n-decane is shown below. The **molecular ion** is seen as a small peak at m/z = 142. Notice the series ions detected that correspond to fragments that differ by 14 mass units, formed by the cleave of bonds at successive -CH_2- units.

The MS of benzyl alcohol is shown in the Fig. 2.36. The **molecular ion** is seen at m/z = 108. Fragmentation via loss of 17 (-OH) gives a common fragment seen for alkyl benzenes at m/z = 91. Loss of 31 (-CH_2OH) from the molecular ion gives 77 corresponding to the phenyl cation. Note the small peaks at 109 and 110 which correspond to the presence of small amounts of 13C in the sample (which has about 1% natural abundance).

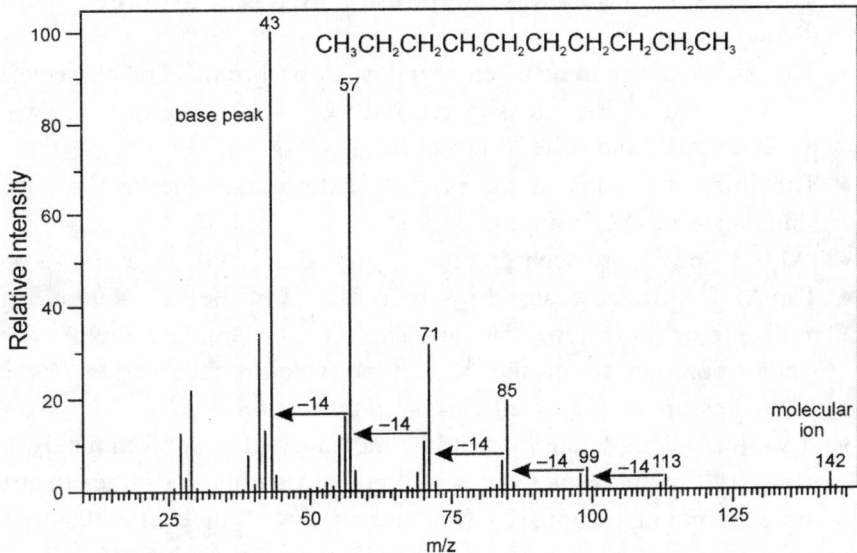

Fig. 2.35.

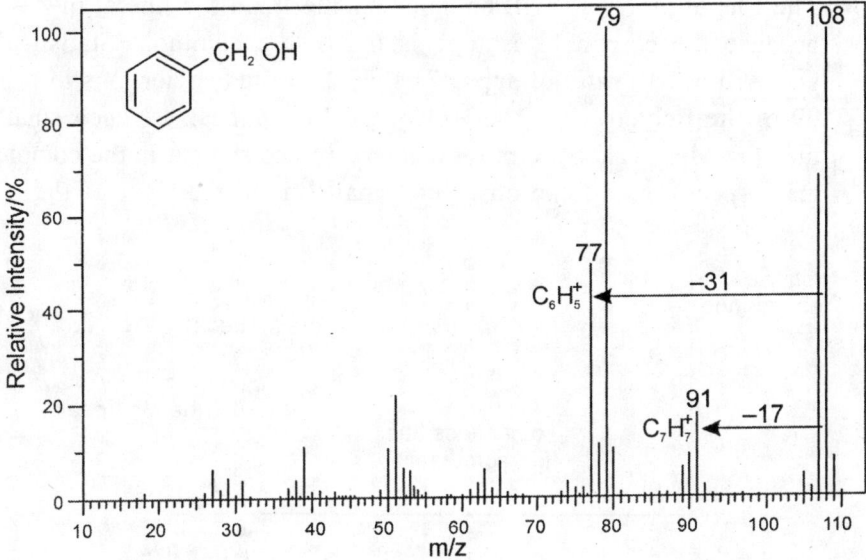

Fig. 2.36.

Isotopic Effect in Mass Spectrum (M + 1 and M + 2 Peaks)

- Mass spectrometers are capable of separating and detecting individual ions even those that only differ by a single atomic mass unit.

- As a result molecules containing different isotopes can be distinguished.
- This is most apparent when atoms such as bromine or chlorine are present (^{79}Br : ^{81}Br, intensity 1:1 and ^{35}Cl : ^{37}Cl, intensity 3:1) where peaks at "M" and "M+2" are obtained.
- The intensity ratios in the isotope patterns are due to the natural abundance of the isotopes.
- "M + 1" peaks are seen due the presence of C OR H in the sample.
- The M + 1 peak is caused by the presence of the ^{13}C isotope in the molecule or ^{2}H isotope of hydrogen. ^{13}C is a stable isotope of carbon - don't confuse it with the ^{14}C isotope which is radioactive. Carbon-13 makes up 1.11% of all carbon atoms.
- If we had a simple compound like methane, CH_4, approximately 1 in every 100 of these molecules will contain carbon-13 rather than the more common carbon-12. That means that 1 in every 100 of the molecules will have a mass of 17 (13 + 4) rather than 16 (12 + 4).
- The mass spectrum will therefore have a line corresponding to the molecular ion $[^{13}CH_4]^+$ as well as $[^{12}CH_4]^+$.
- The line at m/z = 17 will be much smaller than the line at m/z = 16 because the carbon-13 isotope is much less common. Statistically you will have a ratio of approximately 1 of the heavier ions to every 99 of the lighter ones. That's why the M + 1 peak is much smaller than the M + peak. Spectra for methane is also shown. In the complete mass spectrum, we can observe a small line to the right of the

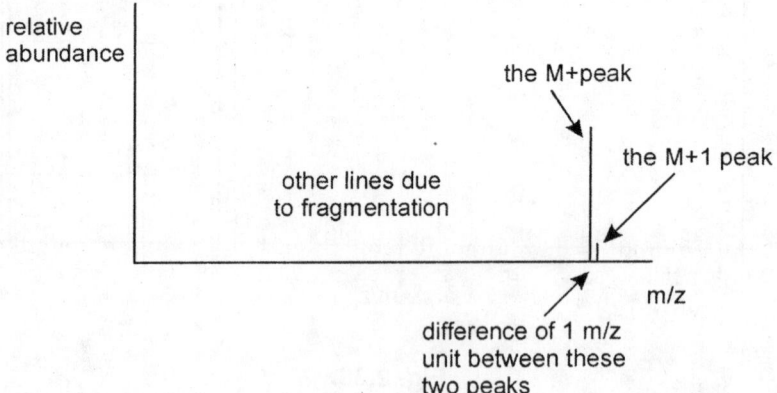

Fig. 2.37.

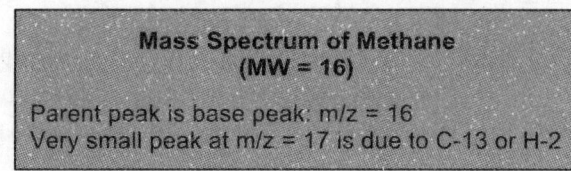

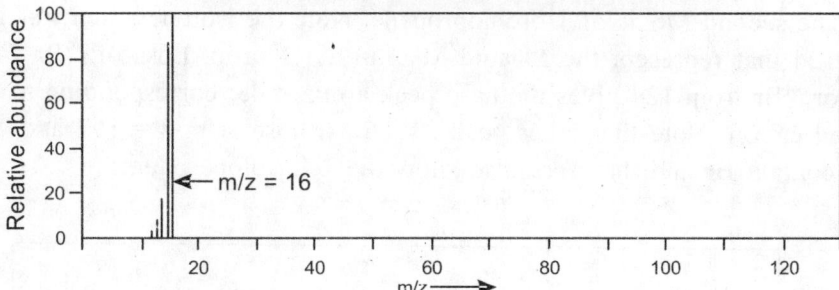

Mass Spectra—The M + 2 Peak

- M + 2 peak in a mass spectrum arises from the presence of chlorine or bromine atoms in an organic compound which is due to presence of isotope of chlorine or bromine, like ^{17}Cl isotope.

The following two mass spectra show examples of haloalkanes with characteristic isotope patterns.

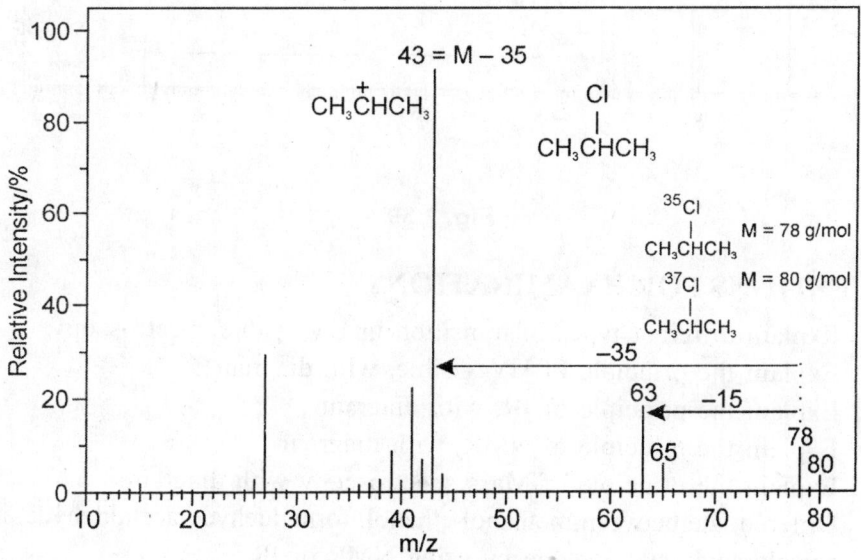

Fig. 2.38.

The first MS is of 2-chloropropane. Note the isotope pattern at 78 and 80 that represent the M amd M + 2 in a 3 : 1 ratio.

Loss of ^{35}Cl from 78 or ^{37}Cl from 80 gives the base peak a m/z = 43, corresponding to the secondary propyl cation. Note that the peaks at m/z = 63 and 65 still contain Cl and therefore also show the 3 : 1 isotope pattern.

The second MS is of 1-bromopropane. Note the isotope pattern at 122 and 124 that represent the M amd M+2 in a 1:1 ratio. Loss of ^{79}Br from 122 or ^{81}Br from 124 gives the base peak a m/z = 43, corresponding to the propyl cation. Note that other peaks, such as those at m/z = 107 and 109 still contain Br and therefore also show the 1:1 isotope pattern.

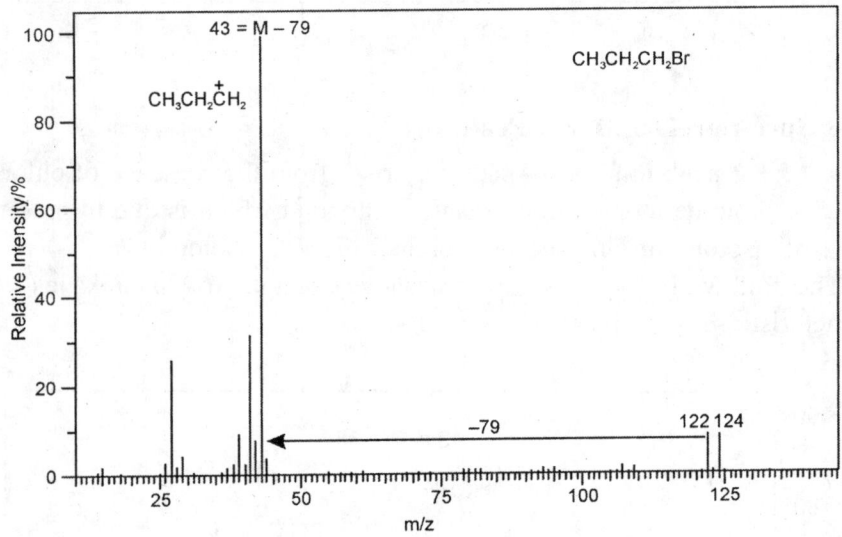

Fig. 2.39.

QUESTIONS FOR EXAMINATIONS

1. Explain different types of transition in UV-visible spectroscopy.
2. Explain the principle of UV-Visible, with diagram
3. Explain the principle of IR, with diagram
4. Explain the principle of NMR, with diagram
5. Explain the principle of Mass spectroscopy with diagram.
6. Differentiate between methanol-ethanol, formaldehyde-acetaldehyde and acetaldehyde and acetone by using NMR or IR.

Chapter 3
CHEMICAL KINETICS

> ➤ Rate of reaction, Moleculairy and order
> ➤ Zero, 1st and 2nd Order derivations
> ➤ Order determination methods
> ➤ Arhenius and Collision theory
> ➤ Numerical Problems
> ➤ Surface Chemistry—Adsorption, absorption and isotherms

Chemical kinetics is the branch of chemistry which addresses the question: "how fast do reactions go?" Chemistry can be thought of, at the simplest level, as the science that concerns itself with making new substances from other substances. Or, one could say, chemistry is taking molecules apart and putting the atoms and fragments back together to form new molecules. If Chemistry is making new substances out of old substances (i.e., chemical reactions), then there are two basic questions that must be answered:

1. Does the reaction want to go? This is the subject of chemical thermodynamics.
2. If the reaction wants to go, how fast will it go? This is the subject of chemical kinetics.

Here are some examples. Consider the reaction,

$$2 H_2(g) + O_2(g) \rightarrow 2 H_2O(l).$$

We can calculate $\Delta_r G^o$ for this reaction from tables of free energies of formation (actually this one is just twice the free energy of formation of liquid water). We find that $\Delta_r G^o$ for this reaction is very large and negative, which means that the reaction wants to go very strongly. A more scientific way to say this would be to say that the equilibrium constant for this reaction is very very large.

However, we can mix hydrogen gas and oxygen gas together in a bulb or other container, even in their correct stoichiometric proportions, and they will stay there for centuries, perhaps even forever, without reacting. (If we drop in a catalyst - say a tiny piece of platinum - or introduce a spark, or even illuminate the mixture with sufficiently high frequency uv light, or compress and heat the mixture, the mixture will explode.).

RATE OF REACTION (Average and Instantaneous Rate)

We are all familiar with processes in which something changes with time. Rate is usually expresses as the ratio of the amount of change in some quantity to the time required to produce that change.

$$\text{Rate} = \frac{\text{(Change in some quantity)}}{\text{(Time taken for the change)}} = \Delta X / \Delta t$$

The term ΔX means $X_{final} - X_{initial}$ and Δt is the amount of time elapsed. For example, a car driver starts his journey at 9.0 a.m. with odometer reading x miles. At 11.a.m. he reached his destination. The odometer reading at destination is y miles. The rate of his travel can be calculated as

$$\text{Rate} = (\Delta(\text{distance}))/(\Delta(\text{time}))$$
$$= (\text{distance}_{(f)} - \text{distance}_{(in)})/(\text{time}_{(f)} - \text{time}_{(in)})$$
$$= (y - x)/(11.0\text{-}9.0) = (y - x)/2 \quad \text{miles h}^{-1}$$

The above example indicates that the car has been driven with uniform rate but actually it has been driven sometimes faster and sometimes slower depending upon the conditions of the road. Thus, the overall rate is an average rate and the rate at which the car was moving at any instant, i.e., instantaneous rate was changeable.

The rate measured over a long time interval is called average rate and the rate measured for an infinitesimally small time interval is called instantaneous rate.

In a chemical change, reactants and products are involved. As the chemical reaction proceeds, the concentration of the reactants decreases, i.e., products are produced. The rate of reaction (average rate) is defined as the change of concentration of any one of its reactants (or products) per unit time.

Average rate of reaction,

r_{av} = (Change of concentration one of the reactants or products)/(Time taken for the change)

Consider a common hypothetical reaction,

$$A \rightarrow B$$

The average rate of reaction may be expressed either in terms of decrease in concentration of A (reactants) or in terms of increase in concentration of B (product).

or Average rate of reaction = (Decrease in concentration of A)/(Time taken)

Average rate of reaction = (Increase in concentration of B)/(Time taken)

Reaction rate has the units of concentration or molarity divided by time. Therefore, the units of rate of reaction may be expressed as:

mole/litre sec (mol L^{-1} s^{-1})

or mole/litre min (mol L^{-1} min^{-1}) or mole/litre time

MOLECULARITY OF A REACTION

In general, molecularity of simple reactions is equal to the sum of the number of molecules of reactants involved in the balanced stoichiometric equation.

OR

The molecularity of a reaction is the number of reactant molecules taking part in a single step of the reaction.

e.g., $PCl_5 \rightarrow PCl_3 + Cl_2$ (Unimolecular)

$2HI \rightarrow H_2 + I_2$ (Bimolecular)

$2SO_2 + O_2 \rightarrow 2SO_3$ (Trimolecular)

$NO + O_3 \rightarrow NO_2 + O_2$ (Bimolecular)

$2CO + O_2 \rightarrow 2CO_2$ (Trimolecular)

$2FeCl_3 + SnCl_2 \rightarrow SnCl_2 + 2FeCl_2$ (Trimolecular)

The minimum number of reacting particles (molecules, atoms or ions) that come together or collide in a rate determining step to form product or products is called the molecularity of a reaction.

For example, decomposition of H_2O_2 takes place in the following two steps:

$$H_2O_2 \rightarrow H_2O + 1/2O_2 \quad \text{(overall reaction)}$$

Step 1: $H_2O_2 \rightarrow H_2O + [O]$ (Slow)

Step 2: $[O] + [O] \rightarrow O_2$ (fast)

The slowest step is rate-determining. Thus from step 1, reaction appears to be unimolecular.

Note:

    (i) Molecularity is a theoretical concept.

    (ii) Molecularity cannot be zero, –ve, fractional, infinite and imaginary.

    (iii) Molecularity cannot be greater than three because more than three molecules may not mutually collide with each other.

There are some chemical reactions whose molecularity appears to be more than three from stoichiometric equations, e.g. in

$$4HBr + O_2 \rightarrow 2H_2O + 2Br_2$$

$$2MNI_4^- + 16H^+ + 5C_2O_4^{2-} \rightarrow 2Mn^{2+} + 10CO_2 + 8H_2O$$

In the first reaction molecularity seems to be '5' and in the second reaction molecularity seems to be '23'. Such reactions involve two or more steps; each step has its own molecularity not greater than three, e.g., in first reaction.

$$HBr + O_2 \rightarrow HOOBr$$

$$HOOBr + HBr \rightarrow 2HOBr$$

$$\underline{[HOBr + HBr \rightarrow H_2O + Br_2] \times 2}$$

$$\overline{4HBr + O_2 \rightarrow 2H_2O + Br_2}$$

Molecularity of each of the above steps is 2.

Expression of Rate

Consider the following reaction between CO and NO_2

$$CO + NO_2 \rightarrow CO_2 + NO$$

The equation shows that when one mole of CO reacts with one mole of NO_2, one mole each of CO_2 and NO are formed. The average rate of reaction can be expressed either by decrease of concentration of any one of the reactants (CO or NO_2) or by the increase in concentration of any one of the products (CO_2 or NO).

Thus, $-\Delta[CO]/\Delta t = -\Delta[NO_2]/\Delta t = \Delta[CO_2]/\Delta t = \Delta[NO]/\Delta t$

However, for the reaction,

$$2H_2O_2 \rightarrow 2H_2O + O_2$$

it is observed that when 2 moles of H_2O_2 decompose, one mole of O_2 is formed in the same time interval. The rate of increase in the concentration of O_2, therefore, is half that of the disappearance of the concentration of H_2O_2 in the same time interval;

So $\Delta[O_2]\Delta t = -1/2 \ \Delta[H_2O_2]/\Delta t$

In general, for a reaction,

$$n_1A + n_2B \rightarrow m_1C + m_2D$$

the rate expression may be expressed as

$$-1/n_1\Delta[A]/\Delta t = -1/2\Delta[B]/\Delta t = 1/m_1\Delta[C]/\Delta t = 1/m_2\Delta[D]/\Delta t$$

Thus, for the reaction,

$$H_2 + I_2 \rightarrow 2HI$$

the rate may be expressed as

$$- \Delta[H_2]/\Delta t = \Delta[I_2]/\Delta t = 1/2 \ \Delta[HI]/\Delta t$$

Similarly, for the decomposition of N_2O_5 in CCl_4 medium, the rate may be expressed as

$$2N_2O_5 \rightarrow 4NO_2 + O_2$$
$$-1/2\Delta[N_2O_5]/\Delta t = 1/4 \ \Delta[NO_2]/\Delta t = \Delta[O_2]/\Delta t$$

Example 2: Decomposition of N_2O_5 is expressed by the equilibrium

$$N_2O_5 \rightarrow 4NO_2 + O_2$$

If during a certain time interval the rate of decomposition of N_2O_5 is 1.8×10^{-3} mol litre^{-1} min^{-1}, what will be the rates of formation of NO_2 and O_2 during the same interval?

Solution: The rate expression for the decomposition of N_2O_5 is

$$- \Delta[N_2O_5]/\Delta t = 1/2\Delta[NO_2]/\Delta t = 2\cdot\Delta[O_2]/\Delta t$$

So $\quad \Delta[NO_2]/\Delta t = 2 \ \Delta[N_2O_5]/\Delta t = 2 \times 1.8 \times 10^{-5}$

$$= 3.6 \times 10^{-3} \text{ mol litre}^{-1} \text{ min}^{-1}$$

and $\quad \Delta[O_2]/\Delta t = 1/2 \ \Delta[N_2O_5]/\Delta t = 1/2 \times 1.8 \times 10^{-3}$

$$= 0.9 \times 10^{-3} \text{ mol litre}^{-1} \text{ min}^{-1}$$

[Rate is always positive and hence $^-\Delta[N_2O_5]/\Delta t$ is taken positive.]

In order to determine changes in concentration of reactants or products, it is customary to take small portions of the reaction mixture at suitable intervals of time and freeze them rapidly to about 0°C as to stop the reaction. The concentration is then measured with the help of a suitable method. In several cases concentration changes are measured by observing changes in certain physical propertied which are proportional to it such as optical densities, electrical conductivity, optical rotation, etc. A curve is plotted between concentration and time. A tangent is drawn to the curve at the point corresponding to time interval 't'. The slope of this tangent gives the instantaneous rate of reaction

Instantaneous rate of reaction = Slope of curve

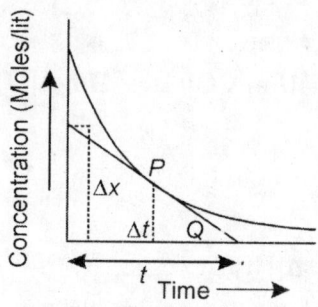

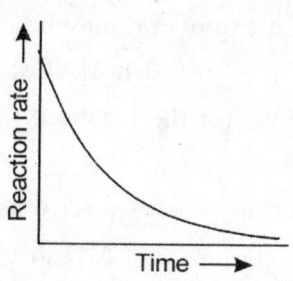

Fig. 3.1 (a): Determination of
rate of reaction

Fig. 3.1 (b): Variation of rate

(Intercept along ordinate)/(Intercept along abscissa) = $\Delta x / \Delta t$

LAW OF MASS ACTION

(Goldberg and Waage, 1864)

This law relates rate of reaction with active mass or molar concentration of reactants.

At a given temperature, the rate of a reaction at a particular instant raised to powers which are numerically equal to the numbers of their respective molecules in the stoichiometric equation describing the reaction.∞

Active mass = molar concentration of the substance

= (number of gram moles at the substance)/

(volume in litres)

= (w/M)/V = n/V

where w = mass of substance and 'M' is the molecular mass in grams. 'n' is the number of g moles and V is volume in litres.

Example: 4 g of hydrogen and 128 g of hydrogen iodide are present in a 2 litre flask. What are their active masses?

Solution: Mass of hydrogen = 4 g

Mol. mass of hydrogen = 2

Volume of the flask = 2 litres

Active mass of hydrogen = 4/2*2 = 1 mol L^{-1}

Mass of HI = 128 g

Mol. mass of HI = 128 g

Volume of the flask = 2 litre

Active mass of hydrogen iodide = 128/(128*2) = 0.5 mol L^{-1}

RATE CONSTANT

Consider a simple reaction A → B.

If C_4 is the molar concentration or active mass of A at a particular instant, then

$$(dx/dt) \propto C_A \text{ or } dx/dt = KC_A$$

where k is a proportionality constant, called velocity constant or rate constant or specific reaction rate.

At a fixed temperature, if $C_A = 1$, then

$$\text{Rate} = dx/dt = k \qquad \qquad ....(i)$$

Let us consider a general reaction.

$$aA + bB \rightarrow \text{product}$$
$$\text{Rate} = (dx/dt) \propto [A]^a [B]^b$$
$$\text{Rate} = k[A]a[B]b \qquad \qquad ....(ii)$$

When $[A] =[B] = 1 \text{ mol/litre}$, then

$$\text{Rate} = k$$

Rate of a reaction at unit concentration of reactants is called rate constant.

The volume of rate constant depends on:

(i) Nature of reactant

(ii) Temperature

(iii) Catalyst

Unit of rate constant

Rate constant has different units for reactions of different order. General rule for rate of reaction may be given as:

$$\text{Unit of rate constant} = [1/(\text{unit of concentration})]^{n-1} \times \text{time}^{-1}$$
$$= [1/(\text{mol/litre})]^{n-1} \times \text{sec}^{-1}$$
$$= [\text{litre/mol}]^{n-1} \times \text{sec}^{-1}$$

where n = order of reaction

S.No.	Rate of reaction	Reaction rate constant
1.	It is speed with which reactants are converted into products.	It is proportionally constant.
2.	It is measured as the rate of decrease concentration of reactants or the rate of increase of concentration of products with time.	It is equal to the rate of reaction when the concentration of each of the reactants in unity.
3.	It depends upon the initial concentration of reactants	It is independent of the initial concentration of the reactants. It has a constant value at fixed temperature.

Order of Reaction

Let us consider a good reaction:

$m_1A + m_2B + m_3C \rightarrow$ product

Let active moles of 'A', 'B' and 'C' be 'α', 'β' and 'γ' respectively. Then, rate of reaction may be given as:

$$\text{Rate} = k[A]^\alpha [B]^\beta [C]^\gamma$$

Sum of powers of concentration terms involved in rate law expression is called order of reaction.

$\alpha + \beta + \gamma$ order.

When $\alpha + \beta + \gamma = m_1 + m_2 + m_3$, then

Order of reaction = molecularity of reaction

Order is an experimentally determined quantity. It may be equal to zero, positive, negative, fractional and greater than three. Infinite and imaginary values are not possible.

Examples:

(i) $2H_2O_2 \rightarrow 2H_2O + O_2$

(observed from law of mass action)

Step 1: $H_2O_2 \rightarrow H_2O + [O]$ [slow]

Step 2: $[O] + [O] \rightarrow O_2$ (fast)

Actual rate $- dx/dt = k[H_2O_2]$

Thus, order of reactions in unity

(ii) $2NO_2 + F_2 \rightarrow 2NO_2F$

Rate law from law of mass action:

$$- dx/dt = k[NO_2][F_2]$$

Experimentally observed rate law:

$$- dx/dt = k[NO_2][F_2]$$

Slowest step is $NO_2 + F_2 \rightarrow NO_2F + [F]$

Thus, order of reaction = $1 + 1 = 2$

(iii) $CH_3CHO \rightarrow CH_4 + CO$

The rate equation derived from experimental data is found to be

$$-dx/dt = k[CH_3CHO]^{1.5}$$

The order of reaction is 1.5

Order of Reaction

Some typical linear plots for the reactions of different orders:

(a) Plots rate vs concentrations [Rate = k(conc.)^n]

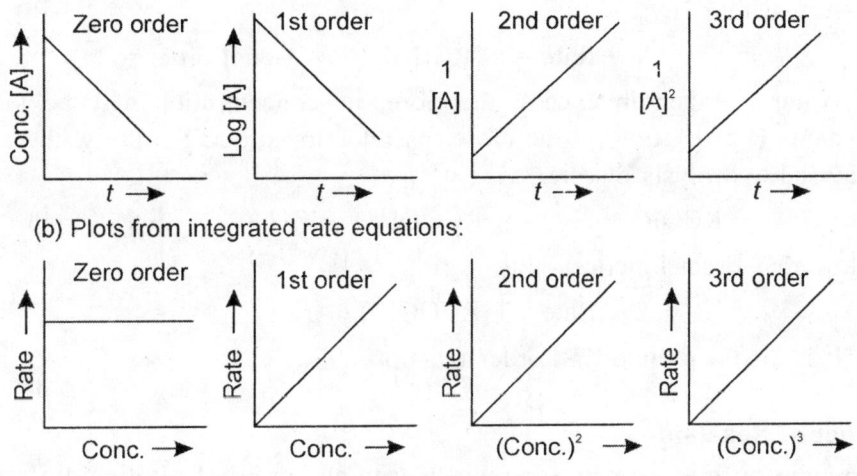

(b) Plots from integrated rate equations:

Fig. 3.2

From the study of the kinetics of many simple reactions, it is observed that for a large number of reactions, the molecularity and order are the same. Some examples are given below to justify this point.

1. Dissociation of N_2O_5.

   $N_2O_5 \rightarrow N_2O_4 + O_2$

   Order = 1, Molecularity = 1

2. Dissociation of H_2O_2.

   $H_2O_2 \rightarrow H_2O + 1/2O_2$

   Order = 1, Molecularity = 1

3. Dissociation of HI,

   $2HI \rightarrow H_2 + I_2$

   Order = 2, Molecularity = 1

4. Formation of NO_2.

   $2NO + O_2 \rightarrow 2NO_2$

   Order = 3, Moelcularity =3

Pseudo-order Reaction

Reactions whose actual order is different from that expected using rate law expression are called pseudo-order reactions; e.g.,

(i) $RCl + H_2O \rightarrow ROH + HCl$

Expected rate law:

$$Rate = k[RCl]\ [H_2O] \quad \text{Expected order} = 1 + 1 = 2$$

Actual rate law:

$$Rate = k'[RCl]; \qquad \text{Actual order} = 1$$

Water is taken in excess; therefore, its concentration may be taken constant. The reaction is, therefore, pseudo first order. Similarly, the acid catalysed hydrolysis of ester, viz.,

$$RCOR' + H_2O \leftrightarrow RCOOH + R'OH$$

follow first order kinetics:

$$Rate = k[RCOOR']$$

It is also a pseudo-first order reaction.

Order of Reaction

The main differences between molecularity and order of reaction are given below:

Molecularity	Order of reaction
1. It is the total number of reacting species (molecules, atoms or ions) which bring the chemical change.	1. It is the sum of powers of molar concentration of the reacting species in the rate equation of the reaction.
2. It is always a whole number.	2. It may be a whole number, zero, fractional, positive or negative.
3. It is a theoretical concept.	3. It is experimentally determined.
4. It is meaningful only for simple reactions or individual steps of a complex reaction. It is meaningless for overall complex reaction.	4. It is meant for the reaction anf not for its individual steps.

Factors Affecting Rate of Reaction

(i) Nature of the reactants:

(a) Physical state of reactants: This has considerable effect over rate of reaction.

(Gaseous state > Liquid state > Solid state)/
(Decreasing rate of reaction)

Similarly in a heterogeneous system collision is not so effective as in homogenous system. Thus, reactions in liquid phase or solution phase will be faster in comparison to heterogeneous conditions when same concen-trations of the reactants are taken.

(b) **Physical size of the reactants**-Among the solids, rate increases with decrease in particle size. In powdered state rate of reaction is maximum because in powdered state, surface area is maximum.

(c) **Chemical nature of reactants:** Consider the following two reactions:

$$2NO\ (g) + O_2(g) \rightarrow 2NO_2(g) \qquad \qquad ...(i)$$

$$CH_2(g) + 2O_2(g) \rightarrow CO_2(g) + 2H_2O \qquad \qquad ...(ii)$$

The first reaction is faster than the second because in the first reaction only N ∞ O bond is to be broken where as in the second reaction four (C-H) bonds are to be broken.

Similarly consider another example of two similar reactions:

$$2NO(g) + O_2(g) \rightarrow 2NO_2(g) \qquad \qquad ...(iii)$$

$$2CO(g) + 2O_2(g) \rightarrow 2CO_2(g) \qquad \qquad ...(iv)$$

No bond is weaker than CO bond, hence broken easily. Thus reaction (iii) is faster than (iv).

(ii) Concentration of reactants

Let us consider the reaction:

$$A + B \rightarrow C + D; \quad Rate = k[A][B]$$

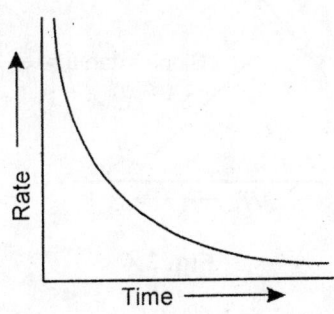

Fig. 3.3

Rate of the above reaction decreases with the passage of time because the concentration of reactants A and B will decrease as time pass on.

Effect of temperature

The rate of reaction increases considerably with an increase in temperature. The rates of many reactions are approximately doubled or tripled for every 10°C rise in temperature. The temperature coefficient of a chemical reaction is defined as the ratio of the specific reaction rates of a reaction at two temperature differing by 10°C.

$$\mu = \text{Temperature coefficeint} = k_{(r+10)}/k_t$$

Let temperature coefficient of a reaction be 'μ' when temperature is raised from T_1 to T_2; then the ratio of rate constants or rate may be calculated as

$$k_{T2}/k_{T1} = (\mu)^{(T_2 - T_1)/10} = \mu^{\Delta T/10}$$

$$\log_{10}(k_{T2}/k_{T1}) = \Delta T/10 \, \log_{10}\mu$$

$$k_{T2}/k_{T1} = \text{antilog} \, [\Delta T/10 \, \log_{10}\mu]$$

Its value lies generally between 2 and 3.

Arrhenius Equation

When the temperature is increased, heat energy is supplied which increases the kinetic energy of the reacting molecules. This will increase the number of collisions and ultimately the rate of reaction will be enhanced. Arrhenius suggested an equation which describes k as a function of temperature, i.e.,

$$k = Ae^{-E_a/RT}$$

where k $\rightarrow$ rate constant

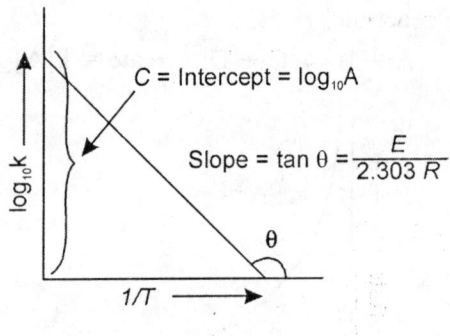

Fig. 3.4

A $\rightarrow$ a constant (frequency factor)

$E_a \rightarrow$ energy of activation

At two temperature T_1 and T_2, taking log of Arrhenius equation, we get

$$\log_e k_1 = \log A - E_a/RT_1 \, \log_e e \qquad \ldots \text{(i)}$$

and

$$\log_e k_2 = \log A - E_a/RT_2 \, \log_e e \qquad \ldots \text{(ii)}$$

subtracting Eq. (ii) from Eq. (i) and converting the log to the base 10, we get

$$\log_{10} k_1/k_2 = -E_a/(2.303 \, R) \, [(T_2 - T_1)/(T_1 T_2)] \quad \text{or}$$

$$\log_{10} k_2/k_1 = E_a/(2.303 \, R) \, [(T_2 - T_1)/(T_1 T_2)]$$

This equation can be used for calculation of energy of activation. Logarithmic Arrhenius equation is:

$$\log_{10} k = \log_{10} A - E_a/(2.303\ R)\ [1/T]$$

$$Y = C + M\ X$$

It is the equation of straight line with negative slope. On plotting $\log_{10}k$ against $[1/T]$ we get a straight line as shown in Fig. 3.4. The graph gives two kinetic parameters.

The slope gives activation energy and intercept gives frequency factor.

Presence of a positive catalyst

The function of a positive is to lower down the activation energy. The greater the decrease in the activation energy caused by the catalyst, higher will be the reaction rate. In the presence of a catalyst, the reaction follows a path of lower activation energy. Under this condition, a large number of reacting molecules are able to cross over the energy barrier and thus the rate of reaction increases. Fig. 3.5 shows how the activation energy is lowered in presence of a catalyst.

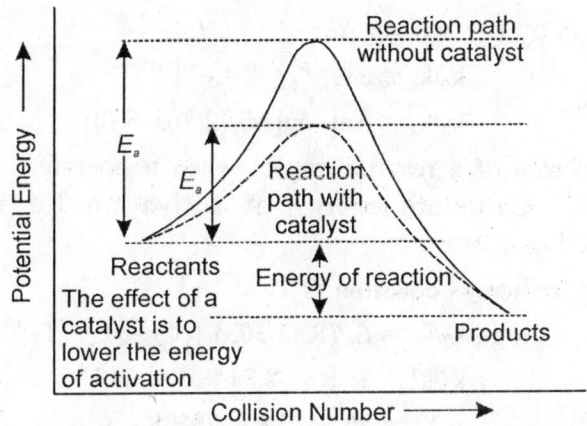

Fig. 3.5: A catalyst changes the reaction path (Positive catalyst)

Presence of negative catalyst

A negative catalyst increases the activation energy of reaction by forming a new intermediate of high energy, i.e., by changing the reaction mechanism.

Due to increased activation energy, some active molecules become inactive, therefore, rate of reaction decreases.

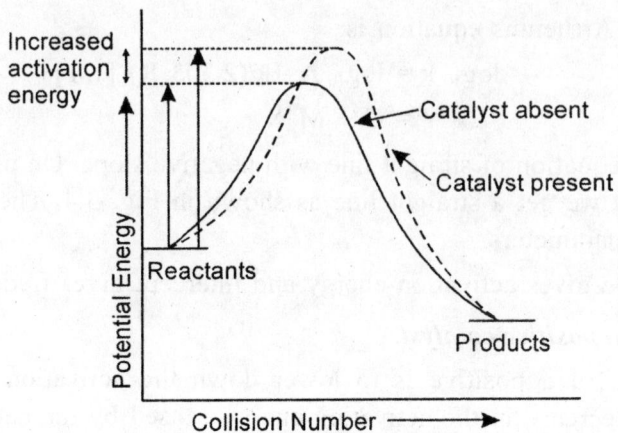

Fig. 3.6: Negative Catalyst

Let 'p' denote presence of catalyst and 'a' denote absence of catalyst.

$$k_p = Ae^{-E_p/RT} \qquad \qquad ... \text{(i)}$$

$$k_a = Ae^{-E_a/RT} \qquad \qquad ... \text{(ii)}$$

Dividing (1) by (2), we get Ae

$$k_p/k_a = e^{(E_a - E_p)/RT} = e^{\Delta E/RT}$$

$$k_p/k_a = \text{Antilog}[\Delta E/(2.303\ RT)]$$

Example: The rate of a reaction triples when temperature changes from 20°C to 50°C. Calculate energy of activation for the reaction (R = 8.314 JK^{-1} mol^{-1}).

Solution: The Arrhenius equation is

$$\log_{10} k_2/k_1 = E_a/(R \times 2.303)\ [(T_2 - T_1)/(T_1 T_2)]$$

Given: $k_2/k_1 = 3$; R = 8.314 JK^{-1} mol^{-1};

$$T_1 = 20 + 273 = 293\ K$$

and $T_2 = 50 + 273 = 323\ K$

Subtracting the given values in the Arrhenius equation,

$$\log_{10} 3 = E_a/(8.314 \times 2.303)\ [(323 - 293)/(323 \times 293)]$$

$$E_a = (2.303 \times 8.314 \times 323 \times 293 \times 0.477)/30$$

$$= 28811.8\ J\ mol^{-1}$$

$$= 28.8118\ kJ\ mol^{-1}$$

Factors Affecting Rate of Reaction

Example: In Arrhenius equation for a certain reaction, the value of A and E_a(activation energy) are 5×10^{13} sec^{-1} and 98.6 kJ mol^{-1} respecti-vely. At what temperature, the reaction will have specific rate constant 1.1×10^{-3} sec^{-1} ?

Solution: According to Arrhenius equation

$$k = Ae^{-E_a/RT}$$

or

$$\log_e k = \log_e A - E_a/RT \log_e e$$

or

$$2.303 \log 10\ k = 2.303 \log 10\ A - E_a/RT$$

or

$$2.303 \log (1.1 \times 10^{-3}) = 2.303 \log(4 \times 10^{13}) - (98.6 \times 10^3)/(8.314 \times T)$$

$$T = (98.6 \times 10^3)/(8.314 \times 2.303 \times 16.56)\ K$$

$$= 310.96\ K$$

Example : The rate constant is given by Arrhenius equation

$$k = Ae^{-E_a/RT}$$

Calculate the ratio of the catalyst and uncatalysed rate constants at 25°C if the energy of activation of a catalysed reaction is 162 kJ and for the uncatalysed reaction the value is 350 kJ.

Solution: Let k_{ca} and k_{un} be the rate constants for catalysed and uncatalysed reactions.

$$2.303 \log_{10} k_{ca} = 2.303 \log_{10} A - (162 \times 10^3)/RT \qquad ...\ (i)$$

and

$$2.303 \log_{10} k_{un} = 2.303 \log_{10} A - (350 \times 10^3)/RT \qquad ...\ (ii)$$

Subtracting Eq. (ii) from Eq. (i)

$$\log_{10} k_{ca}/k_{un} = 10^3/(2.303\ RT)\ (350 - 162)$$

$$= (188 \times 10^3)/(2.303 \times 8..314 \times 298) = 32.95$$

$$k_{ca}/k_{un} = 8.88 \times 10^{32}$$

Example: Calculate the rate constant of a reaction at 293 K when the energy of activation is 103 kJ mol^{-1} and the rate constant at 273 K is 7.87×10^{-7} s^{-1}. $(R = 8.314 \times 10^{-3}$ kJ mol^{-1} $K^{-1})$.

Solution: The Arrhenius equation is

$$\log_{10} k_2/k_1 = E_a/2.303R[(T_2 - T_1)/T_1 T_2]$$

Given:

$$k_1 = 7.87 \times 10^{-7}\ s^{-1};\ E^a = 103\ kJ\ mol^{-1}$$

$$R = 8.314 \times 10^{-3}\ kJ\ mol^{-1}\ K^{-1}$$

$$T = 273\ K\ and\ T_2 = 293\ K$$

Substituting the values in Arrhenius equation

$$\log_{10} = k_2/(7.87 \times 10^{-7})$$
$$= (10.3 \times 20)/$$
$$(2.303 \times 8.314 \times 10^{-2} \times 293 \times 273)$$
$$= 1.345$$
$$k_2 = 1.74 \times 10^{-5} \text{ s}^{-1}$$

Example : At 407 K, the rate constant of a chemical reaction is 9.5×10^{-5} s^{-1} and at 420 K, the rate constant is 1.9×10^{-4} s^{-1}. Calculate the frequency factor of the reaction.

Solution: The Arrhenius equation is,

$$\text{Log}_{10} = k_2/k_1 = E_a/(2.303 \times R) [(T_2 - T_1)/(T_1 T_2)]$$

Given: $k_1 = 9.5 \times 10^{-5}$ s^{-1}; $k_2 = 1.9 \times 1.4$ s^{-1}.

$$R = 8.314 \text{ J mol}^{-1} \text{ K}^{-1}$$

$$T_1 = 407 \text{ K and } T_2 = 420 \text{ K}$$

Substituting the values in Arrhenius equation

$$\log_{10}(1.9 \times 10^{-4})/(9.5 \times 10^{-5}) = E_a/(2.303 \times 8.314) [(420 - 407)/$$
$$(420 \times 407)]$$

$$E_a = 75782.3 \text{ J mol}^{-1}$$

Applying now $\log k_1 = \log A - E_a/(2.303 RT_1)$

$$\log 9.5 \times 10^{-5} = \log A - 75782.3/(2.303 \times 8.314 \times 407)$$

or $\log A/(9.5 \times 10^{-5}) = 75782.3/(2.303 \times 8.314 \times 407) = 9.7246$

$$A = 5.04 \times 10^5 \text{ s}^{-1}$$

Example: The energy of activation for a reaction is 100 kJ mol^{-1}. Presence of a catalyst lowers the energy of activation by 75%. What will be effect on rate of reaction at 20°C, other things being equal?

Solution: The Arrhenius equation is

$$k = Ae^{-E_a/RT}$$

In absence of catalyst, $k_1 = Ae^{-100/RT}$

In presence of catalyst, $k_2 = Ae^{-25/RT}$

So $k_2/k_1 = e^{75/RT}$ or $2.303 \log k_2/k_1 = 75/RT$

or $2.303 \log k_2/k_1 = 75/(8.314 \times 10^{-3} \times 293)$

or $\log k_2/k_1 = 75/(8.314 \times 10^{-3} \times 293 \times 2.303)$

or $k_2/k_1 = 2.34 \times 10^{13}$

As the things being equal in presence or absence of a catalyst.

k_2/k_1 must be = (rate of presence of catalyst)/(rate in absence of catalyst)

i.e., $\qquad\qquad\qquad r_2/r_1 = k_2/k_1 = 2.34 \times 10^{13}$

Solved Examples for Molecularity and Order of Reaction

Example: The experimental data for the reaction

$$2A + B_2 \rightarrow 2AB$$

is as follows:

Expt. No.	[A] (mol L^{-1})	[B$_2$] (mol L^{-1})	Rate (mol $L^{-1} s^{-1}$)
1.	0.50	0.50	1.6×10^{-4}
2.	0.50	1.00	3.2×10^{-4}
3.	1.00	1.00	3.2×10^{-4}

Write the most probable equation for the rate of reaction giving reason for your answer.

Solution: From an examination of above data, it is clear that when the concentration of B_2 is doubled, the rate is doubled. Hence the order of reaction with respect to B_2 is one.

Further when concentration of A is doubled, the rate remain unaltered. So, order of reaction with respect to A is zero.

The probable rate law for the reaction will be $-dx/dt = k[B_2][A]^0 = k[B_2]$

$$\text{Alternatively Rate} = k[B_2]^\alpha$$
$$1.6 \times 10^{-4} = k[0.5]^\alpha$$
$$3.2 \times 10^{-4} = k[1]^\alpha$$

On dividing we get $\quad \alpha = 1$

$\therefore \qquad\qquad$ Rate $= k[A]^0[B_2]^1 = k[B_2]$

Example: For the reaction

$$A + 2B \rightarrow 2C$$

the following data were obtained.

Expt. No.	Initial concentration (mol L^{-1})		Initial reaction rates (mol L^{-1}min^{-1})
	[A]	[B]	
1.	1.0	1.0	0.15
2.	2.0	1.0	0.30
3.	3.0	1.0	0.45
4.	1.0	2.0	0.15
5.	1.0	3.0	0.15

Write down the rate law for the reaction.

Solved Examples for Molecularity and Order of Reaction

Solution : Let the rate law be

$$-dx/dt = k[A]^x [B]^y$$

By keeping the concentration of B constant in experiments (1), (2) and (3) and increasing concentration uniformly, the rate also increases uniformly, thus,

Rate ∞ [A], i.e., $\qquad$ x = 1

By keeping the concentration of A constant in experiments (1), (4) and (5) and increasing the concentration of B, the rate remains the same.

Hence, $\qquad$ y = 0

The rate law is $\quad$ $-dx/dt = k[A]$

Alternatively method:

From Expt. (1), $\qquad$ $k[1.0]^x[1.0]^y = 0.15$ $\qquad\qquad\qquad$ ...(i)

From Expt. (2), $\qquad$ $k[2.0]^x[1.0]^y = 0.30$ $\qquad\qquad\qquad$ ... (ii)

Dividing Eq. (ii) by Eq. (i),

$$[2.0]^x/[1.0]^x = 0.30/0.15 = 2$$

So, $\qquad\qquad\qquad\qquad\qquad$ x = 1

From Expt. (1), $\qquad$ $k[1.0]^x[1.0]^y = 0.15$ $\qquad\qquad\qquad$ ...(i)

From Expt. (4), $\qquad$ $k[1.0]^x[2.0]^y = 0.15$ $\qquad\qquad\qquad$ ... (iii)

Dividing Eq. (iii) by Eq. (i),

$$[2.0]^y/[1.0]^y = 1$$

So, $\qquad\qquad\qquad\qquad\qquad$ y = 0,

Hence, the rate law is $\qquad$ $-dx/dt = k[A]$.

Example: For the reaction:

2NO + Cl$_2$ → 2NOCl, at 300 K following data are obtained.

Expt. No.	Initial concentration		Initial rates
	[NO]	**[Cl$_2$]**	
1.	0.010	0.010	1.2 × 10^{-4}
2.	0.010	0.020	2.4×10^{-4}
3.	0.020	0.020	9.6×10^{-4}

Write rate of law for the reaction. What is the order of the reaction? Also calculate the specific rate constant.

Solution: Let the rate law for the reaction be

$$\text{Rate} = k[NO]^x[Cl_2]^y$$

From Expt. (1), $1.2 \times 10^{-4} = k[0.010]^x[0.010]^y$ ... (i)

From Expt. (2), $2.4 \times 10^{-4} = k[0.010]^x[0.020]^y$ ... (ii)

Dividing Eq. (ii) by Eq. (i),

$$(9.6 \times 10^{-4})/(2.4 \times 10^{-4}) = ([0.020]^x)/[0.010]^x$$

or $$2 = (2)^y$$

$$y = 1$$

From Expt. (2), $2.4 \times 10^{-4} = k[0.010]^x[0.020]^y$ .... (ii)

From Expt. (3), $9.6 \times 10^{-4} = k[0.020]^x[0.020]^y$ .... (ii)

Dividing Eq. (ii) by Eq. (ii),

$$(9.6 \times 10^{-4})/(2.4 \times 10^{-4}) = ([0.020]^x)/[0.010]^x$$

or $$4 = 2^x$$

$$x = 2$$

Order of reaction = $x + y = 2 + 1 = 3$

Rate law for the reaction is

$$\text{Rate} = k[NO]^2[Cl_2]$$

Considering Eq. (i) again,

$$1.2 \times 10^{-4} = k[0.010]^2[0.010]$$

$$k = (1.2 \times 10^{-4})/[0.010]^3$$

$$= 1.2 \times 10^2 \text{ mol}^{-2} \text{ litre}^2 \text{ sec}^{-1}$$

Example: For the hypothetical reaction

$$2A + B \rightarrow \text{products}$$

the following data are obtained.

Expt. No.	Initial conc. of (A) (mol L$_{-1}$)	Initial conc. of (B) (mol L^{-1})	Initial rates L^{-1} s^{-1})
1.	0.10	0.20	3×10^2
2.	0.30	0.40	3.6×10^3
3.	0.30	0.80	1.44×10^4
4.	0.10	0.40	—
5.	0.20	0.60	—
6.	0.30	1.20	—

Find out how the rate of the ration depends upon the concentration of A and B and fill in the blanks.

Solution: From Expt. (2) and (3), it is clear that when concentration of A is kept constant and that of B is doubled, the rate increases four times. This shows that the reaction is of second order with respect to B.

Similarly, from Expt. (1) and (2), it is observed that when concentration of A is increased three times and that of B two times, the rate becomes twelve times. Hence, the reaction is first order with respect to A.

Thus the rate law for the reaction is

$$\text{Rate} = k[A][B]^2$$

FILL IN THE BLANKS

Substituting the values of Expt. (1) in the rate equation.

$$3 \times 10^2 = k[0.10][0.40]^2$$

or
$$k = (3 \times 10^2)/([0.10] \, [0.20]^2)$$
$$= 7.50 \times 10^4 \, L^2 \, s^{-1}$$

Expt. (4): $\text{Rate} = k[0.10][0.40]^2$;
$$= 7.5 \times 10^4 \times 0.10 \times 0.40 \times 0.40$$

Expt. (5): $\text{Rate} = k[0.20][1.20]^2$
$$= 7.5 \times 10^4 \times 0.30 \times 1.20 \times 1.20$$
$$= 3.24 \times 104 \text{ mol } L^{-1} \, s^{-1}$$

Zero order reactions

A reaction is said to be of zero order if its rate is independent of the concentration of the reactants, i.e., the rate is proportional to the zeroth power of the concentration of the reactants.

For the reaction

$$A \rightarrow \text{products}$$

to be of zero order,

$$-dx/dt = k[A]^0 = k$$

Some photochemical reaction and a few heterogeneous reactions are zero-order reactants. Such reactions are not common.

Example:

1. Photochemical reaction between hydrogen and chlorine:

$$H_2(g) + Cl_2(g) \xrightarrow{\ h\nu\ } 2HCl(g)$$

This photochemical reaction is zero-order reaction. The reaction is studied by placing H_2 and Cl_2 gases over water. the rate of reaction is studied by nothing the rate at which water rises in the vessel due to dissociation of HCl formed. the rate of rise of water is the same as the rate of disappearance of H_2 and Cl_2, i.e., the concentration of the gases phase will not change with time, although the quantities will change.

2. Decomposition of N_2O on hot platinum surface:

$$N_2O \rightarrow N_2 + 1/2\ O_2$$
$$\text{Rate } [N_2O]^0 = k[N_2O]^0 = k$$
$$d[N_2O]/dt = k$$

3. Decomposition of NH_3 in presence of molybdenum or tungsten is a zero-order reaction.

$$2NH_3 \xrightarrow{\ [Mo]\ } N_2 + 3H_2$$

The surface of the catalyst is almost completely covered by NH_3 molecules. The adsorption of gas on the surface cannot change by increasing the pressure or concentration of NH_3. Thus, the concentration of gas phase remains constant although the product is formed. Therefore, this reaction zero order kinetics.

Other examples of zero order are:

4. Decomposition of NI on the gold surface.

5. Iodations of acetone in presence of H^+ ions.

$$CH_3COCH + I_2 \xrightarrow{\ H^+\ } ICH_2COCH_3 + HI$$

The rate equation of this reaction does not include $[I_2]$ factor, i.e.,

$$-dx/dt = k[CH_3 COCH][H^+]$$

Characteristics of zero order reaction

(a) The concentration of reactant decreases linearly with time.

$$[A]_t = [A]_0 - kt$$

(b) The time required for the reaction to be complete, i.e., time at which [A] is zero.

$$t_{completion} = [A]_0/k = \text{(Initial concentration)/(Rate constant)}$$

(c) The units of k are mol L^{-1} time^{-1}.

First order reactions

A reaction is said to be first order if its rate is determined by the change of one concentration term only.

Consider the reaction

$$A \rightarrow products$$

Let α be the concentration of A at the start and after time t, the concentration becomes (a − x), i.e, x has been changed into products. The rate of reaction after time 't' is given by the expression

$$dx/dt = k(a - x)$$

or $$dx/((a - x)) = k \, dt$$

Upon integration of above equation,

$$\int dx/(a - x) = k + \int dt$$

or $$-\log_e (a - x) = kt + c$$

where c is integration constant.

When $\qquad t = 0 , \quad x = 0,$

$\therefore \qquad c = -\log_e a$

Putting the value of 'c',

$$-\log_e (a - x) = kt - \log_e a$$

or $$\log_e a - \log_e (a - x) = kt$$

or $$\log_e a/(a - x) = kt$$

or $$k = 2.303/t \, \log_{10} a/(a - x)$$

This is known as the kinetic equation for a reaction of the first order. The following two important conclusions are drawn from this equation:

(i) A change in concentration unit will not change the numerical value of k. let the new unit

So $$k = 2.303/t \, \log_{10} na/n(a - x)$$

or $\qquad k = 2.303/t \log_{10} a/(a-x)$

Thus for first order reaction, any quantity which is proportional to concentration can be used in place of concentration for evaluation of 'k'.

(ii) The time taken for the completion of same fraction of change is independent of initial concentration. For example, for half change,

$$x = 0.5a \text{ and } t = t_{1/2}$$

So $\qquad k = 2.303/t_{1/2} \log_{10} a/0.5a = 2.303/t_{1/2} \log_{10} 2$

$$= 0.693/t_{1/2}$$

or $\qquad t_{1/2} = 0.693/k$

Thus, $t_{1/2}$ is independent of initial concentration 'a'.

Half life- This time 't' in which the initial concentration becomes half is termed as half life period. Half life period of a first order reaction is independent of the initial concentration of the reactant.

Average life- Reciprocal of rate constant is known as average life ($= 1/k$)

Since the velocity constant is independent of concentration and depends inversely on the time, the unit of k will be $time^{-1}$, i.e., sec^{-1} or min^{-1} or $hour^{-1}$. The equation of the first order can also be written in the following form when initial concentration is not known.

$$k = 2.303/((t_2 - t_1)) \log_{10} ((a - x_1))/((a - x_2))$$

$(a-x_1)$ is the concentration after time t_1 and $(a - x_2)$ the concentration after time t_2 when $t_2 > t_1$.

When the log of the concentration of the reactant at various intervals of time is plotted against the time intervals, a straight line is obtained (Fig. given below). The slope of this line gives the value 2.303/k, from which k can be evaluated.

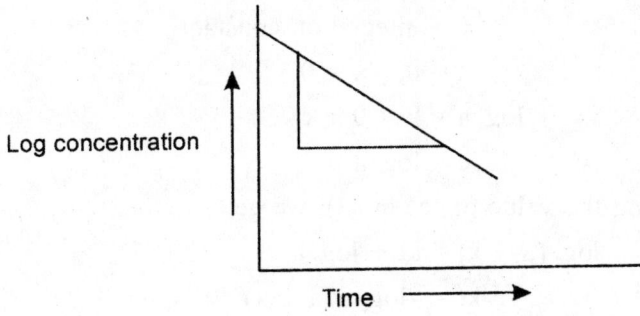

Examples of first order reactions

1. Decomposition of H_2O_2 in aqueous solution

   $H_2O_2 \rightarrow H_2O + 1/2 \; O_2$

2. Hydrolysis of methyl acetate in presence of mineral acids.

   $CH_3COOCH_3 + H_2O \xrightarrow{\quad Acid \quad} CH_3COOH + CH_3OH$

3. Inversion of cane sugar in presence of mineral acids.

   $C_{12}H_{22}O_{11} + H_2O \xrightarrow{\quad Acid \quad} C_6H_{12}O_6 + C_6H_{12}O_6$

4. Decomposition of ammonium nitrite in aqueous solution.

   $NH_4NO_2 \rightarrow N_2 + 2H_2O$

5. Hydrolysis of diazo derivatives.

   $C_5H_5N = NCl + H_2O \rightarrow C_6H_5OH + N_2 + HCl$

Note: In case of gases, pressure can be used in place of concentration.

First Order Growth Kinetics

It is used for population growth and bacteria multiplication, e.g.,

Time	Population
0	a
dt	(a + x)

Growth rate is directly proportional to present population.

$$dx/dt \propto (a + x)$$

$$= k(a + x)$$

$$dx/(a + x) = k \; dt \qquad \qquad ... (i)$$

It is a differential equation of first order and first degree in variable separable form. It may be solved on integration.

$$\int dx/(a + x) = k + \int dt + c$$

$$\log_e (a + x) = kt + c \qquad \qquad ...(ii)$$

Here,   c = integration constant

At $t = 0, \quad x = 0$

$\therefore$ $\log_e a = k \times 0 + c$

$$c = \log_e a \qquad \qquad ...(iii)$$

Substituting the value of 'c' in (ii), we get

$$\log_e (a + x) = kt + \log_e a$$

$$kt = -\log_e a/(a + x)$$

$$k = -2.303/t \ \log_{10} a/(a + x)$$

This is the kinetics for first order growth kinetics

Note:

(1) If volume of reagents are given in volumetric analysis then we use the following equation to determine rate constant.

$$k = 2.303/t \ \log_{10} (V_\infty - C_0)/(V_\infty - V_1)$$

where
V_0 = volume used at zero time,
V_1 = volume used at time 't',
V_∞ = volume used at infinite time

Case I When V_0 is not given, we use

$$k = 2.303/t \ \log_{10} v_\infty/(v_\infty - v_1)$$

Case II When v_∞ is not given, then

$$k = 2.303/t \ \log_{10} (V_0/V_1)$$

(2) if information is given in terms of angle of rotation of optically active compounds, measured by polarimeter with respect to time, then

$$k = 2.303/t \ \log 10 \ \{r_\infty - r_0/r_\infty - r_1\}$$

where
r_0 = angle of rotation at zero time,
r_1 = angle of rotation at time 't',
r_∞ = angle of rotation at infinite time.

Case I If r_0 is not given, then

$$k = 2.303/t \ \log_{10} \ \{r_\infty/r_\infty - r_1\}$$

Case II If r_∞ is not given, then

$$k = 2.303/t \ \log_{10} \ \{r_0/r_1\}$$

(3) if pressure is given in gaseous reaction, then we use the following kinetic equation:

$$k = 2.303/t \ \log_{10} \ \{P_0/(P_0 - x)\}$$

where
P_0 = pressure of reactant at initial stage,

$(P_0 - x)$ = pressure of such a reactant at 't' time

Values of 'P_0' and 'x' can be calculated using the following examples:

$$A(g) \rightarrow B(g) + C(g) + D(g)$$

At $\quad t = 0$	P_0	0	0	0
Pressure after time 't'	$(P_0 - x)$	x	x	x
Pressure after a long time or infinite time	0	P_0	P_0	P_0

Case I. If total pressure of reaction mixture is given in place of pressure of reactant, then

$$P_t = (P_0 - x + x + x + x)$$

where P_1 = pressure of vessel at time 't'.

Case II. If pressure of vessel after a long time or infinite time is given, then

$$P\infty = P_0 + P_0 + P_0$$

2nd order

Second order reactions

A reaction is said to be of second order if its reaction rate is determined by the variation of two concentration terms.

The kinetics of second order reactions are given as follows:

(i) When concentration of both reactants are equal or two molecules of the same reactant are involved in the change, i.e.,

$$A + B \rightarrow products$$

or $$2A \rightarrow products$$

$$dx/dt = k(a - x)^3$$

On solving this equation,

$$k = 1/t. \, x/a(a - x)$$

where a = initial concentration of the reactant or reactants and

x = concentration of the reactant changed in time t.

(ii) When the initial concentrations of the two reactants are different, i.e.,

$$A + B \rightarrow products$$

Initial conc. a b

$$dx/dt = k(a - x)(b - x)$$

$$k = 2.303/t(a - b) \, \log_{10} b(a - x)/a(b - x)$$

(a − x) and (b − x) are the concentrations of A and B after time interval, t.

Characteristics of the second order reactions

(i) The value of k(velocity constant) depends on the unit of concentration. The unit of k is expressed as $(mol/litre)^{-1}$ $time^{-1}$ or litre mol^{-1} $time^{-1}$.

(ii) Half life period $(t_{1/2})$ = 1/k.0.5a/(a×0.5a) = 1/ka

Thus, half life is inversely proportional to initial concentration.

(iii) Second order reaction conforms to the first order when one of the reactants is present in large excess.

Taking k = $2.303/t(a - b) \log_{10} b(a - x)/a(b - x)$; if a>>> b

then $\quad\quad\quad$ (a-x) = a and (a-b) = a

Hence, $\quad\quad\quad$ k = $2.303/ta \log_{10} ba/a(b - x)$

or $\quad\quad\quad$ ka = k' = $2.303/t \log_{10} b/((b - x))$

(since 'a' being very large, may be treated as constant after the change). Thus the reaction follows first order kinetics with respect to the reactant taken relatively in small amount.

Examples of second order reactions

1. Hydrolysis of ester by an alkali (saponification).

$CH_3COOC_2H_5 + NaOH \rightarrow CH_3COONa + C_2H_5OH$

2. The decomposition of NO_2 into NO and O_2.

3. Conversion of ozone into oxygen at 100°C

$2NO_2 \rightarrow 2NO + O_2$

4. Thermal decomposition of chlorine monoxide.

$2Cl_2O \rightarrow 2Cl_2 + O_2$

METHODS FOR DETERMINATION OF ORDER OF A REACTION

The important methods used for the following:

1. Method of integration (Hit and trial method)

The most simple method is the one in which the quantities a, x and t are determined and substituted in the kinetic equations of various orders. The equation which gives the most constant value for the specific rate constant (k) for a series of time intervals is the one corresponding to the order of reaction. If all the reactants are at the same molar concentrations, the kinetic equations are:

k = $2.303/t \log_{10} a/((a - x))$; for first order reactions;

k = $1/t [1/((a - x)) - 1/a]$; for second order reactions;

k = $1/t [1/(a - x)^2 - 1/a^2]$; for third order reactions;

2. Graphical method

A graphical method based on the respective rate laws can also be used.

If the plot of log $(a - x)$ versus 't' is a straight line, the reaction follows second order.

If the plot of $1/(a - x)^2$ versus 't' is a straight line, the reaction follows third order.

In general, for a reaction of nth order, a graph of $1/(a - x)^{n-1}$ versus 't' must be a straight line.

3. Half life method

A general expression for the half life, $(t_{1/2})$, is given by

$$t_{(1/2)} \propto 1/a^{n-1}$$

where 'n' is the order of the reaction.

Starting with different initial concentration a_1 and a_2 for the same reaction, the half lives are $(t_{1/2})_1$ and $(t_{1/2})_2$ respectively are determined. As we know,

$$t_{(1/2)1} \propto 1/a^{n-1}$$

and $$t_{(1/2)2} \propto 1/a_2^{n-1}$$

Dividing (i) by (ii),

$$t_{(1/2)_1}/t_{(1/2)_2} = (a_2/a_1)^{n-1}$$

Methods of Determination of Order of a Reaction

Taking logarithms on both sides,

$$\log_{10} (t_{1/2})_1 - \log_{10}(t_{1/2}) = (n^{-1})(\log_{10} a_2 - \log_{10} a_1)$$

$$n - 1 = (\log_{10} (t_{(1/2)1} - \log_{10} (t_{1/2})_2)/(\log_{10} a_2 - \log_{10}a_1)$$

or $$n = 1 + (\log_{10}(t_{1/2}) - \log_{10}(t_{1/2}))/(\log_{10}a_2 - og_{10}a_1)$$

Plots of half-lives concentration $(t_{1/2} \propto a^{1-a})$:

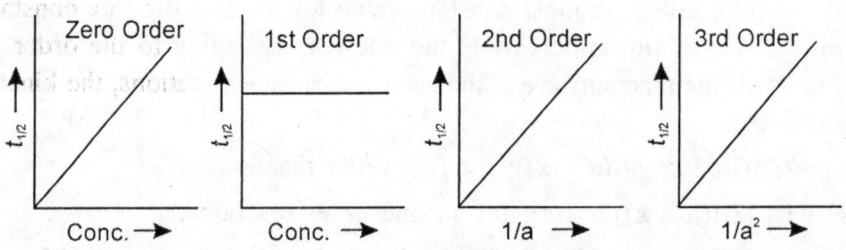

This relation can be used to determine order of reaction 'n'

1. van't Hoff differential method

As we know that, the rate of a reaction varies as the nth power of the concentration of the reactant where 'n' is the order of the reaction. Thus, for twp different initial concentrations C_1 and C_2, equations can be written in the form

$$-(dC_1)/dt = kC_1^n \text{ and } -(dC_2)/dt = kC_2^n$$

Taking logarithms,

$$\log_{10}(-(dC_1)/dt) = \log_{10}k + n\log^{10} C_1 \qquad \text{... (i)}$$

and $\qquad \log10 (-(dC_2)/dt) = \log_{10}k + n\log^{10} C_2 \qquad \text{...(ii)}$

Subtracting Eq. (ii) from (i),

$$\log_{10}(-(dC_1)/dt) - \log_{10}((-dC_2)/dt) = n(\log_{10} C_1 - \log_{10}C_2)$$

or $\qquad n = \log_{10}(-(dC_1)/dt) - \log_{10}((dC_2)/dt)/\log_{10}$

$$C_1 - \log_{10} C_2 \quad \text{...(iii)}$$

$-dc_1/dt$ and $-dc_2/dt$ are determined from concentration vs. time graphs and the value of 'n' can be determined.

Parallel or Competing Reaction

The reaction in which a substance reacts or decomposes in more than one way are called parallel or side reactions.

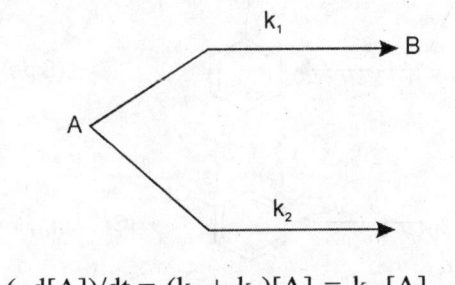

$$(-d[A])/dt = (k_1 + k_2)[A] = k_{av}[A]$$
$$k_1 = \text{fractional yield of B} \times k_{av}$$
$$k_2 = \text{fractional yield of C} \times k_{av}$$

If $k_1 \gg k_2$ then

$A \rightarrow B$ main and

$A \rightarrow C$ is side reaction

Let after a definite interval x mol/litre of B and y mol/litre of C are formed.

$$x/y = k_1/k_2$$

i.e.,   d[B]/dt/d[C]/dt = k₁/k₂

$$i.e., \quad d[B]/dt/d[C]/dt = k_1/k_2$$

Fig. 3.7.

Variation of concentration A, B and C with time may be graphically represented as,

Example

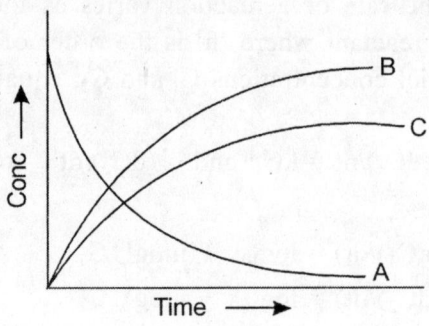

Consecutive Reaction

This reaction is defined as that reaction which proceeds from reactants to final products through one or more intermediate stages. The overall reaction is a result of several successive or consecutive steps.

A → B → C and so on

Example

(i) Decomposition of ethylene oxide

$$(CH_2)_2O \xrightarrow{\ k_1\ } CH_3CHO$$

$$CH_3CHO \xrightarrow{\ k_2\ } CO + CH_4$$

(ii) The pyrolysis of acetone

$$(CH_3)_2CO \rightarrow CH_4 + CH_2 = C = O$$
$$\text{Ketene}$$
$$CH_2 = C = O \rightarrow C_2H_4 + CO$$

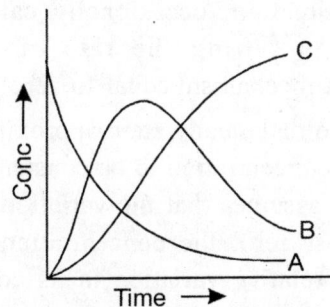

Fig. 3.8 : Variation of concentration of various substances during the progress of reaction (A → B → C)

$$A \xrightarrow{\ k_1\ } B \xrightarrow{\ k_2\ } C$$

Let initially (t = 0), [B] = 0 and $k_1 < k_2$ then maximum concentration of [B] may be calculated as,

$$[B]max = [A]0 \ [k_1/k_2]^{k_2/k_1 - k_2}$$

where $[A]_0$ = Initial concentration of A

Time in which B attains maximum concentration may be given as,

$$t_{max} = 2.303/(k_2 - k_1) \ \log (k_2/k_1)$$

Concentration of [B] after time 't' may be calculates as,

$$[B]_t = (k_1 [A]_0)/(k_2 - k_1) \ [e^{-k_1 t} - e^{-k_2 t}]$$

Parallel or Competing Reaction

Reversible Reaction

The reactions is which the products of chemical change react together to form the original reactants, are called reversible reactions. They are also called opposing or counter reactions.

Let us consider a reversible reaction in which both forward and backward reactions are of first order.

$$A \xrightarrow[k_2]{k_1} B$$

Initial state (t = 0)	a	0
Conc. at time (t)	(a − x)	x
Equilibrium conc.	(a − x_c)	x_e

$$k_1 + k_2 = 2.303/t \, \log_{10} \{x_e/(x_e - x)\}$$

Steady state approximation in chemical kinetics

The steady state approximation, occasionally called the stationary-state approximation, involves setting the rate of change of a reaction intermediate in a reaction mechanism equal to zero.

It is important to note that steady state approximation does not assume the reaction intermediate concentration to be constant (and therefore its time derivative being zero), it assumes that the variation in the concentration of the intermediate is almost zero: the concentration of the intermediate is very low, so even a big relative variation in its concentration is small, if considered quantitatively.

Its use facilitates the resolution of the differential equations that arise from rate equations, which lack an analytical solution for most mechanisms beyond the most simple ones. The steady state approximation is applied, for example in Michaelis-Menten kinetics.

As an example, the steady state approximation will be applied to two consecutive, irreversible, homogeneous first order reactions in a closed system. (For heterogeneous reactions, see reactions on surfaces.) This model corresponds, for example, to a series of nuclear decompositions like $^{239}U \rightarrow ^{239}Np \rightarrow ^{239}Pu$.

If the rate constants for the following reaction are k_1 and k_2; (A → B → C) combining the rate equations with a mass balance for the system yields:

Reaction rates

For reactant A: $\dfrac{d[A]}{dt} = -k_1[A]$

For reactant B: $\dfrac{d[B]}{dt} = k_1[A] - k_2[B]$

For reactant C: $\dfrac{d[C]}{dt} = k_2[B]$

Analytical Solutions

The analytical solutions for these equations (supposing that initial concentrations of every substance except for A are zero) are ;

$[A] = [A]_0 e^{-k_1 t}$

$$[B] = \begin{cases} [A]_0 \dfrac{k_1}{k_2 - k_1}\left(e^{-k_1 t} - e^{-k_2 5}\right); & k_1 \neq k_2 \\ [A]_0 k_1 t e^{-k_1 t} & \text{otherwise} \end{cases}$$

$$[C] = \begin{cases} [A]_0\left(1 + \dfrac{k_1 e^{k_2 t} - k_2 e^{-k_1 t}}{}\right); & k_1 \neq k_2 \\ [A]_0\left(1 - e^{-k_1 t} - k_1 t e^{-k_1 t}\right); & \text{otherwise} \end{cases}$$

Steady State

If the steady state approximation is applied, then the derivative of the concentration of the intermediate is set to zero.

$$\frac{d[B]}{dt} = 0 = k_1[A] - k_2[B]$$

$$\Rightarrow \qquad \frac{d[C]}{dt} = [C] = [A]_0(1 - e^{k_1 t})$$

Collision Theory of Reaction Rate (Arrhenius Theory of Reaction Rate)

(1) A chemical reaction takes place due to collision among reactant molecules. The number of collisions taking place per second per unit volume of the reaction mixture is known as collision frequency (Z). The value of collision frequency is very high, of the order of 10^{25} to 10^{28} in case of binary collisions.

(2) Every collision does not bring a chemical change. The collisions that actually produce the products are effective collisions. The effective collisions which bring chemical change are few in comparison to the form a product are ineffective elastic collisions, i.e., molecules just collide and disperse in different directions with different velocities. For a collision to be effective, the following two barriers are to be cleared.

Energy barrier

The minimum amount of energy which the colliding molecules must possess as to make the chemical reaction to occur, is known as threshold energy. In the Figs. 3.9 and 3.10 'E' corresponds to minimum or threshold energy for effective collision in a hypothetical reaction.

There is an energy barrier for each reaction. The reacting species must be provided with sufficient energy as to cross the energy barrier.

Activation energy: The minimum amount of energy required by reactant molecules to participate in a reaction is called activation energy.

Activation energy = threshold energy

– average kinetic energy of reacting molecules

Threshold energy = initial potential energy of reactant molecules

+ activation energy.

A collision between high energy molecules overcomes the forces of repulsion and brings the formation of an unstable molecule cluster, called the activated complex. The life span of an activated complex is very small. Thus, the activated complex breaks either into reactants again or new substances, i.e., products. The activation energy (E_a) depends upon the nature of chemical bonds undergoing rupture and is independent of enthalpies of reactants and products. The energy changes during exothermic and endothermic reactions versus the progress of the reaction are shown in the given Figs. 3.9 and 3.10.

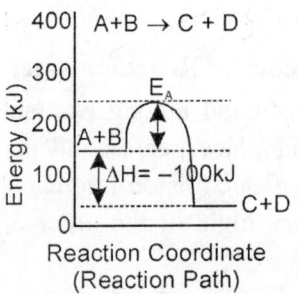 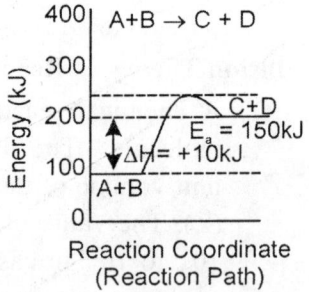

Figs. 3.9 and 3.10: For progress of exothermic and endothermic reaction respectively

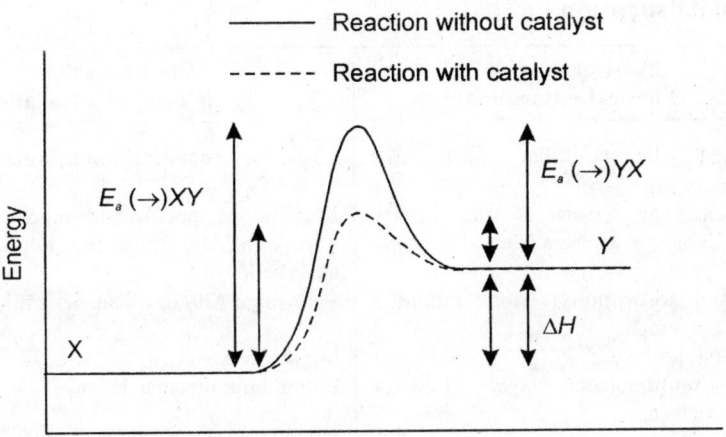

Fig. 3.11: Reaction Path

Effect of catalyst on activation energy(E_a) is shown in the Fig. 3.11 presence of positive catalyst decreases activation energy and more no of molecules pass through the energy barrier and rate of the reaction increases.

SURFACE CHEMISTRY

Adsorption

The phenomenon of existence of a substance in different concentrations at the surface of another substance than in the bulk phases is called **adsorption**.

The substance whose surface **adsorbs** molecular species of another substance is called adsorbent and the substance, which gets adsorbed, is called **adsorbate.**

Difference between Adsorption and Absorption

When a substance is uniformly distributed throughout the bulk of another substance, this shows that absorption has taken place. It occurs at the uniform rate throughout the body of the material. One the contrary, adsorption involves unequal distribution of the molecular species in the bulk and the surface. It is a surface phenomenon. It is rapid in the beginning and gradually slows down at the equilibrium. The forces involves in adsorption are either weak Vander Waal's forces or strong chemical bond forces.

In certain cases, both the adsorption and the absorption take place simultaneously and it is not easy to distinguish them. Such substance is said to be sorbed and the phenomenon is known as sorption.

Types of Adsorption

	Physisorption (Physical adsorption)	Chemisorption (Chemical adsorption)
1.	Caused by intermolecular Vander Waal's forces.	Caused by chemical bond formation.
2.	Depends on nature of gas. Easily liquefiable gases are adsorbed readily.	Much more specific and depends upon the nature of the both the adsorbate and adsorbent.
3.	Heat of adsorption is small (about 5 kcal per mol)	Very large (20-100 kcal per mol).
4.	Reversible	Irreversible
5.	Forms multimolecular layers on adsorbent surface.	Forms unimolecular layer.
6.	Occurs at low temperature; decreases with increase in temperature.	Increases with increase of temperature
7.	Increase of pressure increases adsorption	High pressure is favourable. Decrease of pressure does not cause desorption.
8.	Equilibrium is attained readily and it is reversible.	Equilibrium is attained slowly and mostly not reversible.

Enthalpy of adsorption

The adsorption of one substance on the surface of another leads to the existence of new types of forces between them. Therefore, it is an exothermic process and is accompanied by the release of energy. The enthalpy or heat of adsorption is defined as the heat energy evolved when one mole of adsorbate is adsorbed on the surface of adsorbent. Since physical adsorption involves weak forces of attraction between the molecules of the adsorbent and the adsorbate, the heat of physisorption is generally low, of the order of 20-40 kJ mol^{-1}. Chemical adsorption, on the other hand involves strong chemical bond formation and the heat of chemisorptions is quite high, of the order of 80-400 kJ mol^{-1}.

Adsorption of Gases on Solids

The extent of adsorption of a gas on the surface of a solid depends on the following factors:

(a) Nature of gas

(b) Nature of solid

(c) Specific area of solid

(d) Pressure of gas

(e) Temperature

(f) Activation of solid

(a) Nature of gas: Since physical adsorption is non-specific in nature, any gas will be adsorbed on the surface of a solid to some extent or other. However, under any given conditions of temperature and pressure, easily liquefiable gases such as NH_3, CH_4 HCl, Cl_2, SO_2, CO etc. are adsorbed more than permanent gases like H_2, O_2, N_2 etc. Chemisorption is specific in nature. Therefore, only those gases will be adsorbed which form chemical bonds with it.

(b) Nature of solid: Activated charcoal is the most common adsorbent for easily liquefiable gases. Poisonous gases such as CH_4 and CO fall in this group. Therefore, it is used in gas masks. Other gases such as O_2, H_2 and N_2 adsorb more on metals such as Ni, Pt and Pd.

(c) Specific area of solid: Specific area of an adsorbent is the surface area available for adsorption per gm of adsorbent. Greater the specific area of an adsorbent, greater will be the adsorption. The specific area of an adsorbent can be increased by making the surface rough. The pores must be large enough to allow penetrations of gas molecules.

Adsorption of Gases on Solids

(d) Pressure of a gas: As physical adsorption is reversible, it is accompanied by decrease in pressure. Therefore, it is expected that at a given temperature the extent of adsorption will increase with the increase of pressure of the gas. The extent of adsorption is measured as x/m where m is the mass of adsorbent and x that of adsorbate. If the physical adsorption is limited to unimolecular layer, the plot of x/m vs. equilibrium pressure at a constant temperature is as shown.

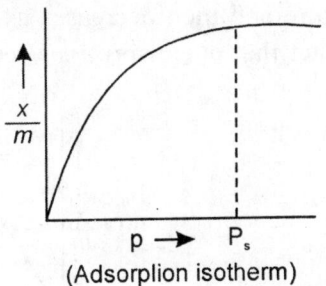

(Adsorplion isotherm)

It is evident from the graph that at a certain pressure the adsorption reaches a maximum value i.e. the adsorption becomes saturated and the corresponding pressure is called saturation pressure (Ps). Beyond this pressure the adsorption remains constant.

At low pressures, x/m varies linearly with p

$\therefore$ $x/m \propto p^1$ or $x/m = kp^1$

At high pressures, x/m is independent of p

$\therefore$ $x/m \propto p^1$ or $x/m = kp^0$

At intermediate pressures, the variation of x/m vs p can be expressed as $x/m \propto p^{(1/n)}$ where

$$n > 1.$$

or $$x/m = k\, p^{(1/n)}$$

or $$\log x/m = \log k + 1/n \log p$$

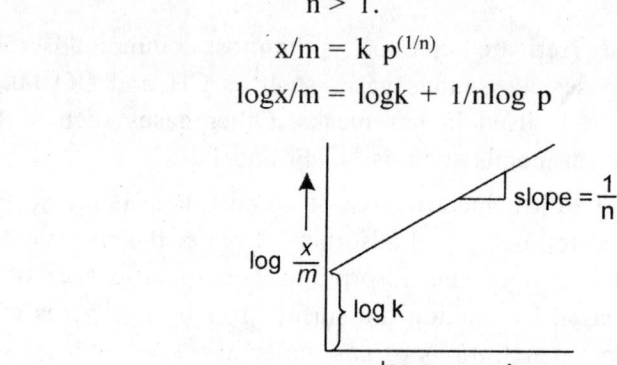

This is called **Freundlich adsorption isotherm.**

Adsorption of Gases on Solids

(e) Temperature: As adsorption is accompanied by release of heat energy, so in accordance with Le-Chatelier's principle, the increase of temperature should decrease the extent of adsorption. This has indeed been found to be so. A plot of x/m vs. temperature at constant pressure is called adsorption isobar. In the case of physical adsorption x/m decreases with increase of temperature. However, in the case of chemisorption x/m initially increases with temperature and then decreases as shown below. The initial increase is due to the fact that chemisorptions require activation energy.

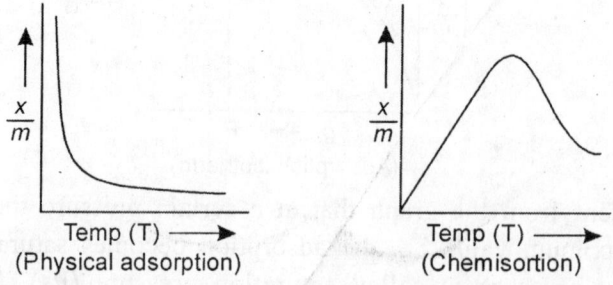

(f) Activation of solid: Activation of adsorbent means increasing its adsorbing power. This is increased by increasing specific area either by making the surface rough or by breaking the solid into smaller particles. But care must be taken so that particles do not become very small, otherwise the inter-particle spaces will be too small to allow penetration of gas molecules.

Competing adsorption

There is always a competition between different adsorbates to adsorb on the adsorbent. A strongly adsorbable substance can easily displace a weakly adsorbed substance. For example, on the surface of activated charcoal, gases such as O_2, N_2 etc. are already adsorbed. But when charcoal comes in contact with poisonous gases such as CH_4, CO which are strongly adsorbable, O_2 and N_2 get displaced. If a mix of gases is allowed to adsorb on a particular adsorbent, the strongly adsorbable adsorbate adsorbs to a greater extent than its partial pressure indicates. For example, moisture though present in small proportion in air is strongly adsorbed by silica gel. Charcoal adsorbs poisonous gases even though they are present in small concentration in air.

Adsorption from Solution

Some solids are capable of adsorbing certain solutes from the solution. This property is made use of in adsorbing colouring matter from solutions of organic substances. Raw cane juice is decolourised by activated charcoal. Similarly, charcoal adsorbs oxalic and acetic acid dyes from their aqueous solutions.

Freundlich adsorption isotherm is also applicable to solutions by replacing the pressure term by the concentration (C) of adsorbates in solutions. The relationship is modified as follows $x/m = kC^{(1/n)}$

Taking logarithm, it becomes

$$\log x/m = \log k + 1/n \log C$$

A graph between log (x/m) and log C is a straight line for small ranges of concentrations.

Applications of Adsorption

Some of the applications of adsorption are as follows:

a. Activates charcoal is used in gas masks to remove poisonous gases such as carbon monoxide, methane etc. Animal charcoal is used to remove colouring matter from sugarcane juice in the manufacture of sugar.

b.   Ion exchange resin is used to remove hardness of water.

c.   Several organic compounds are purified by chromatographic adsorption.

d.   Silica gel is used for removing and controlling humidity.

e.   The catalytic effect of a number of catalysts like spongy iron (in the manufacture of ammonia) and nickel, platinum or palladium (used in the reduction of unsaturated hydrocarbons is based on the principle of adsorption.

f.   Production of high vacuum.

g.   Gas masks-It is a device which consists of activated charcoal. This is used to adsorb poisonous gases.

h.   Humidity control-Silica gel and aluminium gel are used for this purpose.

i.   Removal of colouring matter from solutions-Animal charcoal is used for decolorising cane sugar.

j.   Heterogeneous catalysis

k.   Separation of inert gases by coconut charcoal

l.   Softening of hard water

m.   De-ionising of water

n.   Cleaning agents

o.   Froth floatation process

p.   Adsorption indicators

q.   Chromatographic analysis

r.   In curing many diseases.

Chapter 4

PHASE RULE

➤ **Basic terms**
➤ **Phase rule**
➤ **Phase**
➤ **Component**
➤ **Degree of freedom**
➤ **One component system**
➤ **Two component system**
➤ **Numerical Problems**

DEFINITIONS OF TERMS

1. **Phase:** Phase can be defined as any homogeneous and physical distinct part of a system, which is bounded by a definite surface and is mechanically separable from other parts of the system. Phase has identical thermodynamic properties.

2. **Degree of freedom:** The degree of freedom of a system is defined as the number of independent parameters of state such as temperature, pressure and concentration, which must be specified in order to define the system completely.

3. **Phase transition:** A change in the state of substance is called a phase transition. It occurs at a characteristic temperature for a given pressure. A phase transition proceeds until an equilibrium is attained.

4. **Phase Equilibrium:** Phase equilibrium is an equilibrium in a system in which phase transitions occur in addition to a chemical process.

5. **Component:** Components of a system at equilibrium is defined as the smallest number of independent variable constituents by means of which the composition of any phase of the system can be expressed either directly or indirectly in the form of a chemical equation.

6. **Phase Rule:** Phase rule is a mathematical relation that exists between the number of independent components, the number of phases and the number of degree of freedom of system. For any equilibrium thermodynamic system, the sum of degree of freedom f and number of phases P is equal to the sum of number of independent components C and number of external factors n affecting the physical state of the system

$$F + P = C + 2$$

7. **Triple Point:** Triple point is the point, where all the three phases i.e. solid liquid and vapours coexist in equilibrium.

8. **Transition Temperature:** The transition temperature is the temperature at which one crystalline phase changes into another phase.

9. **Phase boundaries:** The phase diagram' of a substance shows the region of pressure and temperature at which its various phases are thermodynamically stable, the lines separating the regions are called phase boundaries.

10. **Colligative Properties:** Colligative properties of a dilute solution are those properties which depend entirely upon the number of-particles of the solute contained in a known volume of given solvent and not at all upon the nature -of the solute.

Gibbs Phase rule

J.W. Gibbs deduced the phase rule, which is the relationship between the degree of freedom F, the number of components C and number of phases at eqm. P for a system of any composition. It is represented as $F = C - P + 2$

Phase: A part of the system which is homogeneous and separable from other parts of the system by a definite boundary physically and chemically different from other parts of the systems and separable from other parts of the system by mechanical means.

Component: Smallest number of independent variable constituents by which composition of each phase can be expressed either directly or in the form of chemical equation. In expressing the composition of a phase in the form of chemical equation +ve, −ve and zero as coefficients are used,

Example

Water exists in three phases but having one component i.e. water

ice $\rightleftharpoons$ liquid vapour one component system.

Degrees of Freedom (D): Number of independent variables like temperature pressure and conc. which must be specified in order to define the system completely For example state of a pure gas can be expressed by two variable P and T or Press and volume so it has two degrees of freedom

$$F = C - P + 2$$
$$C = \text{Component}$$
$$P = \text{Phases}$$

DERIVATION OF GIBBS PHASE RULE

Consider a system in equilibrium containing P phases and C components. Assume that the passage of a component from one phase to another does not contribute a chemical reaction. The state of each phase of the system is completely specified by the two variables, temperature and pressure and also by composition of each phase. So we have to describe the mole fraction of each component. If C is the number of components required to describe the composition of a phase, then the total number of composition variables for the P phases are PC. Besides, there are two more variables, temperature and pressure, which have to be considered. The total number of independent variables is PC + 2.

However, all the variables are not independent since in each phase, sum of the mole fractions must equal to unity:

$$X_1 + X_2 + X_3 + \ldots\ldots X_C = 1$$
$$\sum X_i = 1$$

Therefore the total numbers of independent variables to be specified are:

$$CP + 2 - P$$
$$P(C - 1) + 2$$

When a heterogeneous system is in equilibrium at a constant temperature and pressure, the chemical potential of a particular component must be the same in all the phases in which it appears. For a one-component system having two phases α and β, the equality of chemical potential implies

$$\mu(\alpha) = \alpha\ (\beta)$$

Similarly, in a one component system having three phases a, p and y, we have,

$$\mu\ (\alpha) = \mu(\beta) = \mu(\gamma)$$

Similarly, for a system containing C number of components and P phases, the requirement that the chemical potential of any component is same in all P phases at equilibrium leads to the equations for the C components in P phases.

$$\mu_1 (\alpha) = \mu_1 (\beta) = \mu_1 (\gamma) = \ldots\ldots\ldots = \mu_1 (P)$$

$$\mu_2 (\alpha) = \mu_2 (\beta) = \mu_2 (\gamma) = \ldots\ldots\ldots = \mu_2 (P)$$

$$\mu_3 (\alpha) = \mu_3 (\beta) = \mu_3 (\gamma) = \ldots\ldots\ldots = \mu_3 (P)$$

$$\ldots\ldots\ldots\ldots\ldots\ldots\ldots\ldots\ldots\ldots\ldots\ldots\ldots\ldots\ldots\ldots\ldots\ldots\ldots$$

$$\mu_C (\alpha) = \mu_c (\beta) = \mu_c (\gamma) = \ldots\ldots\ldots = \mu_c (P)$$

In general, for each component in P phases, $(P - 1)$ relations are possible. Since there are C components, the total number of these equations are $C(P - 1)$.

$$F = \text{total number of variables} -$$
$$\text{total number of relations among the variables}$$
$$= PC + 2 - P - C(P - 1)$$
$$= C - P + 2$$
$$F + P = C + 2$$

Another way of Derivation of the Phase Rule

It is important to recognize that the simple formulation of Gibbs' Phase Rule is derivative from fundamental thermodynamic principles. The Gibbs-Duhem equation establishes the relationship between the intensive parameters temperature (T) and pressure (P) and the chemical potential of all components (μ_i) in the system:

$$dG = Vdp - Sdt + \Sigma N_i d\mu_i$$

This means that there are

- $C + 2$ independent variables that describe the system: P, T and one each for the chemical potential for all components, and
- P independent equations (of the Gibbs-Duhem form) that describe the energetic of the system—one equation for each phase.

  In mathematical terms, the variance (F) is determined by the difference between $(C + 2)$ variables and (P) equations. Thus,

  $F = C + 2 - P$ or as originally written, $P + F = C + 2$

Counting the number of phases

(a) Liquid water, pieces of ice and water vapour are present together.

The number of phases is 3 as each form is a separate phase. Ice in the system is a single phase even if it is present as a number of pieces.

(b) Calcium carbonate undergoes thermal decomposition.

The chemical reaction is: $CaCO_3(s)$ $CaO(s) + CO_2(g)$, Number of phases = 3

This system consists of 2 solid phases, $CaCO_3$ and CaO and one gaseous phase, that of CO_2.

(c) Ammonium chloride undergoes thermal decomposition.

The chemical reaction is: $NH_4Cl(s) = NH_3(g) + HCl (g)$

Number of phases = 2. This system has two phases, one solid, NH_4Cl and one gaseous, a mixture of NH_3 and HCl.

(d) A solution of NaCl in water Number of phases = 1

(e) A system consisting of monoclinic sulphur, rhombic sulphur and liquid sulphur

Number of phases = 3   This system has 2 solid phases and one liquid. Monoclinic and rhombic sulphur, polymorphic forms, constitute separate phases.

Counting the number of components

(a) The sulphur system is a one component system. All the phases, monoclinic, rhombic, liquid and vapour – can be expressed in terms of the single constituent   sulphur.

(b) A mixture of ethanol and water is an example of a two component system. We need both ethanol and water to express its composition.

(c) An example of a system in which a reaction occurs and an equilibrium is established is the thermal decomposition of solid $CaCO_3$. In this system, there are three distinct phases: solid $CaCO_3$, solid CaO and gaseous CO_2. Though there are 3 species present, the number of components is only two, because of the equilibrium:

$$CaCO_3 (s) \quad CaO(s) + CO_2(g)$$

Any two of the three constituents may be chosen as the components. If CaO and CO_2 are chosen, then the composition of the phase $CaCO_3$ is expressed as one mole of component CO_2 plus one mole of component CaO. If, on the other hand, $CaCO_3$ and CO_2 were chosen, then the composition of the phase CaO would be described as one   mole of $CaCO_3$ minus one mole of CO_2.

(d) A system in which ammonium chloride undergoes thermal composition.

$$NH_4Cl(s) \: NH_3(g) + HCl \: (g)$$

There are two phases, one solid-NH4Cl and the other gas – a mixture of NH_3 and HCl. There are three constituents. Since NH_3 and HCl can be prepared in the correct stoichiometric proportions by the reaction:

$$NH_4Cl \rightarrow NH_3 + HCl$$

The composition of both the solid and gaseous phase can be expressed in terms of NH_4Cl. Hence the number of components is one.

If additional HCl (or NH_3) were added to the system, then the decomposition of NH_4Cl would not give the correct composition of the gas phase. A second component, HCl (or NH_3) would be needed to describe the gas phase.

Systems of different variance

The degrees of freedom or variance of a system is defined as the minimum number of variables such as temperature, pressure, concentration, which must be arbitrarily fixed in order to define the system completely.

Examples

(a) A gaseous mixture of CO_2 and N_2. Three variables: pressure, temperature and composition are required to define this system. This is, hence, a trivariant system.

(b) A system having only liquid water has two degrees of freedom or is bivariant. Both temperature and pressure need to be mentioned in order to define the system.

(c) If to the system containing liquid water, pieces of ice are added and this system with 2 phases is allowed to come to equilibrium, then it is an univariant system. Only one variable, either temperature or pressure need to be specified in order to define the system. If the pressure on the system is maintained at 1 atm, then the temperature of the system gets automatically fixed at 0°C, the normal melting point of ice.

SOME SIMPLE ONE-COMPONENT EXAMPLES

Water system

Water exists in three phases but having one component i.e. water

Ice $\rightleftharpoons$ liquid $\rightleftharpoons$ vapour one component system.

Degrees of Freedom (D): Number of independent variables like temperature, pressure and cone. which must be specified in order to define the system completely. For example state of a pure gas can be expressed by two variable P and T or Press and volume so it has two degrees of freedom.

$$F = C - P + 2$$
$$C = Component$$
$$P = Phases.$$

Phase-Equilibrium for water system: This system has three phases and one component. It is represented in Fig. 4.1.

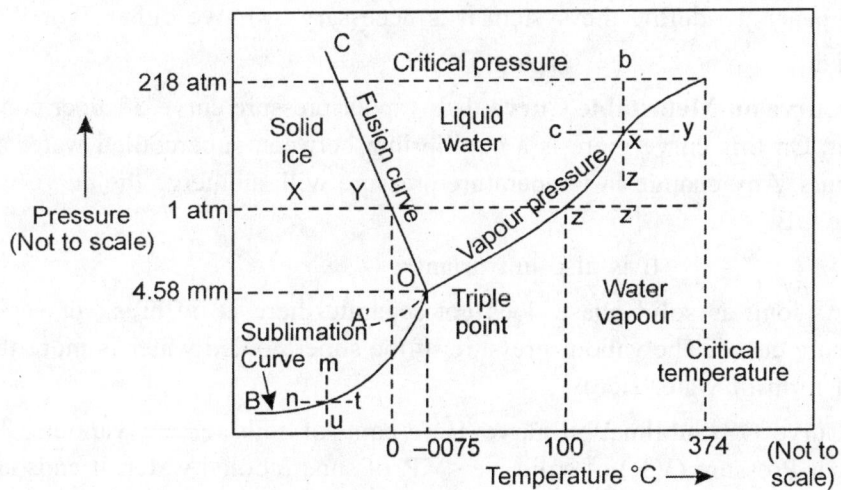

Fig. 4.1

Ice (s) $\rightleftharpoons$ water (I) $\rightleftharpoons$ vapours (g)

The three phases may occur in four combinations

$$Liquid \rightleftharpoons vapour$$
$$solid \rightleftharpoons vapour$$
$$solid \rightleftharpoons liquid$$
$$solid \rightleftharpoons liquid \rightleftharpoons vapour$$

The number of phases which exists at equilibrium can be expressed by certain temperature and pressure conditions. The conditions can be determined experimentally and phase diagram is as shown

It has (i) Three stable curves and one metastable curve (ii) Three areas (iii) Point O (Triple point).

Curves: Curve OA vaporization curve starts from O. On this liquid $\rightleftharpoons$ water vapours lies at different temperature. Point A is called critical point and at this critical temperature is 374°C and critical press is 218 atm.

$$F = C - P + 2$$
$$= 1 - 2 + 2 = 1.$$

So curve is univariant Beyond A two phases merge into each other.

On any point of this curve if we fix pressure value then temperature is automatically fixed. (By keeping P constant if we increase temperature then liquid phase will disappear and if temperature is lowered then vapour phase disappear). To define the system it is necessary to move either T or P

i.e. $F = 1$

Curve on Metastable Curve: It is vapour pressure curve of super cooled water. On this curve there is a equilibrium between supercooled water and vapours. Any change in temperature/pressure will submerge the curve with curve OB.

It is also univariant.

As long as solid phase does not separate there is no break in vapour pressure curve. The vapour pressure of the super cooled water is more than solid form of water (ice).

Curve OS Sublimation curve: Here eqm. of solid $\rightleftharpoons$ vapours. The Vapour Pressure (V.R) of solid ice <V.P, of super cooled water. It ends at B (–273°C). Here also system is univariant. For a particular temperature value of P gets fixed

$$F = C - P + 2$$
$$= 1 - 2 + 2 = 1$$

System is univariant.

Curve OC Fusion Curve: It is eqn. of $\underset{\text{ice}}{(s)} \rightleftharpoons \underset{\text{water}}{(\ell)}$. It starts from O and ends at C (2000atm, –20°C). Beyond this two phases merge into each. The slope of OC indicates that melting point gets lowered by increasing pressure. It is univariant

$$F = C - P + 2$$
$$= 1 - 2 + 2 = 1$$

Areas: Three areas

Area AOB: It is bivariant. It is vapour phase area

$$F = C - P + 2$$
$$= 1 - 1 + 2 = 2$$

Area AOC: It is liquid water area

It is also bivariant

$$F = C - P + 2$$
$$= 1 - 1 + 2 = 2$$

Area BOC: It is solid water (ice) area

$$F = C - P + 2$$
$$= 1 - 1 + 2 = 2$$

It is also bivariant.

Triple point O: At this point three phases are in equilibrium OA, OB, OC meet at this point

$$F = C - P + 2$$
$$= 1 - 3 + 2 = 0$$

It is non variant. If T or P is changed then one of the phases will disappear. It 0 corresponds at 0.0098°C and 4.58 mm pressure.

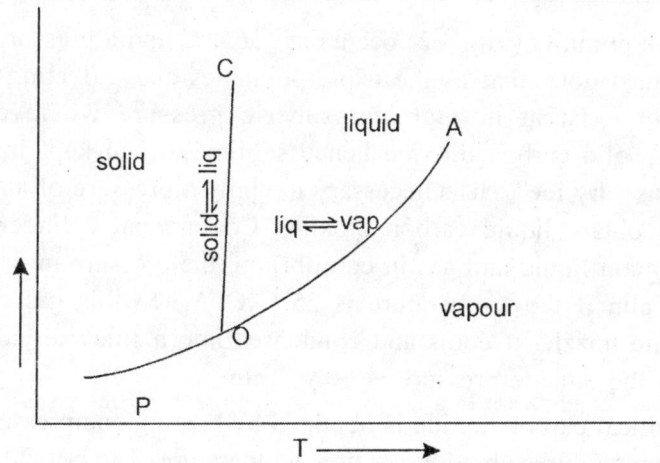

Fig. 4.2: Phase diagram for CO_2 system

The phase diagram for carbondioxide

The system of CO_2 (Fig. 4.2) is very similar to the water system except that the solid – liquid line OC slopes to the right, away from the pressure axis. This indicates that the melting point of solid carbon dioxide rises as the pressure increases. The slope of this line follows the clapeyron equation:

$$\left(\frac{dp}{dT}\right)_{s,l} = \frac{\Delta H_{m,fus}}{T(V_{m,l} - V_{m,s})}$$

(1)	BO	sublimation curve	solid vapour	P = 2, F = 1	T or P
(2)	OA	Vaporization curve	Liquid vapour	P = 2, F = 1	T or P
(3)	OC	Fusion curve	Solid Liquid	P = 2, F = 1	T or P
(4)	Area left of BOC		Solid phase	P = 2, F = 1	T & P
(5)	Area AOC		Liquid phase	P = 2, F = 1	T & P
(6)	Area below		Vapour phase	P = 2, F = 1	T & P
(7)	Point O (−56.4°C, ~5 atm)	Tripal point	Solid Liquid vapour	F = 3 F = 0	
(8)	Point A (31.1°C, 73 atm)	Critical temperature, critical pressure			

The triple point, O (Fig. 4.2) occurs at −56.4°C and a pressure of about 5 atm. We must note, that as the triple point lies above 1 atm, the liquid phase cannot exist at normal atmospheric pressure whatever be the temperature. Solid carbon dioxide hence sublimes when kept in the open (referred to as "dry ice"). It is necessary to apply a pressure of about 5 atm or higher to obtain liquid carbon dioxide. Commercial cylinders of CO_2 generally contain liquid and gas in equilibrium, the pressure in the cylinder is about 67 atm if the temperature is 25°C C. When this gas comes out through a fine nozzle, it cools and condenses into a finely divided snow-like solid as the outside pressure is only 1 atm.

Super critical carbondioxide is obtained by heating compressed carbon-dioxide to temperatures above its critical temperature. The critical constants of CO_2 are: Tc = 304.1K and Pc = 73.8 bar which are not far from ambient conditions. It is inexpensive and easily available in large quantities. It is non toxic, nonflammable and inert to most materials. It has good dissolving properties and hence used as a super critical solvent. It is thus an ideal eco friendly substitute for hazardous and toxic solvents. It is used for extracting flavours, decaffeination of coffee and tea, recrystallization of pharmaceuticals etc. It is also used in supercritical fluid chromatography, a form of chromatography in which the supercritical fluid is used as the mobile phase.

THE SULPHUR SYSTEM

Sulphur can exists in four possible phases

Two solid polymorphic phase ,Rhombic Sulphur (S_R m.p. 114°C), Monoclinic Sulphur (S_M m.p. 120°C), Sulphur Liquid and Sulphur Vapours the rhombic form stable at ordinary temperatures and the monoclinic form at higher temperatures. Substances that can exist in more than one crystalline form, each form having its own characteristics vapour pressure curve, are said to exhibit the phenomenon of polymorphism. Two types of polymorphism are observed, enantiotropy (Greek: opposite change) and monotropy (Greek: one change).

Enantiotropy

Two crystalline modifications of a substance are said to be enantiotropic (or to exhibit enantiotropy) when each has a definite range of stability and conversion from one modification to the other takes place at a definite temperature in either direction. This temperature is the transition point and it is the only temperature at which the two modifications can coexist in equilibrium at a given pressure. A change in this temperature results in the complete transformation of one modification into the other, one being stable above the transition point and the other below it.

We represent, say, the two enantiotropic forms by α and β and we assume that the α form is stable at lower temperatures while the β form at higher temperatures.

Figure 4.3 gives the phase diagram of sulphur. As mentioned earlier, rhombic and monoclinic are the two enantiotropic forms of sulphur, rhombic being stable at lower temperatures. If the temperature of the system, rhombic sulphur in equilibrium with sulphur vapour, represented by the point A is raised at constant volume, the vapour pressure increases along the curve AB. The curve AB, sublimation curve of rhombic sulphur, gives the temperatures and pressures at which rhombic sulphur and its vapour exist in equilibrium.

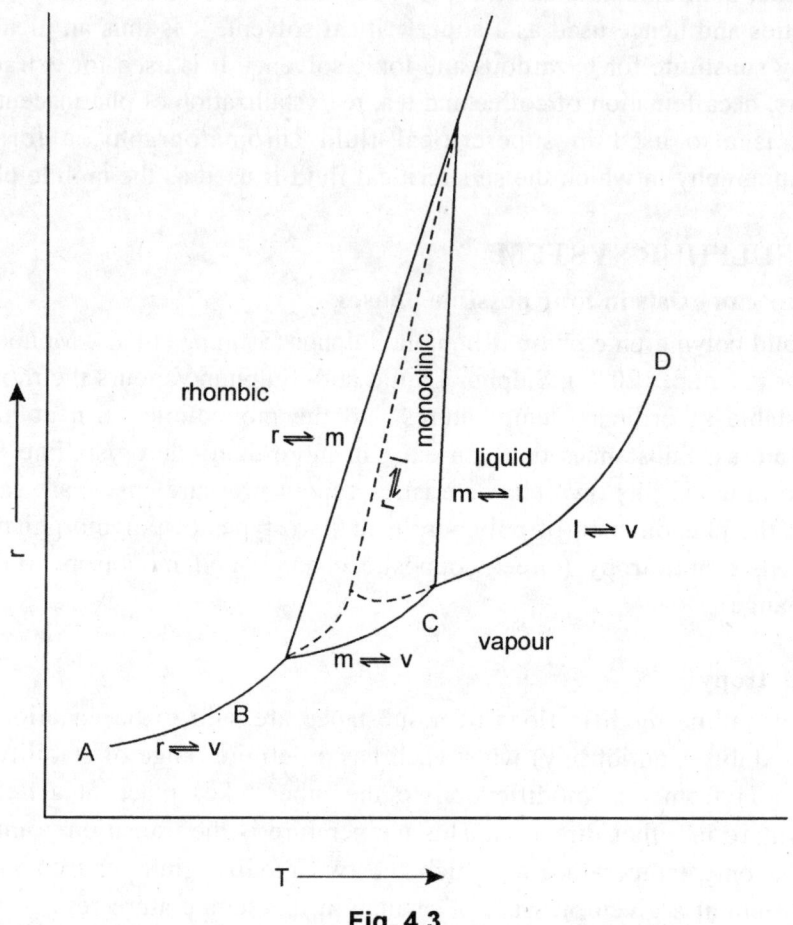

Fig. 4.3

If a system on the curve AB is allowed to expand keeping temperature constant, more of solid sulphur will sublime to keep the vapour pressure at a constant value. If this process in continued, then the solid phase will disappear and the system will be all vapour. If on the other hand the same system is subjected to an isothermal compression, then vapour will condense to keep the vapour pressure at a constant value. On the continuation of the process, vapour phase will disappear and the system will be all solid rhombic sulphur. Hence, we conclude that the phases above and below the curve AB comprise of rhombic sulphur and vapour sulphur respectively. As the heating of the system, rhombic sulphur in equilibrium with vapour, is continued at constant volume, the vapour pressure of rhombic sulphur increases along AB and at the point B becomes equal to that of monoclinic sulphur. Then the rhombic form undergoes transition into the monoclinic form and the system at the point B has three phases, rhombic, monoclinic and vapour. This is an invariant system (P = 3 and F = 0) and the temperature and pressure of the system remain unchanged as long as the three phases coexist. These variables remain constant as the heating at constant volume is continued till the entire rhombic sulphur gets converted into the monoclinic sulphur. The system then has only 2 phases, monoclinic and vapour in equilibrium. with each other. If the heating at constant volume is continued, then the monoclinic in equilibrium with vapour moves along BC, the sublimation curve of monoclinic sulphur. The slope of the curve AB is larger than that of the curve BC at the triple point B as can be seen by applying the Clapeyron equation at the point B.

The vapour pressure of monoclinic sulphur increases as heating at constant volume is continued and becomes equal to that of liquid sulphur at the point C. At C, a triple point, three phases coexist, monoclinic sulphur, liquid sulphur and vapour. As the heating is continued, all the solid melts to give liquid, temperature and pressure remaining constant. The vapour pressure of liquid sulphur in equilibrium with vapour moves along CD with heating and reaches D, the critical temperature. It can be seen that the slope of the curve BC is larger than that of the curve CD at the point C in accordance with the Clapeyron equation. It can also be shown by subjecting a system on the curve CD to isothermal expansion and compression that the phase below CD is vapour and that above CD is liquid sulphur . When a system consisting of rhombic sulphur at some high pressure is gradually heated, a temperature is reached when rhombic gets converted to monoclinic sulphur. This temperature known as the transition point, remains constant till all the rhombic form gets converted to the monoclinic form. The transition temperature depends on the pressure of the system and the transition line BE gives the dependence. The line BE has a positive slope because rhombic sulphur is more dense than monoclinic. Rhombic sulphur exists to the left of the line BE and monoclinic sulphur to the right. As the monoclinic form is heated, a temperature is reached when it starts melting and the system, monoclinic S liquid S, is represented by a point on the line CE. The temperature remains constant till the change of phase is completed. Along the line CE, the equilibrium between monoclinic and liquid sulphur exists whereas only solid exists to the left of the line and only the liquid to the right of the line. The two lines BE and CE meet at E, a triple point where rhombic, monoclinic and liquid sulphur coexist in equilibrium. If the pressure of the system is higher than the triple point pressure, then the rhombic form gets converted directly to the liquid along the line EF.

Metastable equilibria in the sulphur system—Heating a system on the curve AB rapidly may not result in the conversion of rhombic to monoclinic at B and the vapour pressure curve may continue along BG. There exists a metastable equilibrium between rhombic and vapour along BG. Similarly cooling rapidly a system on DC may not result in the formation of solid monoclinic form at C and the system may continue along CG. Liquid and vapour sulphur coexist in a state of metastable equilibrium along CG. The point G where the curves BG and CG meet is a triple point (metastable) where rhombic, liquid and vapour sulphur coexist in equilibrium.

If a system consisting of rhombic sulphur at some high pressure is heated rapidly, then transition to monoclinic form may not occur on the line BE. Rhombic form may continue until the system meets the dotted line GE when it would melt to give liquid sulphur. Along the line GE, rhombic sulphur would exist in a state of metstable equilibrium with liquid sulphur. In the area BGEB, rhombic sulphur exists in a metastable state. Similarly in the area CGEC, liquid sulphur exists in a metastable state. These metastable states are formed only if rhombic form fails to undergo transition to monoclinic form on the line BE and liquid sulphur does not pass over to monoclinic form on the line CE. As the monoclinic form is the stable form in this region BCEB, any other form has a metastable existence and has a tendency to spontaneously change over to the monoclinic form. Table given below describes, in brief, the phase diagram of sulphur.

Brief Description of sulphur system

AB	sublimation curve of rhombic sulphur	r v	$P = 2$	$F = 1$
BC	sublimation curve of monoclinic sulphur	m v	$P = 2$	$F = 1$
CD	vaporization curve of liquid sulphur	l v	$P = 2$	$F = 1$
BE	Transition line of rhombic to monoclinic	r m	$P = 2$	$F = 1$
CE	Fusion line of monoclinic sulphur	m l	$P = 2$	$F = 1$

NUMERICAL PROBLEMS

Q.1. What is the degree of freedom of the following system in equilibrium.

$$NaCl(s) \rightleftharpoons NaCl\ water\ (aq) \rightleftharpoons water\ vap.(g)$$

Ans. In this system,

$$NaCl(s) \rightleftharpoons NaCl\ water\ (aq) \rightleftharpoons water\ vap.(g)$$

Three phases co-exist and it is a one component system.

So, $\qquad\qquad\qquad F = C - P + 2$
$$= 1 - 3 + 2 = 0$$

It is invariant system. When three phases of a component exist at a particular point at a particular temperature and under a particular pressure then that point is called triple point.

Q..2. **A substance Z has triple point at 18°C and 0.5 atm., its normal melting and boiling points are 20°C and 300°C respectively sketch the schematic phase diagram for Z.**

Ans. Schematic phase diagram

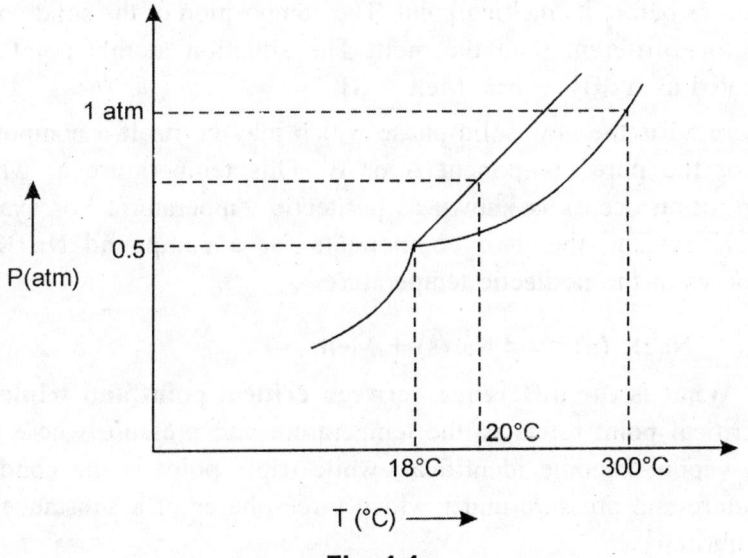

Fig. 4.4

Q.3. **What is critical solution temperature? How does it very for phenol water and trimethyl qruine water system?**

Ans. Critical solution temp (CST). The temp. at which two partially miscible liquids becomes completely miscible in all proportions is called critical solution temperature. In some cases the solubility of two partially miscible liquids increases with increase in temperature and in some case decreases. For phenol water-system, the solubility increases with increase in temperature. It UCST is 68°C

For trimethyl amine water system, the solubility decreases with increase of temperature i.e. LCST for this solution 18.5°C.

Q.4. **What is condensed Phase Rule? When is it applied?**

Ans. Condensed phase rule:

It is used to designate a vapour that is in equilibrium with a nearby condensed phase. It is applied to vapour and liquid water as well as ice because of intramolecular vibration.

Q.5.   Distinguish between Eutectic point and Peritectic point.
Ans. Eutectic point: It represents the lowest temperature at which a liquid phase can exist in the system or it is the maximum temperature upto which a solid phase can exist. Phase temperature at which a binary mixture of definite composition exists in the solid as well as liquid state is called eutectic temperature. For e.g. Pb-Ag system, KI-water system etc.

Peritectic point: A compound is said to have peritectic point if it decomposes before its melting point. The composition of the solid compound is therefore different than the melt. The situation at this point may be represented as Ax By $\rightleftharpoons$ Melt + S1

Here S1 is the new solid phase which may be itself a compound like Ax By or the pure component A or B. This temperature at which the decomposition occurs is known as peritectic temperature. For example in Na — K system, the .two components for a compound Na2K which decomposes at the peritectic temperature.

$$Na2K \text{ (a)} \rightleftharpoons Na \text{ (s) + Melt.}$$

Q.6.   What is the difference between critical point and triple point?
Ans. Critical point refers to the temperature and pressure where a liquid and its vapour become identical; while triple point is the condition of temperature and pressure under which three phases of a substance coexist in equilibrium.

Q.7.   Write short notes on the following:
Liquid-liquid Phase Diagram.

Ans. Liquid-liquid Phase Diagram: There are three types of partially miscible liquid, liquid systems depending upon the effect of temperature. These are

1. System in which partial miscibility increases on increasing the temperature. Forexample, phenol-water, aniline-hexane, aniline-water and methanol-carbondisulphide system. These liquid pairs become completely miscible at and above acertain temperature called upper critical solution temperature (UCST).

2. System in which partial miscibility increases on lowering the temperature. Forexample Diethylamine-water and triethylamine-water system. These liquid pairs become completely miscible at and below

a certain temperature called lower critical solution temperature (LCST).

3. System in which partial miscibility increases on both raising as well as lowering the temperature. For example, nicotine-water and picoline-water system. The liquid pairs show complete miscibility both above and below certain temperature. Example of UCST: Phase diagram for Aniline hexane system

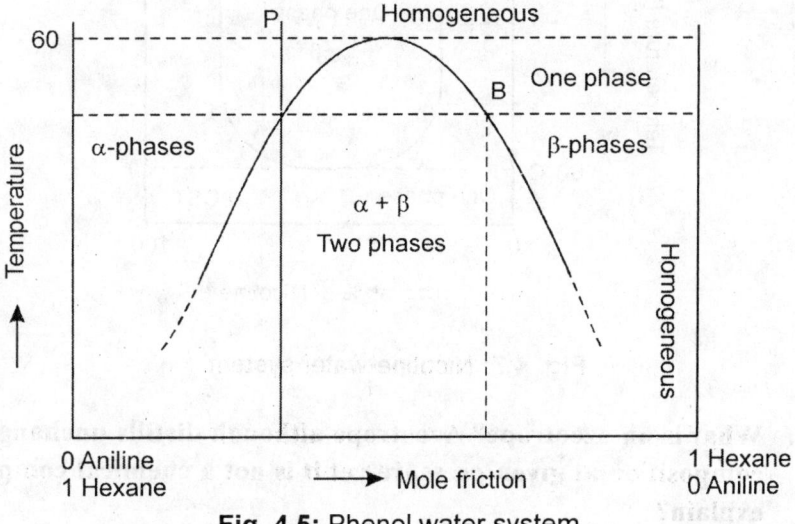

Fig. 4.5: Phenol water system

Example of LCST System:

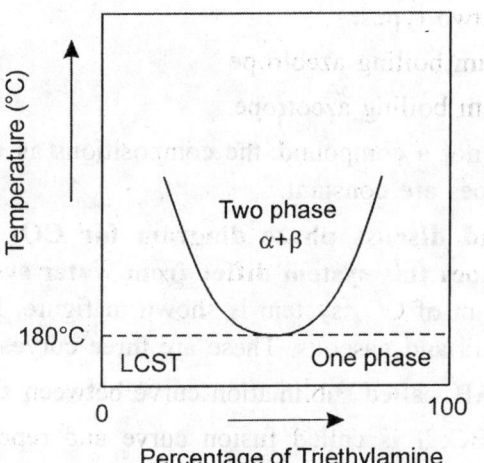

Fig. 4.6: Triethylamine water system

3. System which show both LCST and UCST

Eg: Nicotine-water system

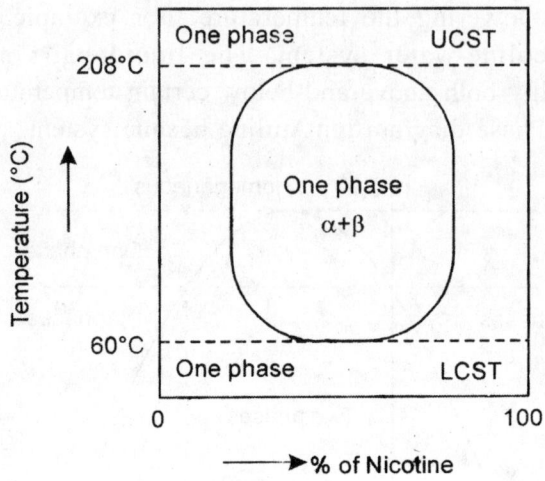

Fig. 4.7: Nicotine-water system

Q.8. **What is an azeotrope? Azeotrope although distills unchanged in composition at given pressure yet it is not a chemical compound explain?**

Ans. Azeotrope: A liquid mixture which behaves like a pure liquid and having constant boiling point. It distills off without any change in composition and in fixed ratio.

These are of two types:

(i) Maximum boiling azeotrope

(ii) Minimum boiling azeotrope.

Azeotrope is not a compound: the compositions as well as the boiling points of azeotropes are constant.

(b) **Draw and discuss phase diagram for CO_2 system. In what respect does this system differ from water system?**

Ans. Phase diagram of CO_2 system is shown in figure. It consists of three phases-solid, liquid and gaseous. These are three curves

(i) Curve AB: called sublimation curve between solid and Gas.

(ii) Curve BC: It is called fusion curve and represents equilibrium between liquid and solid states.

(iii) Curve BD: called vaporization curve which shows an equilibrium between Liquid and Vapour phases.

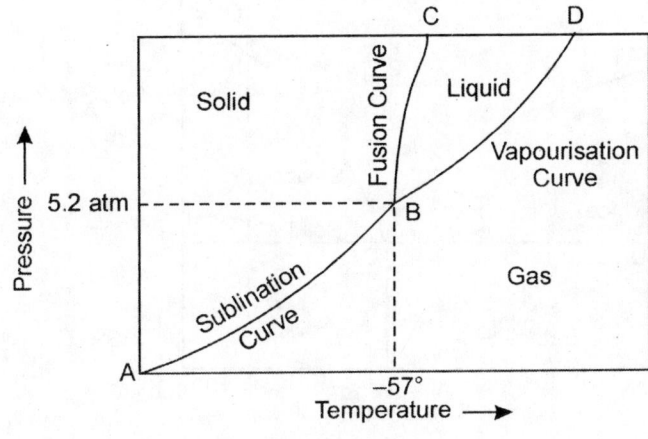

Fig. 4.8

Triple Point B: It is the point where all of three curves meet. The temperature at this point is −57°C and pressure is 5.2 atm. Degrees of freedom at this paint are zero i.e. the system is non variant at this point

Difference from Water System

The main points of difference are:

(a) Fusion curves slopes away from pressure axis.

(b) Vapour pressure of solid-CO_2 at extremely low temperature is very high and many times higher than ice.

(c) Solid CO_2 can exist in equilibrium with liquid CO_2 at very high temperature. While in case of water system, it occurs at very low pressure.

Curves: Curve OA vaporization curve starts from O. On this liquid water $\rightleftharpoons$ vapours lies at diffe

Q.9. Discuss the application of phase rule to potassium iodine water system Explain the formation of freezing mixtures by addition of suitable salts to ice?

Ans. Application of KI water system: KI-water system is a typical binary system involving a salt and water which form a eutectic mixture

The existences of various phases in different regions of equilibrium diagram are shown in Fig. 4.9.

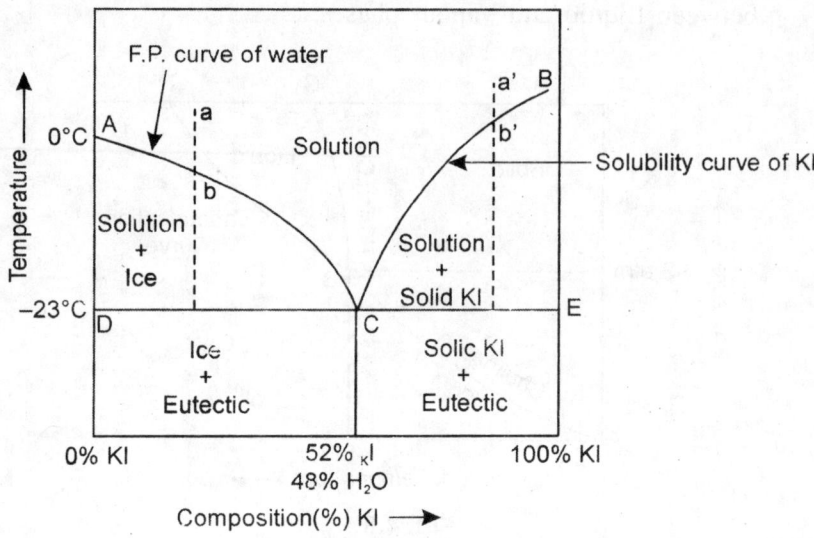

Fig. 4.9

If a solution represented by point a is cooled. The temperature will fall along ab. without any change in composition as the system is bivariant. On reaching b, ice will separate out, The system will now become univariant. Therefore the composition of the solution will change with temperature. Accordingly, on continued cooling the composition of the solution will move along the freezing point. Curve AC until the eutectic point C is reached when KI will separate out. The number of phases now rise to 3 and degrees of freedom at constant pressure falls to zero. Ultimately, the whole of solution will freeze to give the eutectic mixture at a constant temperature. If a solution of composition say a' lying on the right of the eutectic point is cooled, KI will begin to crystallise out as soon as the point b is reached. The composition will change with temperature along b'c and more of KI will continue to separate out until at the eutectic point C, ice also begins to deposit ultimately the whole of the solution will freeze to give the eutectic mixture consisting of 52%, KI and 48% ice at a constant temperature.

Finally, consider a solution of composition represented by C which lies exactly vertically above the eutectic point. When such a solution is cooled, the temperature will continue to fall along cC without any change in composition until the eutectic point C is reached when ice and potassium iodine both begin to separate out simultaneously. It will be seen from the above discussion that all solutions on cooling ultimately show an arrest in temperature at the eutectic point. Also when a solid mixture of same composition as the eutectic mixture is heated, it melts sharply at the eutectic temperature. Hence the mixture of KI and ice deposited at the eutectic point is considered as compound of the form of salt hydrate. This was given name cryohydrate.

However physical properties like density and heat of solution of eutectic solid were almost exactly equal to the mean values of the two constituents namely, KI and ice, indicating that it is a mixture. Both constituents form separate crystals if seen under powerful microscope. So eutectic solid is a mixture not compound. The constant composition and metting point cannot establish that it is a chemical compound.

Formation of freezing mixture on the addition of suitable salts to ice-

If salt is added to ice, it results in the melting of ice and lowering of temperature. The salt goes into water so formed. Mixture of ice and salts are frequently used for getting the low temperatures. Such mixtures are called freezing mixtures: A freezing mixture should have

  (i) low cryohydric point

 (ii) heat of solution of salt should be high

(iii) components should form an intimate mixture

(iv) material used should be economical.

In actual practice freezing mixture is made up of ice and NaCI. Although NaCl is cheap but heat of solution of this salt is very low.

$CaCI_2$ $6H_2O$ and ice forms a good freezing mixture because high heat of solution and low cryohydric point.

Q.10. **Liquid A and B form and ideal solution at 50°C, the vapour pressure of this solution containing 1 mole of A and 4 mole and B is and 420 mm of Hg. After adding X moles of A the vapour pressure of this solution changes to 450 mm of Hg. Find X if the V.R of pure A and B are respectively 600 and 375 mm of Hg.**

Ans. Mole fraction of

$$A (X_A) = \frac{1}{1+4} = \frac{1}{5}$$

$$X_B = \frac{4}{1+4} = \frac{4}{5}$$

$$P = P_A^0 X_A + P_B^0 X_B$$

$$420 = P_A^0 X_A + P_B^0 X_B$$

$$420 = \frac{1}{5} P_A^0 + \frac{4}{5} P_B^0 \qquad \qquad ...(1)$$

When X moles of A are added.

$$X_A = \frac{1+X}{1+X+4} = \frac{1+X}{5+X}$$

$$X_B = 1 - X_A = 1 - \frac{1+X}{5+X}$$

$$= \frac{5+X-1-X}{5+X} = \frac{4}{5+X}$$

Now vapour pressure of solution changes to 450 mm.

$$450 = X_A P_A^0 + X_B P_B^0$$

$$= \frac{1+X}{5+X} P_A^0 + \frac{4}{5+X} P_B^0 \qquad \qquad ... (2)$$

From eqn. no. (1) $420 = \dfrac{1}{5} P_A^0 + \dfrac{4}{5+X} P_B^0$

Multiply overall by 5

$$2100 = P_A^0 + 4P_B^0 \qquad \qquad ... (3)$$

From eqn. no. 2 $450 \times (5 + X) = (1+X)P_A^0 + 4P_B^0$

$$2250 + 450 X = P_A^0 + XP_B^0 + 4P_B^0 \qquad \qquad ... (4)$$

Subtract eqn. no. (3) from eqn. (4) and find X.

Q.11. Write short notes on the following two component systems phenol water and nicotine water.

Ans: Phenol Water System: At ordinary temperature phenol and water are partially miscible into each other i.e. at ordinary temperature on shaking phenol and water, two solutions i.e. phenol in water and water in phenol are formed This type of solution is called conjugate solution With increase in temperature the solubility of one liquid into other increases and at one temperature the conjugate solution changes into homogeneous solution In this case this temperature is 68 1°C (composition is 36 1% phenol and 63 9% water) Above the critical temperature the solution is homogeneous for all the composition If any point above the curve say P is considered as shown in fig it represents homogeneous solution at all the temperature and composition.

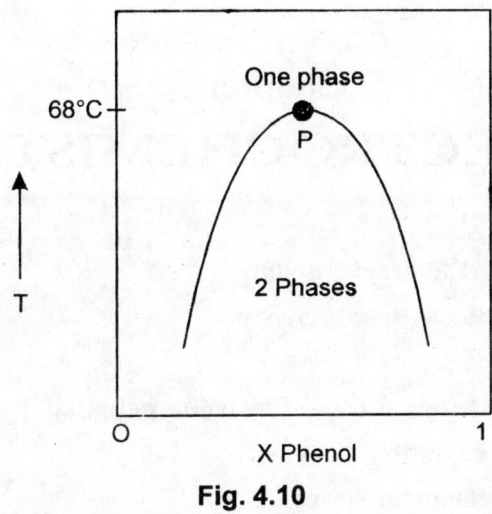

Fig. 4.10

Nicotine Water System

In this system both nicotine and water are partially miscible with each other. The mutual solubility of the two components increases with the increase in temperature as well as with decrease in temp. So this type of system has LCST as well as VCST which is 60.8°C and 208°C.

The phase diagram shows that any point within the closed curve has 2 layers. While any point outside the curve has one layer.

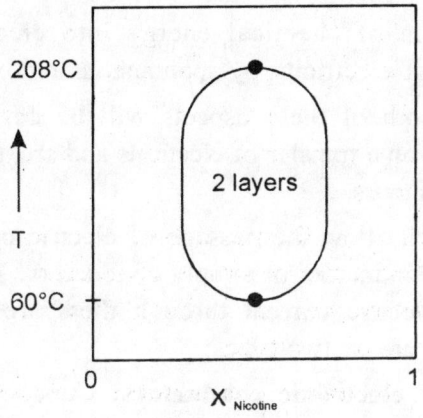

Fig. 4.11

Chapter 5

ELECTROCHEMISTRY

> ➤ **Laws of Electrochemistry**
> ➤ **Conductance, conductivity**
> ➤ **Kohlrausch law**
> ➤ **Electrochemical cell—Electrode potential**
> ➤ **Nernst Equation**
> ➤ **Electrochemical series**
> ➤ **Fuel Cell**
> ➤ **Buffer, Solubility and Solubility Product**
> ➤ **Numerical Problems**

Electrochemistry deals with the interactions of electrical energy with chemical species. It is broadly divided into two categories, namely

(i) Production of chemical change by electrical energy (phenomenon of electrolysis) and

(ii) Conversation of chemical energy into electrical energy, i.e., generation of electricity by spontaneous redox reactions.

In this chapter both of these aspects will be described. All electrochemical reactions involve transfer of electrons and are, therefore, oxidation-reduction (redox) reactions.

Subtractions which allow the passage of electric current through then are called electrical conductors or simply conductors. Those which do not allow the flow of electric current through them are termed insulators. Electrical conductors are of two types:

(i) **Metallic or electronic conductors:** Conductors which transfer electric current by transfer of electrons, without transfer of any matter, are known as metallic or electronic conductors. Metals such as copper, silver, aluminum, etc., non-metals like carbon (graphite - an allotropic form of carbon) and various alloys belong to this class. These materials contain electrons which are relatively free to move. The passage of current though these materials has no observable effect other than a rise in their temperature.

(ii) **Electrolytic conductors:** Conductors like aqueous solutions of acids, bases and salts in which the flow of electric current is accompanied by chemical decomposition are known as electrolytic conductors. The substances whose aqueous solutions allow the passage of electric current and are chemically decomposed, are termed electrolytes.

The substances whose aqueous solutions do not conduct electric current are called non-electrolytes. Solutions of cane sugar, glycerine, alcohol, etc., are examples of non-electrolytes.

In order to pass the current through an electrolytic conductor (aqueous solution or fused electrolyte), two rods or plates (metallic conductors) are always needed which are connected with the terminals of a battery. These rods or plates are known as electrodes. The electrode through which the current enters the electrolytic solution is called the anode (positive electrode) with the electrode through which the current leaves the electrolytic solution is known as cathode (negative electrode). The electrolytic solution conductors electricity not by virtue of the electrolytic as in metallic conductors but as a result of movement of charged particles called ions towards the respective oppositely charged electrodes. The ions which carry positive charge and move towards cathode are termed cations while ions carrying negative charge which move towards anode are called anions. When these ions reach the boundary between a metallic and an electrolytic conductor, electrons are being either attached to or removed from the ions. Removal of electrons is termed oxidation (de-electronation) which occurs at anode while addition of electrons is called reduction (electronation) that takes place at cathode. Hence, flow of electrons through the outer circuit from anode to cathode across the boundary is accompanied by oxidation and reduction.

The process of chemical decomposition of an electrolyte by passage of electric current through its solution is called electrolytes.

or

Chemical change (oxidation and reduction) occurring at electrode s when electric current is passed though electrolytic solution is called elec olysis.

Molecules of an electrolyte when dissolved in water split up in o ions, i.e., into cations and anions. On passing current, these ions move towards oppositely charged electrodes. On reaching the electrodes the ions lose their charge either by accepting electrons or losing electrons and thereby deposited at the respective electrodes or undergo a secondary change. For example, when electric current is passed through a solution of hydrochloric acid, the H^+ ions move towards cathode and Cl^- ions move towards anode.

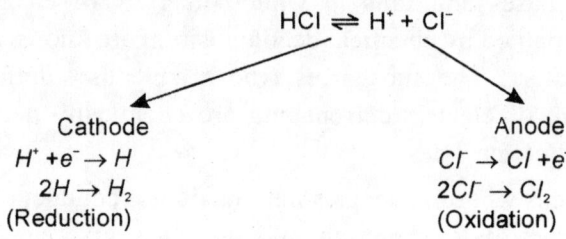

$$HCl \rightleftharpoons H^+ + Cl^-$$

Cathode	Anode
$H^+ + e^- \rightarrow H$	$Cl^- \rightarrow Cl + e^-$
$2H \rightarrow H_2$	$2Cl^- \rightarrow Cl_2$
(Reduction)	(Oxidation)

Fig. 5.1

The decomposition of HCl into H_2 and Cl_2 as a result of passage of current is termed electrolysis of HCl. It is, thus, a process in which electric current brings the chemical change.

The device in which electrolysis (chemical reaction involving oxidation and reduction) is carried out by using electricity or in which conversation of electrical energy into chemical change is done is known as electrolytic cell. An electrolytic cell consists of a vessel for the electrolytic solution or fused electrolyte and two metallic electrodes immersed in the reaction material which are connected to a source of electric current. The metallic electrodes which do not react with ions or final products are called inert electrodes. Inert electrodes are usually used in an electrolytic cell.

FARADAY'S LAWS OF ELECTROLYSIS

The relationship between the quantity of electric charge passed through an electrolyte and the amount of the substance deposited at the electrodes was presented by Faraday in 1834, in the form of laws of electrolysis.

(i) Faraday's First Law

When an electric current is passed through an electrolyte, the amount of substance deposited is proportional to the quantity of electric charge passed through the electrolyte.

If W be the mass of the substance deposited by passing Q coulomb of charge, then according to the law, we have the relation:

$$W \propto Q$$

A coulomb is the quantity of charge when a current of one ampere is passed for one second. Thus, amount of charge in coulombs,

$$Q = \text{current in amperes} \times \text{time in seconds}$$

$$= 1 \times t$$

So $W \propto 1 \times t$

or $W = z \times 1 \times t$

where z is a constant, known as electro-chemical equivalent, and is characteristic of the substance deposited.

When a current of one ampere is passed for one second, i.e., one coulomb (Q = 1), then

$$W = Z$$

Thus, electrochemical equivalent can be defined as the mass of the substance deposited by one coulomb of charge or by one ampere of current passed for one second. For example, when a charge of one coulomb is passed through silver nitrate solution, the amount of silver deposited is 0.001118 g. this is the value of electrochemical equivalent of silver.

Faraday's Second Law

When the same quantity of charge is passed through different electrolytes, then the masses of different substances deposited at the respective electrodes will be in the ratio of their equivalent masses.

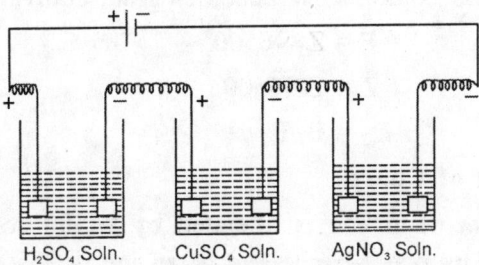

H₂SO₄ Soln.   CuSO₄ Soln.   AgNO₃ Soln.

Fig. 5.2: Voltametres arranged in series

The law can be illustrated by passing same quantity of electric current through three voltametres containing solutions of H_2SO_4, $CuSO_4$ and $AgNO_3$ respectively as shown in Fig. 5.2. In the first voltameter, hydrogen and oxygen will be liberated; in the second, copper will be deposited and in the third, silver will be deposited.

(Mass of hydrogen)/(Mass of copper) = (Equivalent mass of hydrogen)/

(Equivalent mass of copper)

or   (Mass of copper)/(Mass of silver) = (Equivalent mass of copper)/
                                                    (Equivalent mass of silver)

or (Mass of silver)/(Mass of hydrogen) = (Equivalent mass of silver)/
                                                    (Equivalent mass of hydrogen)

It is observed that by passing one coulomb of electric charge.

Hydrogen evolved = 0.00001036 g.

Copper deposited = 0.0003292 g.

and   Silver deposited = 0.001118 g

These masses are in the ratio of their equivalent masses. From these masses, the amount of electric charge required to deposit one equivalent of hydrogen or copper or silver can be calculated.

For hydrogen = 1/0.0001036 = 96500 coulomb ˙

For copper = 31.78/0.0003292 = 96500 coulomb

For silver = 107.88/0.001118 = 96500 coulomb

This follows that 96500 coulomb at electric charge will deposit one g equivalent of any substance. 96500 coulomb us termed as one Faraday and is denoted by F.

Again according to first law,

$$W = Z \times Q$$

Then Q = 96500 coulomb, W becomes gram equivalent mass (E).

Thus, $E = Z \times 96500$

or $Z = E/96500$

$$z_1/z_2 = E_1/E_2$$

Fundamental unit of Charge

As one g-equivalent of an ion is liberated by 96500 coulomb, it follows that charge carried by one g-equivalent of an ion is 96500 coulomb. If the valency of an ion is 'n', then one mole of these ions will carry a charge of nF coulomb. One g-mole of an ion contains 6.02×10^{23} ions.

Then,

The charge carried by an ion = $nF/(6.02 \times 10^{23})$ coulomb

For n = 1,

The fundamental unit of charge = $F/(6.02 \times 10^{23})$

i.e., $96500/(6.02 \times 10^{23}) = 1.6 \times 10^{-19}$ coulomb

or   1 coulomb* = 6.24×10^{18} electrons

The rate of following of electric charge through a conductor is called the electric current.

Coulomb

It is the unit of electric charge. It is the amount of charge that moves past may given point in a circuit when a current of 1 ampere is supplied for one second.

$$1 \text{ coulomb} = 1 \text{ ampere} - \text{second}$$

It is also defined as the amount of charge which is required to deposit by electrolysis 0.001118 g of silver from a solution of silver nitrate.

An electron has 1.6×10^{-19} coulomb of negative charge. Hence, one coulomb of charge is carried by 6.24×10^{18} coulombs. 1 mole of electrons carry a charge of 96500 coulomb. This quantity of charge is called Faraday.

Charge carried by 1 mole of electrons

$$= (6.023 \times 10^{23})(1.6 \times 10^{-19})$$

$$= 96368 \text{ coulomb}$$

$$= 96500 \text{ coulomb}$$

$$\text{Electric current} = (\text{Electric charge})/\text{Time}$$

$$1 \text{ ampere} = (1 \text{ coulomb})/(1 \text{ second})$$

Volt is a unit of electrical potential difference. It is defined as potential energy per unit charge.

$$1 \text{ volt} = (1 \text{ joule})/(1 \text{ coulomb})$$

$$= (1 \text{ newton} \times 1 \text{ metre})/(1 \text{ ampere} \times 1 \text{ second})$$

$$\text{Electrical energy} = \text{Potential difference} \times \text{Quantity of charge}$$

$$= V \times Q$$

$$= V \times 1 \times 1 \qquad (1 = \text{ampere}; 1 = \text{second})$$

$$= \text{Watt-second}$$

CONDUCTANCE, SPECIFIC CONDUCTANCE AND MOLAR CONDUCTANCE

Electrolytic Conductance

The conductance is the property of the conductor (metallic as well as electrolytic) which facilitates the flow of electricity through it. It is equal to the reciprocal of resistance i.e.,

$$\text{Conductance} = 1/\text{Resistance} = 1/R \qquad \text{... (i)}$$

It is expressed on the unit called reciprocal ohm (ohm^{-1} or mho) or siemens.

Specific conductance or conductivity

The resistance of any conductor varies directly as its length (l) and inversely as its cross-sectional area (a), i.e.,

$$R \propto 1/a \text{ or } R = \rho l/a \qquad \ldots \text{(ii)}$$

where ρ is called the specific resistance.

If $l = 1$ cm and $a = 1$ cm^2, then

$$R = \rho \qquad \ldots \text{(iii)}$$

The specific resistance is, thus, defines as the resistance of one centimeter cube of a conductor.

The reciprocal of specific resistance is termed the specific conductance or it is the conductance of one centimeter cube of a conductor.

It is denoted by the symbol . Thus,

$$\kappa = 1/\rho, \ \kappa = \text{kappa} - \text{the specific conductance}$$

$$\ldots \text{(iv)}$$

Specific conductance is also called conductivity.

From Eq. (ii), we have

$$\rho = a/l.R \text{ or } 1/\rho = 1/a.1/R$$

$$K = 1/a \times C \ (1/z = \text{cell constant})$$

or   Specific conductance = Conductance × cell constant

In the case of electrolytic solutions, the specific conductance is defined as the conductance of a solution of definite dilution enclosed in a cell having two electrodes of unit area separated y one centimeter apart as shown in Fig. 5.3.

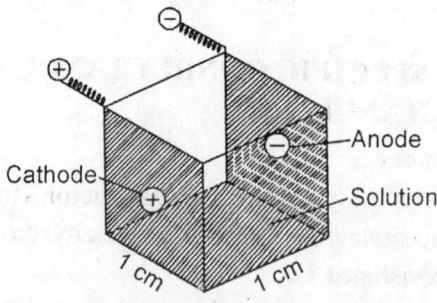

Fig. 5.3 : Representation of specific conductance

The unit of specific conductance is ohm^{-1} cm^{-1}.

Equivalent conductance

One of the factors on which the conductance of an electrolytic solution depends is the concentration of the solution. In order to obtain comparable results for different electrolytes, it is necessary to take equivalent conductance's.

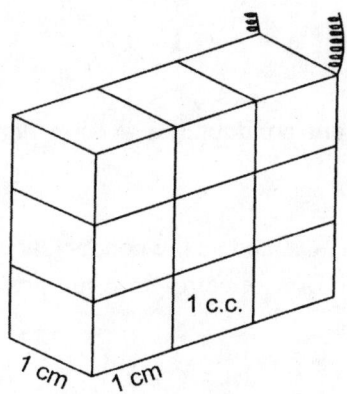

1 c.c.

1 cm   1 cm

Fig. 5.4

¯Equivalent conductance is defined as the conductance of all the ions produced by one gram equivalent of an electrolyte in a given solution. It is denoted by Λ.

To understand the manning of equivalent conductance, imagine a rectangular trough with two opposite sides made of metallic conductor (acting as electrodes) exactly 1 cm apart, If 1 cm^3 (1 mL) solution containing 1 gram equivalent of an electrolyte is places in this container is measured.

According to definitions,

$$\text{Conductance} = \text{Specific conductance (K)}$$

$$= \text{Equivalent conductance } (\Lambda)$$

If the solution is diluted to say (9 cm^3) (9 mL), the conductance of the solution will be the same but specific conductance becomes 1/9th as it contains nine cubes. The conductance is also equal to the equivalent because the solution still has 1 g equivalent of the electrolyte. This is shown in Fig. 5.3. Thus,

Equivalent conductance $(\Lambda) = 9 \times k$

In general,

$$\Lambda = k \times V \qquad \qquad ... \text{(v)}$$

where V is the volume in mL containing 1g equivalent of the electrolyte.

In case, if the concentration of the solution is c g equivalent per litre, then the volume containing 1 g equivalent of the electrolyte will be 1000/e.

So equivalent conductance

$$\Lambda = k \times 1000/c \qquad \qquad ... \text{(vi)}$$

$$\Lambda = k \times 1000/N$$

where N = normality

The unit of equivalent conductance is $ohm^{-1} \, cm^{-2} \, equi^{-1}$.

Molar conductance

The molar conductance is defined as the conductance of all the ions produced by ionization of 1 g mole of an electrolyte when present in V mL of solution. It is denoted by .

Molar conductance $\quad \mu = k \times V \qquad \qquad$ ... (vii)

where V is the volume in mL containing 1 g mole of the electrolyte. If c is the concentration of the solution in g mole per litre, then

$$\mu = k \times 1000/c$$

It units are $ohm^{-1} \, cm^2 \, mol^{-1}$.

Equivalent conductance = (Molar conductance)/n

where $\qquad\qquad\qquad\qquad$ n = (Molecular mass)/(Equivalent mass)

Measurement of conductance

It is now known to us that when the solution of an electrolyte is taken between two parallel electrodes of cross-sectional area 'a' and 'l' cm apart, then the specific conductance, k, should be:

$$k = 1/a.1/R$$

Thus, knowing the values of R, l and a, the specific conductance can be measured. The resistance of the solution between two parallel electrodes is determined by using Wheatstone bridge method. The diagram of the apparatus is shown in Fig. 5.5 AB is a uniform wire and X is a sliding contact which moves over it. C is the conductivity cell containing the solution of the electrolyte and S represents the source of alternating current. R is the resistance box and T is a headphone to detect the flow of current. A suitable resistance is taken out from the resistance box and the sliding contact

X is moves on the wire to search a point of minimum sound in the headphone. At this point, the bridge is balanced.

(Resistance of solution)/(Resistance from resistance box)

$$= \text{(Resistance XB)/(Resistance XA)}$$

$$= \text{(Length XB)/(Length XA)}$$

Thus, resistance of solution can be used because it produces two complications.

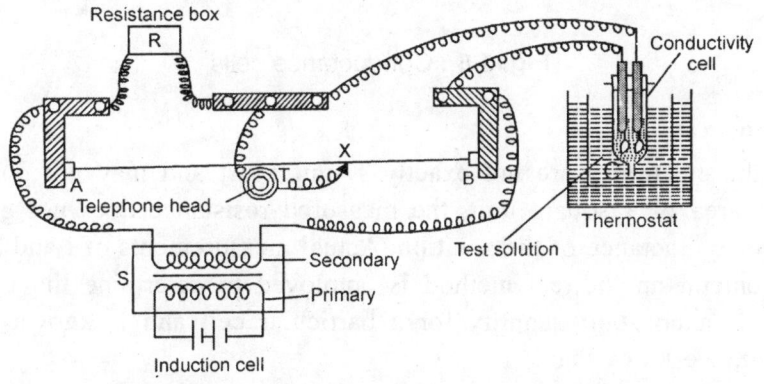

Fig. 5. 5: Determination of conductivity

(i) Change in the concentration of the solution occurs due to electrolysis which will change the resistance.

(ii) Polarisation at the electrodes sets in which also charges the resistance.

Thus, an alternating current (A.C.) is used to overcome the above complications.

The solution whose conductance is to be measured is taken in a special type of cell known as conductivity as conductivity cell. Various types of cells are shown in Fig. 5.6. The electrodes consist of platinum discs coated with finely divided platinum black and welded to platinum wires fused in two glass tubes. The glass tubes contain mercury and are finely fixed in the cover of cells. Contact with the platinum is made by dipping the copper wires of the circuit in the mercury contained in the tubes. As the conductivity changes with temperature, the cell is usually placed in a constant temperature bath during the experiment. Cells with along paths are used for concentrated solution and cells with sort paths and large electrodes are used for dilute solutions.

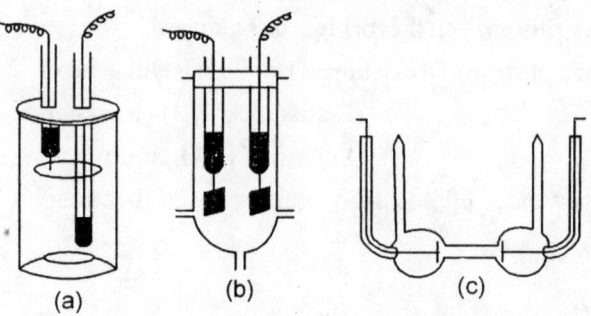

Fig. 5.6 : Conductance cells

Cell constant

Since the electrodes are not exactly 1 unit apart and may not possess a surface area of 1 square unit, the measured resistance does not give the specific conductance of the solution. Actual measurements of l and a being inconvenient, an indirect method is employed to determine the value of which is a constant quantity for a particular cell and is known as cell constant. We know that

(Specific conductance)/Conductance = l/a = cell constant

The resistance of cell, i.e., conductance is measured when filled with a standard solution (say N/10 KCl solution) at a given temperature. The standard values of specific conductance of KCl solutions of various concentrations at different temperature are known. Thus, the cell constant is calculated by using the above equation. The sane cell constant applies to a measurement with any other solution.

The determination of specific conductance of an electrolytic solution, thus, consists of two steps:

(i) Determination of cell constant by using a standard KCl solution of known concentration in the conductivity cell.

(ii) Determination of resistance of he given solution using the same cell. The reciprocal of this gives the value of conductance.

Multiplication of conductance and cell constant gives the value of specific conductance of the solution.

In order to determine equivalent conductance or molar conductance, the concentration of the experimental solution should be known. In conductance measurements, the solutions are always prepared in conductivity water which has no conductance due to dissolved impurities. It is prepared by distilling a number of times the distilled water to which a little $KMnO_4$ and KOH have been added in a hard glass distillation assembly. Such water has very low conductance of the order of 4.3×10^{-8} ohm^{-1}. For ordinary purposes, double distilled water may be used.

Effect of dilution on equivalent conductance

The value of equivalent conductance increases with dilution. This is due to the fact that degree of ionization increases with dilution thereby increasing the total number of ions in solution. Solution which contains large number of ions compared to another solution of the same concentration at the same temperature has more conductance and is said to be stronger electrolyte. The one which has relatively small number of ions is called a weak electrolyte. The number of ions from an electrolyte depends on the degree of dissociation. The curve (Fig. 5.7) shows the variation of the equivalent conductance of some electrolytes with dilution. It shows that electrolytes behave in two ways on dilution.

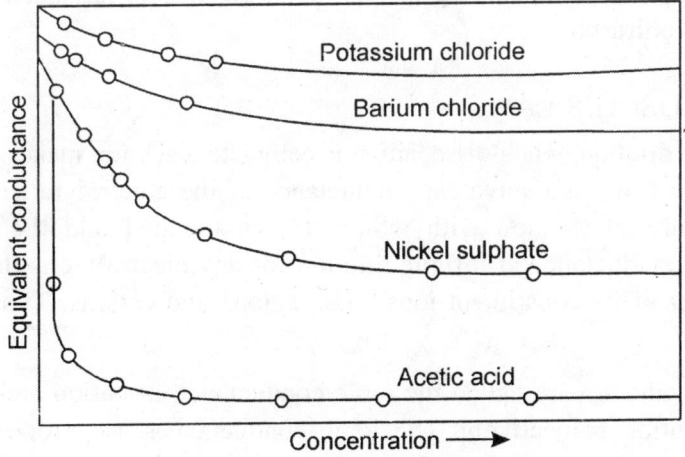

Fig. 5.7 : Conductance curve

(i) Electrolytes like KCl have high value of conductance even at low concentration and there is no rapid increase in their equivalent conductance on dilution. Such electrolytes are termed strong electrolytes. In the case of strong electrolytes, there is a tendency for equivalent conductance to approach a limiting value when the concentration approaches zero. When the whole of the electrolyte has ionized, further addition of the water does not bring any change in the value of equivalent conductance. This stage is called infinite dilution. The equivalent conductance has a limiting value at infinite dilution and is represented by Λ_∞.

(ii) Electrolytes like acetic acid have a low value at high concentration and there is a rapid increase in the value of equivalent conductance with dilution. Such electrolytes are termed weak electrolytes. There is no indication that a limiting value of equivalent conductance can be attained even when the concentration approaches zero. Thus, graphically, Λ_∞ of weak electrolytes cannot be obtained.

It is thus concluded that equivalent conductance of electrolytes whether strong or weak increases with dilution and reaches to a maximum or limiting value which is termed Λ_∞ (equivalent conductance at infinite dilution.) Λ_∞ in the case of strong electrolytes cannot be obtained by extrapolation of the graph of equivalent conductance to zero concentration but in the case of weak electrolytes it cannot be obtained accurately. An indirect method for obtaining Λ_∞ for weak electrolyte has been given by Kohlrusch.

KOHLRAUSCH'S LAW

"At infinite dilution, when dissociation is complete, each ion makes a definite contribution towards equivalent conductance of the electrolyte irrespective of the nature of the ion with which it Is associated and the value of equivalent conductance at infinite dilution for any electrolyte is the sum of contribution of its constituent ions", i.e., anions and cations. Thus,

$$\Lambda_\infty = \lambda_a + \lambda_c$$

The λ_a and λ_c are called the ionic conductance of cation and anion at infinite dilution respectively. The ionic conductances are proportional to their ionic mobilities. Thus, at infinite dilution,

$$\lambda_c = ku_c$$

and $\lambda_a = ku_a$

where u_c and u_a are ionic mobilities of cation and anion respectively at infinite dilution. The value of k is equal to 96500 c, i.e., one Faraday.

Thus, assuming that increase in equivalent conductance with dilution is due to increase in the degree of dissociation of the electrolyte; it is evident that the electrolyte achieves the degree of dissociation as unity when it is completely ionized at infinite dilution. Therefore, at any other dilution, the equivalent conductance is proportional to the degree of dissociation. Thus,

Degree of dissociation

$$\alpha = \Lambda/(\Lambda_\infty)$$

$$= \text{(Equivalent conductance at a given concentration)/}$$

$$\text{(Equivalent conductance at infinite dilution)}$$

Calculation of absolute ionic mobilities

It has been experimentally found that ionic conductance is directly proportional to ionic mobilities.

$$\lambda_+ \propto u_+$$

$$\lambda_- \propto u_-$$

where u_+ and u_- are ionic mobilities of cations and anions.

$$\lambda_+ = Fu_+$$

where $\qquad\qquad F = \text{Faraday}$

$$\lambda_- = Fu_- = 96500 \text{ coulomb}$$

$$\text{Ionic mobility} = \text{(Ionic velocity)/(Potential gradient)}$$

$$= \text{(Ionic velocity (cm/sec))/}$$

$$\text{(Potential gradient (volt)/elctrode seperation)}$$

Relation between equivalent and molar conductance at infinite dilution

$$\Lambda^\infty = \frac{1}{z^+}\lambda_+^\infty + \frac{1}{z^+}\lambda_-^\infty \qquad\qquad \ldots \text{(i)}$$

where $z+$ and $z-$ are cprresponding charges on the ions,

e.g.,

$$\lambda_{BaCl_2}^\infty = \frac{1}{2}\lambda_{Ba^{2+}}^\infty + \frac{1}{1}\lambda_{Cl^-}^\infty \qquad\qquad \ldots \text{(ii)}$$

$$\lambda_{AlCl_3}^\infty = \frac{1}{3}\lambda_{Al^{3+}}^\infty + \frac{1}{1}\lambda_{Cl^-}^\infty \qquad\qquad \ldots \text{(iii)}$$

$$\lambda_{Al_2(SO_4)_s}^\infty = \frac{1}{3}\lambda_{Al^{3+}}^\infty + \frac{1}{2}\lambda_{SO_4^{2-}}^\infty \qquad\qquad \ldots \text{(iv)}$$

Molar conductance at infinite dilution

$$\wedge_m^\infty \text{ or } \mu^\infty = \text{Molar conductance at infinite dilution}$$

$$= m\lambda_+^\infty + n\lambda_-^\infty$$

Where m and n are number of ions formed.

$$\mu^{\infty}_{Al_2(SO_4)_s} = 2\lambda^{\infty}_{Al^3} + 3\lambda^{\infty}_{SO_4^{2-}} = 6 \wedge^{\infty}_{Al_2} (SO_4)_s$$

$$\lambda_{BaCl} = \lambda^{\infty}_{Ba^2} + 2\lambda^{\infty}_{Cl^-} = 2 \wedge^{\infty}_{BaCl}$$

Example: 1.0 N solution of a salt surrounding two platinum electrodes 2.1 cm apart and 4.2 sq.cm in area was found to offer a resistance of 50 ohm. Calculate the equivalent conductivity of the solution.

Solution: Given,   l = 2.1 cm, a = 4.2 sq xm, R = 5–ohm

Specific conductance, k = l/a.1/R

or   k = 2.1/4.2×1/50 = 0.01 ohm^{-1} cm^{-1}

Equivalent conductivity = k = V

                                V = the volume containing 1g equivalent

                                   = 1000 mL

So,

Equivalent conductivity = 0.01 × 1000

                                    = 10 ohm^{-1} cm^{-2} equiv^{-1}

Example: Specific conductance of a decinormal solution of KCl is 0.0112 ohm^{-1} cm^{-1}. The resistance of a cell containing the solution was found to be 56. What is the cell constant?

Solution: We know that

                Sp. conductance = Cell constant × conductance

or   Cell constant = (Sp.conductance)/Conductance

                                  = Sp. conductance × Resistance

                                  = 0.0112 × 56

                                  = 0.06272 cm^{-1}

Example: The specific conductivity of 0.02 M KCl solution at 25°C is 2.768 × 10^{-3} ohm^{-1} cm^{-1}. The resistance of this solution at 25°C when measured with a particular cell was 250.2 ohms. The resistance of 0.01 M CuSO$_4$ solution at 25°C measured with the same cell was 8331 ohms. Calculate the molar conductivity of the copper sulphate solution.

Solution: Cell constant = (Sp.cond.of KCl)/(Conductane of KCl)

                          = (2.768 × 10^{-3})/(I/250.2)

                          = 2.768 × 10^{-3} × 250.2

For 0.01 M CuSO$_4$ solution

Sp. conductivity = Cell constant × conductance

$$= 2.768 \times 10^{-3} \times 250.2 \times 1/8331$$

Molar conductance = Sp. cond. × 1000/c

$$= (2.768 \times 10^{-3} \times 25.2)/8331 \times 1000/(1/100)$$

Example: Specific conductance of a decinormal solution of KCl is 0.0112 ohm^{-1} cm^{-1}. The resistance of a cell containing the solution was found to be 56. What is the cell constant?

Solution: We know that

Sp. conductance = Cell constant × conductance

or　　　　Cell constant = (Sp.conductance)/Conductance

$$= Sp. \ conductance \times Resistance$$

$$= 0.0112 \times 56$$

$$= 0.06272 \ cm^{-1}$$

ELECTRO CHEMICAL CELL

Electrochemical cell is a system or arrangement in which two electrodes are fitted in the same electrolyte or in two different electrolytes which are joined by a salt bridge. Electrochemical cells are of two types:

(a) Electrolytic cell

(b) Galvanic or voltaic cell

Electrolytic cell

It is a device in which electrolysis (chemical reaction involving oxidation and reduction) is carried out by using electricity or in which conversion of electrical energy into chemical energy is done.

Galvanic or voltaic cell

It is a device in which a redox reaction is used to convert chemical energy into electrical energy, i.e., electricity can be obtained with the help of oxidation and reduction reaction. The chemical reaction responsible for production of electricity takes place in two separate compartments. Each compartment consists of a suitable electrolyte solution and a metallic conductor. The metallic conductor acts as an electrode. The compartments containing the electrode and the solution of the electrolyte are called half-cells. When the two compartments are connected by a salt bridge and electrodes are joined by a wire through galvanometer the electricity begins to flow. This is the simple form of voltaic cell.

DANIELL CELL

It is designed to make use of the spontaneous redox reaction between zinc and cupric ions to produce an electric current. It consists of two half-cells. The half-cells on the left contains a zinc metal electrode dipped in $ZnSO_4$ solution.

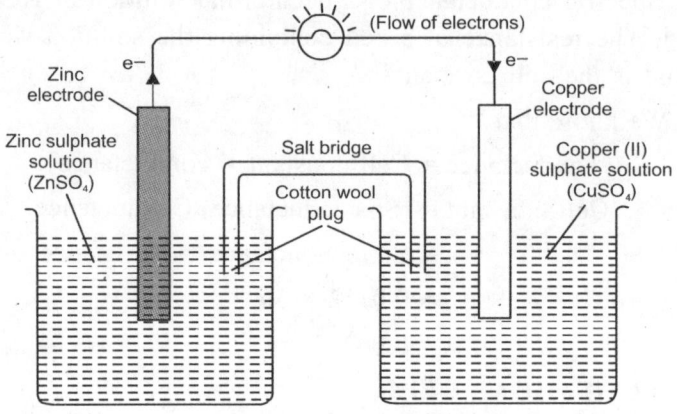

Fig. 5.8: Daniell cell

The half-cell on the right consists of copper metal electrode in a solution $CuSO_4$. The half-cells are joined by a salt bridge that prevents the mechanical mixing of the solution.

When the zinc and copper electrodes are joined by wire, the following observations are made:

(i) There is a flow of electric current through the external circuit.

(ii) The zinc rod loses its mass while the copper rod gains in mass.

(iii) The concentration of ZnSO4 solution increases while the concentration of copper sulphate solution decreases.

(iv) The solutions in both the compartments remain electrically neutral.

During the passage if electric current through external circuit, electrons flow from the zinc electrode to the copper electrode. At the zinc electrode, the zinc metal is oxidized to zinc ions which go into the solution. The electrons released at the electrode travel through the external circuit to the copper electrode where they are used in the reduction of Cu^{2+} ions to metallic copper which is deposited on the electrode. Thus, the overall redox reaction is:

$$Zn(s) + Cu^{2+} \quad Cu(s) + Zn^{2+}(aq)$$

Thus, indirect redox reaction leads to the production of electrical energy.

At the zinc rod, oxidation occurs. It is the anode of the cell and is negatively charged while at copper electrode, reduction takes, place; it is the cathode of the cell and is positively charged.

Thus, the above points van be summed up as:

(i) Voltaic or Galvanic cell consists of two half-cells. The reactions occurring in half-cells are called half-cell reactions. The half-cell in which oxidation taking place in it is called oxidation half-cell and the reaction taking place in it is called oxidation half-cell reaction. Similarly, the half-cell occurs is called reduction half-cell and the reaction taking place in it is called reduction half-cell reaction.

(ii) The **electrode where oxidation occurs is called anode** and the **electrode where reduction occurs is termed cathode.**

(iii) Electrons flow from anode to cathode in the external circuit

(iv) Chemical energy is converted into electrical energy.

(v) The net reaction is the sum of two half-cell reactions. The reaction is Daniel cell can be represented as

Oxidation half reaction, $Zn(s) \rightarrow Zn^{2+}(aq) + 2e^-$

Reduction half reaction, $Cu^{2+}(aq) + 2e^- \rightarrow Cu(s)$

Net reaction $\qquad Zn(s) + Cu^{2+}(aq) \rightarrow Zn^{2+}(aq) + Cu(s)$

Electrode Signs

The signs of the anode and cathode in the voltaic or galvanic cells are opposite to those in the electrolytic cells in the Fig. 5.9.

Electrolytic Cell	**Voltaic Or Galvanic Cell**
(e.m.f. is applied to cell)	(e.m.f. is generated by cell)

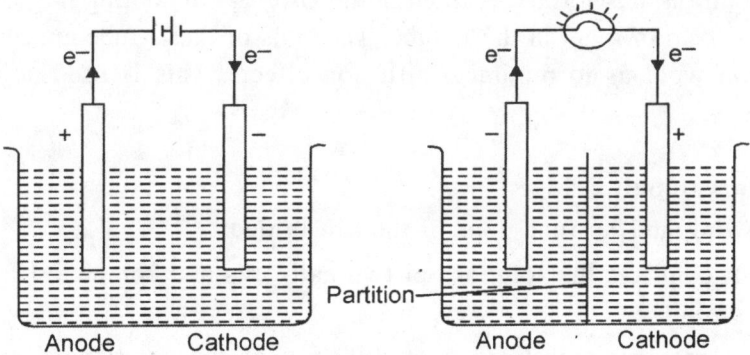

Fig. 5. 9.

Table 5. 1

	Electrolytic cell		Voltaic or Galvanic cell	
	Anode	Cathode	Anode	Cathode
Sign	+	−	−	+
Electron flow	Out	in	Out	in
Half-reaction	Oxidation	reduction	Oxidation reduction	

Table 5.2: Difference in electrolytic cell and galvanic cell

Electrolytic cell	Galvanic cell
1. Electrical energy is converted into chemical energy.	Chemical energy is converted into electrical energy.
2. Anode positive electrode. Cathode negative electrode.	Anode negative electrode. Cathode positive electrode.
3. Ions are discharged on both the electrodes.	Ions are discharged only on the cathode.
4. If the electrodes are inert, concentration of the electrolyte decreases when the electric current is circulated.	Concentration of the anodic half-cell increases while that of cathodic half-cell decreases when the two electrodes are joined by a wire.
5. Both the electrodes can be fitted in the same compartment.	The electrodes are fitted in different compartments.

SALT BRIDGE AND ITS SIGNIFICANCE

Salt bridge is usually an inverted U-tube filled with con-centrated solution of inert electrolytes. An inert electrolyte is one whose ions are neither involved in any electrochemical change nor do they react chemically with the electrolytes in the two half-cells. Generally salts like KCl, KNO_3, NH_4NO_3, etc., are used. For the preparation of salt bridge, gelatin or agar-agar is dissolved in a hot concentrated aqueous solution of an inert electrolyte and the solution thus formed is filled in the U-tube. On cooling the solution sets in the form of a gel in the U-tube. The ends of the U-tube are plugged with cotton wool as to minimize diffusion effects. This is used as a salt bridge.

Significance of Salt Bridge
The following are the func-tions of the salt bridge:

(i) It connects the solutions of two half-cells and completes the cell circuit.

(ii) It prevents transference or diffusion of the solutions from one half-cell to the other.

(iii) It keeps the solutions in two half-cells electrically neutral. In anodic half cell, positive ions pass into the solution and there shall be accumulation of extra positive charge in the solution around the anode which will prevent the flow of electrons from anode. This does not happen because negative ions are provided by salt bridge. Similarly, in cathodic half-cell negative ions will accumulate around cathode due to deposition of positive ions by reduction. To neutralize these negative ions, sufficient number of positive ions is provided by salt bridge. Thus, salt bridge maintains electrical neutrality.

(iv) It prevents liquid-liquid junction-potential, i.e., the potential difference which arises between two solutions when in contact with each other.

A broken vertical line or two parallel vertical lines in a cell reaction indicates the salt bridge.

$$Zn|Zn^{2+}||Cu^{2+}|Cu$$

Salt bridge can be replaced by a porous partition which allows the migration of ions without allowing the solutions to intermix.

REPRESENTATION OF AN ELECTRO-CHEMICAL CELL (GALVANIC CELL)

The following universally accepted conventions are followed in representing an electrochemical cell:

(i) The anode (negative electrode) is written on the left hand side and cathode (positive electrode) on the right hand side.

(ii) A vertical line or semicolon (;) indicates a contact between two phases. The anode of the cell is represented by writing metal first and then the metal ion present in the electrolytic solution. Both are separated by a vertical line or a semicolon. For example,

$$Zn|Zn^{2+} \quad or \quad Zn;Zn^{2+}$$

The molar concentration or activity of the solution is written in brackets after the formula of the ion. For example:

$$Zn|Zn^{2+}(1\ M) \quad or \quad Zn \mid Zn^{2+}(0.1\ M)$$

(iii) The cathode of the cell is represented by writing the cation of the electrolyte first and then metal. Both are separated by a vertical line or semicolon. For example,

$$Cu^{2+}|Cu \quad or \quad Cu^{2+};Cu \quad or \quad Cu^{2+}(1\ M)|Cu$$

(iv) The salt bridge which separates the two half-cells is indicated by two parallel vertical lines.

(v) Sometimes negative and positive signs are also put on the electrodes.

The Daniell cell can be represented as:

$$Zn|ZnSO_4(aq)||CuSO_4(aq)|C^+u$$

Anode   Salt bridge   Cathode

Oxidation half-cell   Reduction half-cell

or $Zn|Zn^{2+}||Cu^{2+}|Cu$

or $Zn|Zn^{2+}(1\ M)||Cu^{2+}(1\ M)|Cu$

ELECTRODE POTENTIAL

When a metal is placed in a solution of its ions, the metal acquires either a positive or negative charge with respect to the solution. On account of this, a definite potential difference is developed between the metal and the solution. This potential difference is called electrode potential. For example,

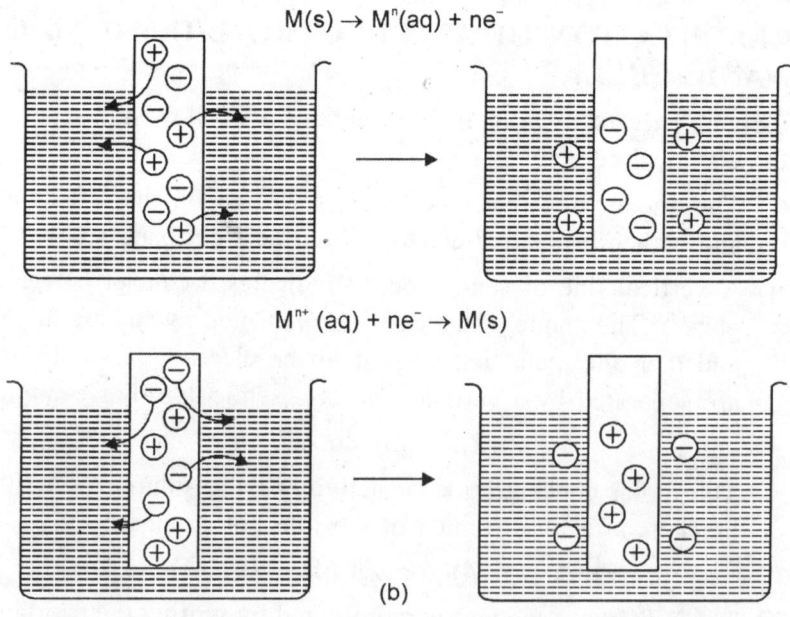

Fig. 5.10

when a plate of zinc is placed in a solution having Zn^{2+} ions, it becomes negatively charged with respect to solution and thus a potential difference is set up between zinc plate and the solution. This potential difference is termed the electrode potential of zinc. Similarly, when copper is placed in a solution having Cu^{2+} ions, it becomes positively charged with respect to solution. A potential difference is set up between the copper plate and the solution. The potential difference thus developed is termed as electrode potential of copper. The potential difference is estab-lished due to the formation of electrical double layer at the

$$M(s) \rightarrow M^n + ne^-$$

(a) **Oxidation:** Metal ions pass from the electrode into solution leaving an excess of electrons and thus a negative charge on the electrode.

(b) **Reduction:** Metal ions in solution gain electrons from the electrode leaving a positive charge on the electrode. Interface of metal and the solution. The development of negative charge (as on zinc plate) or positive charge (as on copper plate) can be explained in the following manner. When a metal rod is dipped in its salt solution, two changes occur:

   (i) The conversion of metal atoms into metal ions by the attractive force of polar water molecules.

$$M \rightarrow M^n + ne^-$$

   The metal ions go into the solution and the electrons remain on the metal making it negatively charged. The tendency of the metal to change into ions is known as electrolytic solution pressure.

   (ii) Metal ions start depositing on the metal surface leading to a positive charge on the metal.

$$M^{n+} + ne^- \rightarrow M$$

   This tendency of the ions is termed **osmotic pressure.**

   In the beginning, both these changes occur with different speeds but soon an equilibrium is established.

$$M \leftrightarrow M^{n+} + ne^-$$

In practice, one effect is greater than the other, if first effect is greater than the second, the metal acquires a negative charge with respect to solution and if the second is greater than the first, it acquires positive charge with respect to solution, thus in both the cases a potential difference is set up.

The magnitude of the electrode potential of a metal is a measure of its relative tendency to lose or gain electrons, i.e., it is a measure of the relative tendency to undergo oxidation (loss of electrons) or reduction (gain of electrons). The mag-nitude of potential depends on the following factors:

   (i) Nature of the electrode,

  (ii) Concentration of the ions in solution,

 (iii) Temperature.

Depending on the nature of the metal electrode to lose or gain electrons, the electrode potential may be of two types:

   (i) Oxidation potential: When electrode is negatively charged with respect to solution, i.e., it acts as anode. Oxidation occurs.

$$M \rightarrow M^{n+} + ne^-$$

  (ii) Reduction potential: When electrode is positively charged with respect to solution, i.e., it acts as cathode. Reduction occurs.

$$M^{n+} + ne^- \rightarrow M$$

It is not possible to measure the absolute value of the single electrode potential directly. Only the difference in potential between two electrodes can be measured experimentally. It is, therefore, necessary to couple the electrode with another electrode whose potential is known. This electrode is termed as **reference electrode**. The emf of the resulting cell is measured experimentally. The emf of the cell is equal to the sum of potentials on the two electrodes.

$$\text{Emf of the cell} = E_{Anode} + E_{Cathode}$$
$$= \text{Oxidation potential of anode}$$
$$+ \text{Reduction potential of cathode}$$

Knowing the value of reference electrode, the value of other electrode can be determined.

STANDARD ELECTRODE POTENTIAL

In order to compare the electrode potentials of various electrodes, it is necessary to specify the concentration of the ions present in solution in which the electrode is dipped and the temperature of the half-cell. The potential difference developed between metal electrode and the solution of its ions of unit molarity (1M) at 25°C (298 K) is called **standard electrode potential.**

According to the IUPAC convention, the reduction potential alone be called as the electrode potential ($E°$), i.e., the given value of electrode potential be regarded as reduction potential unless it is specifically mentioned that it is oxidation potential. Standard reduction potential of an electrode means that reduc-tion reaction is taking place at the electrode. If the reaction is reversed and written as oxidation reaction, the numerical value of electrode potential will remain same but the sign of standard potential will have to be reversed. Thus

Standard reduction potential = – (Standard oxidation potential)

or Standard oxidation potential = – (Standard reduction potential)

REFERENCE ELECTRODE
(STANDARD HYDROGEN ELECTRODE, SHE OR NHE)

Hydrogen electrode is the primary standard electrode. It con-sists of a small platinum strip coated with platinum black as to adsorb hydrogen gas. A platinum wire is welded to the platinum strip and sealed in a glass tube as to make contact with the outer circuit through mercury. The platinum strip and glass tube is surrounded by an outer glass tube which has an inlet for hydrogen gas at the top and a number of holes at the base for the escape of excess of hydrogen gas. The platinum strip is placed in an acid solution which has H^+ ion concentration 1 M. Pure hydrogen gas is circulated at one atmospheric pressure. A part of the gas is adsorbed and the rest escapes through holes. This gives an equilibrium between the adsorbed hydrogen and hydrogen ions in the solution.

$$H_2 \leftrightarrow 2H^+ + 2e^-$$

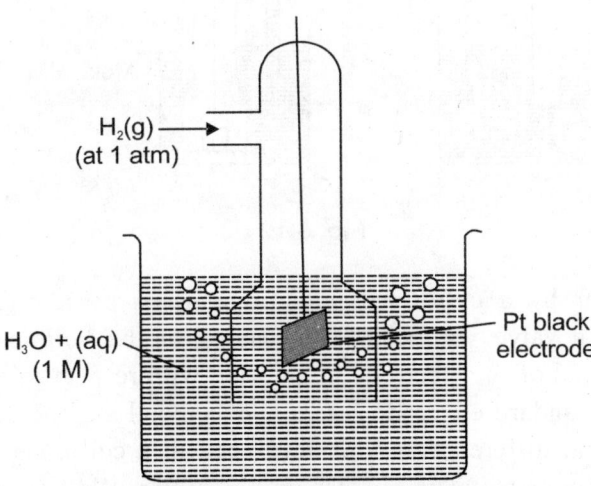

Fig. 5.11: Hydrogen electrode

The temperature of the cell is maintained at 25°C. By international agreement the standard hydrogen electrode is arbitrarily assigned a potential of exactly ± 0.000. .. volt.

The hydrogen electrode thus obtained forms one of two half-cells of a voltaic cell. When this half-cell is connected with any other half-cell, a voltaic cell is constituted. The hydrogen electrode can act as cathode or anode with respect to other electrode.

SHE half reaction	Electrode potential
$H_2 \rightarrow 2H^+ + 2e^-$	0.0 V (Anode)
$2H^+ + 2e^- \rightarrow H_2$	0.0 V (Cathode)

MEASUREMENT OF ELECTRODE POTENTIAL

The measurement of electrode potential of a given electrode is made by constituting a voltaic cell, i.e., by connecting it with a standard hydrogen electrode (SHE) through a salt bridge. 1 M solution is used in hydrogen half-cell and the temperature is maintained at 25°C. The emf of the cell is

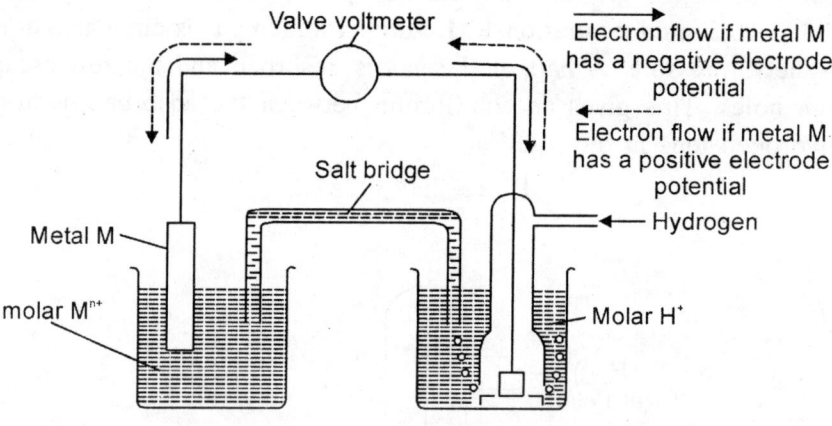

Fig. 5.12

measured either by a calibrated potentiometer or by a high resistance voltmeter, i.e., a valve voltmeter. The reading of the voltmeter gives the electrode potential of the electrode in question with respect to the hydrogen electrode. The standard electrode potential of a metal may be determined as it is the potential difference in volt developed in a cell consisting of two electrodes: the pure metal is contact with a molar solution of one of its ions and the standard hydrogen electrode.

Determination of standard electrode potential of Zn/Zn²⁺ electrode

A zinc rod is dipped in 1 M zinc sulphate solution. This half-cell is combined with a standard hydrogen electrode through a salt bridge. Both the electrodes are con-nected with a voltmeter as shown in Fig. 5.13. The deflection of the voltmeter indicates that current is flowing from hydrogen electrode to metal electrode or the electrons are moving from zinc rod to hydrogen electrode. The zinc electrode acts as an anode and the hydrogen electrode as cathode and the cell can be represented as

$$Zn \mathbb{Z}n^{2+} (aq)/Anode(-) \parallel 2H(aq)| H_2(g)/Cathode (+)$$

$$Zn \rightarrow Zn^{2+} + 2e^-; 2H^+ + 2e^- \rightarrow H_2\uparrow$$

(Oxidation)   (Reduction)

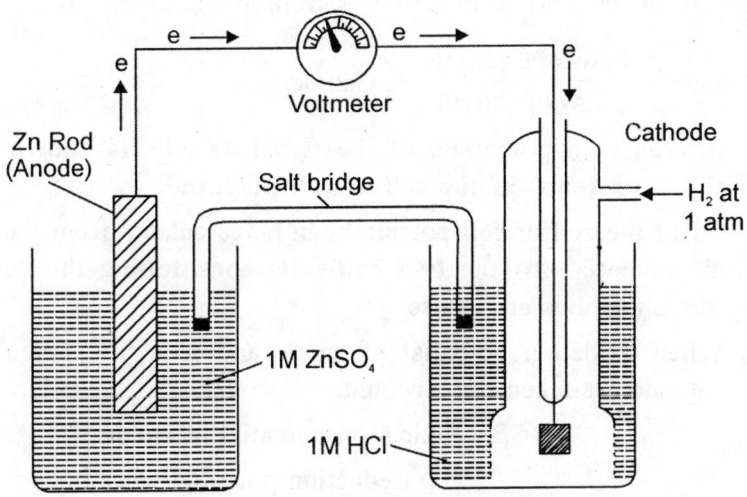

Fig. 5.13: Zn–H₂ electro-chemical cell

The emf of the cell is 0.76 volt

$$E_{Cell} = E^0_{Anode} + E^0_{Cathode}$$

$$0.76 = E^0_{Anode} + 0 \text{ or } E^0_{Anode} = +0.76 \text{ V}$$

As the reaction on the anode is oxidation, i.e.,

$$Zn \rightarrow Zn^{2+} + 2e,$$

E^0_{Anode} is the standard oxidation potential of zinc. This potential is given the positive sign.

$$E^0_{0x} (Zn/Zn^{2+}) = +0.76 \text{ volt}$$

So standard reduction potential of Zn, i.e.,

$$E^0 (Zn/Zn^{2+}) = E^0_{0x} = -(+0.76) = -0.76 \text{ volt}$$

The emf of such a cell gives the positive value of standard oxidation potential of metal M. The standard reduction potential (E^0) is obtained by reversing the sign of standard oxidation potential.

Emf of a Galvanic Cell

Every galvanic or voltaic cell is made up of two half-cells, the oxidation half-cell (anode) and the reduction half-cell (cathode). The potentials of these half-cells are always different. On account of this difference in electrode potentials, the electric current moves from the electrode at higher potential to the electrode at lower potential, i.e., from cathode to anode. The direction of the flow of electrons is from anode to cathode.

$$\text{Anode} \xleftarrow{\quad \text{Flow of electrons} \quad} \text{Cathode}$$
$$\xrightarrow{\quad \text{Flow of current} \quad}$$

The difference in potentials of the two half-cells is known as the electromotive force **(emf) of the cell or cell potential**.

The emf of the cell or cell potential can be calculated from the values of electrode potentials of the two half-cells constitut-ing the cell. The following three methods are in use:

(i) When oxidation potential of anode and reduction poten-tial of cathode are taken into account:

$$E_{Cell}^0 = \text{Oxidation potential of anode}$$
$$+ \text{ Reduction potential of cathode}$$
$$= E_{0x}^0 \text{ (anode)} + E_{red}^0 \text{ (cathode)}$$

(ii) When reduction potentials of both electrodes are taken into account:

$$E_{Cell}^0 = \text{Reduction potential of cathode}$$
$$- \text{ Reduction potential of anode}$$
$$= E_{Cathode}^0 - E_{Anode}^0 \text{ or}$$
$$= E_{right}^0 - E_{left}^0$$

(iii) When oxidation potentials of both electrodes are taken into account:

$$= \text{Oxidation potential of anode}$$
$$- \text{ Oxidation potential of cathode}$$

$$E_{Cell}^{\circ} = E_{ox}^{\circ} \text{ (anode)} - E_{red}^{\circ} \text{ (cathode)}$$

Difference between Emf and Potential Difference

The potential difference is the difference between the electrode potentials of the two electrodes of the cell under any condition while emf is the potential generated by a cell when there is zero electron flow, i.e., it draws no current. The points of difference are given below:

Emf	Potential difference
1. It is the potential difference between two electrodes when no current is flowing in the circuit.	1. It is the difference of the electrode potentials of the two electrons two electrodes when the cell is under operation.
2. It is the maximum voltage that the cell can deliver.	2. It is always less than the maximum the cell can deliver.
3. It is responsible for the steady flow of current in the cell.	3. It is not responsible for the steady flow of current in the cell.

Reversible and Irreversible Cells

Daniell cell has the emf value 1.09 volt. If an opposing emf exactly equal to 1.09 volt is applied to the cell, the cell reaction, stops but if it is increased

$$Zn + Cu^{2+} \rightarrow Cu + Zn^{2+}$$

infinitesimally beyond 1.09 volt, the cell reaction is reversed.

$$Cu + Zn^{2+} \rightarrow Zn + Cu^{2+}$$

Such a cell is termed a **reversible cell**. Thus, the following are the two main conditions of reversibility:

(i) The chemical reaction of the cell stops when an exactly equal opposing emf is applied.

(ii) The chemical reaction of the cell is reversed and the current flows in opposite direction when the opposing emf is slightly greater than that of the cell.

Any other cell which does not obey the above two conditions is termed as irreversible. A cell consisting of zinc and copper electrodes dipped into the solution of sulphuric acid is **irre-versible**. Similarly, the cell

$$Zn|H_2SO_4(aq)|Ag$$

is also irreversible because when the external emf is greater than the emf of the cell, the cell reaction,

$$Zn + 2H^+ \rightarrow Zn^{2+} + H_2$$

is not reversed but the cell reaction becomes

$$2Ag + 2H^+ \rightarrow 2Ag^+ + H_2$$

Concentrations Cells

If two plates of the same metal are dipped separately into two solutions of the same electrolyte and are connected with a salt bridge, the whole arrangement is found to act as a galvanic cell. In general, there are two types of concentration cells:

(i) Electrode concentration cells: In these cells, the potential difference is developed between two like electrodes at different concentrations dipped in the same solution of the electrolyte. For example, two hydrogen electrodes at different has pressure in the same solution of hydrogen ions constitute a cell of this type.

$$(Pt, H_2 \text{ (Pressure } p_1))/\text{Anode} |H^+| (H_2 \text{ (Pressure } p_2)Pt)/\text{Cathode}$$

If p_1, p_2 oxidation occurs at L.H.S. electrode and reduction occurs at R.H.S. electrode.

$$E_{cell} = 0.0591/2 \ \log(p_1/p_2) \ \text{at } 25° C$$

In the amalgam cells, two amalgams of the same metal at two different concentrations are interested in the same electrolyte solution.

Prediction for Occurance of a Redox Reaction

Any redox reaction would occur spontaneously if the free energy change (ΔG) is negative. The free energy is related to cell emf in the following manner:

$$\Delta G° = -nFE°$$

where n is the number of electrons involved, F is the value of Faraday and $E°$ is the cel emf. ΔG can be negative if $E°$ is positive.

When $E°$ is positive, the cell reaction is spontaneous and serves as a source of electrical energy.

To predict whether a particular redox reaction will occur or not, write down the redox reaction into two half reactions, one involving reduction oxidation reaction and the other involving reduction reaction. Write the oxidation reaction and reduction potential value for reduction reaction. Add these two values, if the algebraic summation gives a positive value, the reaction will occur, otherwise not.

Electrode and Cell Potentials/Nernst Equation

The electrode potential and the emf of the cell depend upon the nature of the electrode, temperature and the activities (concentrations) of the ions in solution. The variation of electrode and cell potentials with concentration of ions in solution can be obtained from thermodynamic considerations. For a general reaction such as

$$M_1A + m_2B \ ..... \ n_1X + n_2Y + \ ....$$ ...(i)

occurring in the cell, the Gibbs free energy change is given by the equation

$$G = \Delta G^o + 2.303RT \ \log_{10}(a_x{}^n{}_1 \times a_y{}^n{}_2)/(a_A{}^m{}_1 \times a_B{}^m{}_2) \ ... \text{(ii)}$$

where 'a' represents the activities of reactants and products under a given set of conditions and ΔG^o refers to free energy change for the reaction when the various reactants and products are present at standard conditions. The free energy change of a cell reaction is related to the electrical work that can be obtained from the cell, i.e., $\Delta G^o = -nFE_{cell}$ and $\Delta G^o = -nFE^o$. On substituting these values in Eq. (ii) we get

$$-nFE_{cell} = -nFE^o + 2.30eRT \ \log_{10}(a_x{}^n{}_1 \times a_y{}^n{}_2)/(a_A{}^m{}_1 \times a_B{}^m{}_2)$$
$$... \text{(iii)}$$

or $$E_{cell} = E_{cell}{}^o - 2.303RT/nF \ \log_{10}(a_x{}^n{}_1 \times a_y{}^n{}_2)/(a_A{}^m{}_1 \times a_B{}^m{}_2)$$
$$... \text{(iv)}$$

This equation is known as Nearnst equation.

Putting the values of $R = 8.314 \ JK^{-1} \ mol^{-1}$, $T = 298K$ and $F = 96500 \ C$, Eq. (iv) reduces to

$$E = E^o - 0.0591/n \ \log_{10}(a_x{}^n{}_1 \times a_y{}^n{}_2)/(a_A{}^m{}_1 \times a_B{}^m{}_2) \ ... \text{(v)}$$
$$= E_o - 0.0591/n \ \log_{10}([Products])/([Reactants]) \ ... \text{(vi)}$$

Potential of single electrode (Anode): Consider the general oxidation reaction,

$$M \rightarrow M^{n+} + ne^-$$

Applying Nernst equation,

$$E_{ox} = E_{ox}{}^o - 0.0591/n \ \log_{10}[M^{n+}]/[M]$$

where E_{ox} is the oxidation potential of the electrode (anode), is the standard oxidation potential of the electrode.

[**Note:** The concentration of pure solids and liquids are taken as unity.]

$$E_{ox} = E_{ox}{}^o - 0.0591/n \ \log_{10}[M^{n+}]$$

Let us consider a Daniell cell to explain the above equations. The concentrations of the electrolytes are not 1M.

$$Zn(s) + Cu^{2+}(aq) \leftrightarrow Zn^{2+}(aq) + Cu(s)$$

Zn(s)|Zn²⁺(aq) ‖ Cu²⁺(aq)|Cu

Potential at zinc electrode (Anode)

$$E_{ox} = E_{ox}{}^o - 0.0591/n \; log_{10} \, [Zn^{++}]$$

Potential at copper electrode (Cathode)

$$E_{red} = E_{red}{}^o - 0.0591/n \; log_{10} \, [Cu^{2+}]$$

Emf of the cell

$$E_{cell} = E_{ox} + E_{red}$$
$$= (E_{ox}{}^o + E_{red}{}^o) - 0.0591/n \; [Zn^{2+}/Cu^{2+}]$$

The value of n = 2 for both zinc and copper.

Let us consider an example, in which the values of n for the two ions in the two half-cells are not same. For example, in the cell

Cu|Cu²⁺ ‖ Ag⁺|Ag

The cell reaction is

$$Cu(s) + 2Ag^+ \rightarrow Cu^{2+} + 2Ag$$

The two half-cell reaction are:

$$Cu \; \rightarrow Cu^{2+} + 2e^-$$
$$Ag^+ + e^- \rightarrow Ag$$

The second equation is multiplied by 2 to balance the number of electrons.

$$2Ag^+ + 2e^- \rightarrow 2 \, Ag$$
$$E_{ox} = E_{ox}{}^o - 0.0591/2 \; log_{10}[Cu_{2+}]$$
$$E_{red} = E_{red}{}^o - 0.0591/2 \; {}^log_{10}[Ag^+]^2$$
$$E_{cell} = E_{ox} + E_{red}$$
$$= E_{ox}{}^o - 0.0591/2 \; log_{10} \, [Cu^{2+}]/[Ag^+]^2$$
$$= E_{cell} = 0.0591/2 \; log_{10} \, [Cu^{2+}]/[Ag^+]^2$$

Example: Construct the cells in which the following reactions are taking place. Which of the electrodes shall act as anode (negative electrode) and which one as cathode (positive electrode)?

(a) $Zn + CuSO_4 = ZnSO_4 + Cu$

(b) $Cu + 2AgNO_3 = Cu(NO_3)_2 + 2 \, Ag$

(c) $Zn + H_2SO_4 = ZnSO_4 + H_2$

(d) $Fe + SnCl_2 = FeCl_2 + Sn$

Solution: It should always be kept in mind that the metal which goes into solution in the form of its ions undergoes oxidation and thus acts as negative electrode (anode) and the element which comes into the free state undergoes reduction and acts as positive electrode (cathode):

(a) In this case Zn is oxidized to Zn^{2+} and thus acts as anode (negative electrode) while Cl^{2+} is reduced to copper and thus acts as cathode (positive electrode). The cell can be represented

as $\qquad$ $Zn \mid ZnSO_4 \| CuSO_4 \mid Cu$

or $\qquad$ $Zn \mid Zn^{2+} \| Cu^{2+} \mid Cu$

Anode (−) Cathode (+)

(b) In this case Cu is oxidized to Cu^{2+} and Ag^+ is reduced to Ag. The cell can be represented as

$$Cu \mid Cu(NO_3)_2 \| AgNO_3 \mid Ag$$

or $\qquad$ $Cu \mid Cu^{2+} \| Ag^+ \mid Ag$

Anode (−) Cathode (+)

(c) In this case Zn is oxidized to Zn^{2+} and H^+ is reduced to H_2. The cell can be represented as

$$Zn \mid ZnSO_4 \| H_2SO_4 \mid Cu$$

or $\qquad$ $Zn \mid Zn^{2+} \| 2H^+ \mid H_2(Pt)$

Anode (−) Cathode (+)

(d) Here Fe is oxidized to Fe^{2+} and Sn^{2+} is reduced to Sn. The cell can be represented as

$$Fe \mid FeCl_2 \| SnCl_2 \mid Sn$$

or $\qquad$ $Fe \mid Fe^{2+} \| Sn^{2+} \mid Sn$

Anode (−) Cathode (+)

Example: Consider the reaction,

$$2Ag^+ + Cd \rightarrow 2Ag + Cd^{2+}$$

The standard electrode potentials for $Ag^+ \rightarrow Ag$ and $Cd^{2+} \rightarrow Cd$ couples are 0.80 volt and −0.40 volt, respectively.

(i) What is the standard potential E^o for this reaction?

(ii) For the electrochemical cell in which this reaction takes place which electrode is negative electrode?

Solution: (i) The half reactions are:

$2Ag^+ + 2e^- \rightarrow 2Ag$.Reduction $\qquad$ (Cathode)

$E^o_{Ag^+/Ag} = 0.80$ volt $\qquad$ (Reduction potential)

$$Cd \rightarrow Cd^{2+} + 2e^-, \qquad \text{Oxidation (Anode)}$$

$$E^o_{Cd^+/Cd} = -0.40 \text{ volt} \qquad \text{(Reduction potential)}$$

or $\qquad E^o_{Cd^+/Cd^2} = +0.40 \text{ volt}$

$$E^o = E^o_{Cd^+/Cd^2} + E^o_{Ag^+/Ag} = 0.40 + 0.80 = 1.20 \text{ volt}$$

(ii) The negative electrode is always the electrode whose reduction potential has smaller value or the electrode where oxidation occurs. Thus, Cd electrode is the negative electrode.

Example: Consider the cell,

$$Zn|Zn^{2+} \text{ (aq)}(1.0M)\|Cu^{2+}\text{(aq)}(1.0M)|Cu$$

The standard electrode potentials are

$$Cu^{2+} + 2e^- \rightarrow Cu\text{(aq)} \qquad E^o = 0.350 \text{ volt}$$

$$Zn^{2+} + 2e^- \rightarrow Zn\text{(aq)} \qquad E^o = -0.763 \text{ volt}$$

(i) Write down the cell reaction.

(ii) Calculate the emf of the cell

Solution:

(i) Reduction potential of Zn is less than copper, hence Zn acts as anode and copper as cathode.

At anode $\qquad Zn \rightarrow Zn^{2+} + 2e^- \qquad$ (Oxidation)

At cathode $\qquad Cu^{2+} + 2e^- \rightarrow Cu \qquad$ (Reduction)

Cell reaction $\qquad Zn + Cu^{2+} \rightarrow Zn^{2+} + Cu$

(ii) $\qquad E^o_{Cell} = E^o_{Zn/Zn^{2+}} + E^o_{Cu^{2+}/Cu}$

$\qquad\qquad$ = Oxi. Potential of zinc + Red. Potential of copper

$E^o_{Zn/Zn^{2+}} = -0.763 \qquad$ (Reduction potential)

$E^o_{Zn^{2+}/Zn} = +0.763 \qquad$ (Oxidation potential)

and

$E^o_{Cu^{2+}/Cu} = 0.350 \qquad$ (Reduction potential)

So $\quad E_{cell}^o = 0.763 + 0.350 = 1.113 \text{ volt}$

Oxidation potential is $E^o_{M/M^{a+}}$ while reduction potential is represented as $E^o_{M^{a+}/M}$. The value of $E^o_{Zn/Zn^{2+}}$ (oxidation potential of Zn) is +0.76 volt and the value of $E^o_{Cu^{2+}/Cu}$ (reduction potential of copper) is +0.34 volt. The electrode having lower value of reduction potential acts as an anode while that having higher value of reduction potential acts as cathode.

Example: Will Fe be oxidiesed to Fe^{2+} by reaction with 1.0M HCl? E^o for Fe/Fe^{2+} = +0.44 volt.

Solution: The reaction will occur if Fe is oxidized to Fe^{2+}.

$$Fe + 2HCl \rightarrow FeCl_2 + H_2$$

Writing two half reaction,

$Fe \rightarrow Fe^{2+} + 2e^-$	Oxidation $E^o_{Fe/Fe^{2+}} = 0.44$ volt
$2H^+ + 2e^- \rightarrow H2$	Reduction $E^o_{H^+/H} = 0.0$ volt

Adding, emf = 0.44 volt

Since emf is positive, the reaction shall occur.

Example: The values of Eo of some of the reactions are given below:

$I_2 + 2e^- \rightarrow 2I^-$;	$E^o = +0.54$ volt
$Cl_2 + 2e^- \rightarrow 2Cl^-$;	$E^o = +1.36$ volt
$Fe^{3+} + e^- \rightarrow Fe^{2+}$;	$E^o = +0.76$ volt
$Ce^{4+} + e^- \rightarrow Ce^{3+}$;	$E^o = +1.60$ volt
$Sn^{4+} + 2e^- \rightarrow Sn^{2+}$;	$E^o = +0.15$ volt

On the basis of the above data, answer the following questions:

(a) Whether Fe^{3+} oxidizes Ce^{3+} or not?

(b) Whether I_2 displaces chlorine form KCl?

(c) Whether the reaction between $FeCl_3$ and $SnCl_2$ occurs or not?

Solution:

(a) Chemical reaction,

$$Fe^{3+} + Ce^{3+} \rightarrow Ce^{4+} + Fe^{2+}$$

	Two half reactions,
$Fe^{3+} + e \rightarrow Fe^{2+}$	Reduction $E^o = 0.76$ volt
$Ce^{3+} \rightarrow Ce^{4+} + e^-$	Oxidation $E^o_{ox} = -1.60$ volt
	Adding $= -0.84$ volt

Since, emf is negative the reaction does not occur, i.e., Fe^{3+} does not oxidise Ce^{3+}.

(b) Chemical reaction

$$I_2 + 2KCl = 2Kl + Cl_2$$

Half reactions

$I_2 + 2e^- \rightarrow 2I^-$	Reduction $E^o = 0.54$ volt
$2Cl^- \rightarrow Cl_2 + 2e^-$	Oxidation $E^o_{ox} = -1.36$ volt
	Adding $= -0.82$ volt

Since, emf is negative, the reaction does not occur, i.e., I_2 does not displace Cl_2 from KCl.

(c) Chemical reaction

$$SnCl_2 + 2FeCl_3 \rightarrow SnCl_4 + 2FeCl_2$$

Half reactions

$Fe^{3+} + eFe^{2+}$	Reduction $E^o = 0.76$ volt
$Ce^{2+} Sn^{4+} + 2e^-$	Oxidation $E^o = -0.15$ volt
	Adding $\quad = +0.61$ volt

Since, emf is positive, the reaction will occur.

Example: Calculate the electrode potential at a copper electrode dipped in a 0.1M solution of copper sulphate at 25°C. The standard electrode potential of Cu^{2+}/Cu system is 0.34 volt at 298 K.

Solution: We know that

$$E_{red} = E^o_{red} + 0.0591/n \ log_{10}[ion]$$

Putting the values of

$$E^o_{red} = 0.34V, n = 2 \ and \ [Cu^{2+}] = 0.1 \ M$$
$$E^o_{red} = 0.34 + 0.0591/2 \ log_{10}[0.1]$$
$$= 0.34 + 0.02955 \times (-1)$$
$$= 0.34 - 0.02955 = 0.31045 \ volt$$

Example: What is the single electrode potential of a half-cell foe zinc electrode dipping in 0.01 M $ZnSO_4$ solution at 25° C? The standard electrode potential of Zn/Zn^{2+} system is 0.763 volt at 25° C.

Solution: We know that

$$E_{ox} = E^o_{red} - 0.0591/n \ log_{10}[ion]$$

Putting the value of

$$E^o ox = 0.763 \ V, n=2 \ and$$
$$[Zn^{2+}] = 0.01 \ M$$
$$E^o ox = 0.763 - 0.0591/2 \ log\_10 \ [0.01]$$
$$= 0.763 - 0.02955 \times (-2)$$
$$= (0.763 + 0.0591) \ volt = 0.8221 \ volt$$

Example 41: Calculate the e.m.f of the cell.

$$Mg(s)|Mg^{2+}(0.2M)||Ag^+(1 \times 10^{-3})|Ag$$
$$E^o_{Ag+/Ag} = +0.8 \ volt, \quad E^o_{Mg2+/Mg} = -2.37 \ volt$$

What will be the effect on e.m.f. if concentration of Mg^{2+} ion is decreased to 0.1 M?

Solution: $E^o_{cell} = E^o_{Cathode} - E^o_{anode}$

$$= 0.80 - (-2.37) = 3.17 \text{ volt}$$

Cell reaction

$$Mg + 2Ag^+ \rightarrow 2Ag + Mg^{2+}$$

$$E_{cell} = E_{cell}^o - 0.0591/n \log(Mg^{2+})/[Ag^+]^2$$

$$= 3.17 - 0.0591/2 \log 0.2/[1 \times 10^{-3}]^2$$

$$= 3.17 - 0.1566 = 3.0134 \text{ volt}$$

when $Mg^{2+} = 0.1 \text{ M}$

$$E_{cell} = E^o_{cell} - 0.0591/n \log(0.1)/[1 - 10^{-3}]^2$$

$$= (3.17 - 0.1477) \text{ volt}$$

$$= 3.0223 \text{ volt}$$

Example: To find the standard potential of M^{3+}/M electrode, the following cell is constituted:

$$Pt|M|M^{3+}(0.0018 \text{ mol}^{-1}L)\|Ag^+(0.01 \text{ mol}^{-1}L)|Ag$$

The emf of this cell is found to be 0.42 volt. Calculate the standard potential of the half reaction $M^{3+} + 3e^- M^{3+} = 0.80$ volt.

Solution: The cell reaction is

$$M + 3Ag^+ \rightarrow 3Ag + M^{3+}$$

Applying Nernst equation,

$$E_{cell} = E_{cell}^o - 0.0591/n \log(Mg^{2+})/[Ag^+]^3$$

$$0.42 = E_{cell}^o - 0.0591/n \log (0.0018)/(0.01)^3 = E_{cell}^o - 0.064$$

$$E_{cell}^o = (0.042 + 0.064) = 0.484 \text{ volt}$$

$$E^o_{cell} = E^o_{cathode} - E^o_{anode}$$

or $\quad E^o_{anode} = E^o_{cathode} - E^o_{cell}$

$$= (0.80 - 0.484) = 0.32 \text{ volt}$$

ELECTROCHEMICAL SERIES

By measuring the potentials of various electrodes versus stand-ard hydrogen electrode (SHE), a series of standard electrode potentials has been established. When the electrodes (metals and non-metals) in contact with their ions are arranged oh the basis of the values of their standard reduction potentials or standard oxidation potentials, the resulting series is called the **electrochemical** or **electromotive** or **activity series** of the elements.

By international convention, the standard potentials of electrodes are tabulated for reduction half reactions, indicating the tendencies of the electrodes to behave as cathodes towards SHE. Those with positive $E°$ values for reduction half reactions do in fact act as cathodes versus SHE, while those with negative $E°$ values of reduction half reactions behave instead as anodes versus SHE. The electrochemical series is shown in the following table.

Table 5.3: Standard Aqueous Electrode Potentials at 25°C 'The Electrochemical Series'

Element	Electrode Reaction (Reduction)	Standard Electrode Reduction potential $E°$, volt
Li	$Li^+ + e^- = Li$	−3.05
K	$K^+ + e^- = K$	−2.925
Ca	$Ca^{2+} + 2e^- = Ca$	−2.87
Na	$Na^+ + e^- = Na$	−2.714
Mg	$Mg^{2+} + 2e^- = Mg$	−2.37
Al	$Al^{3+} + 3e^- = Al$	−1.66
Zn	$Zn^{2+} + 2e^- = Zn$	−0.7628
Cr	$Cr^{3+} + 3e^- = Cr$	−0.74
Fe	$Fe^{2+} + 2e^- = Fe$	−0.44
Cd	$Cd^{2+} + 2e^- = Cd$	−0.403
Ni	$Ni^{2+} + 2e^- = Ni$	−0.25
Sn	$Sn^{2+} + 2e^- = Sn$	−0.14
H_2	$2H^+ + 2e^- = H_2$	0.00
Cu	$Cu^{2+} + 2e^- = Cu$	+0.337
I_2	$I_2 + 2e^- = 2I^-$	+0.535
Ag	$Ag^+ + e^- = Ag$	+0.799
Hg	$Hg^{2+} + 2e^- = Hg$	+0.885
Br_2	$Br_2 + 2e^- = 2Br^-$	+1.08
Cl_2	$Cl_2 + 2e^- = 2Cl^-$	+1.36
Au	$Au^{3+} + 3e^- = Au$	+1.50
F_2	$F_2 + 2e^- = 2F^-$	+2.87

Characteristics of Electrochemical series

(i) The negative sign of standard reduction potential indicates that an electrode when joined with SHE acts as anode and oxidation occurs on this electrode. For example, standard reduction potential of zinc is −0.76 volt. When zinc electrode is joined with SHE, it acts as anode (−ve electrode) i.e., oxidation occurs on this electrode. Similarly, the +ve sign of standard reduction potential indicates that the electrode when joined with SHE acts as cathode and reduction occurs on this electrode.

(ii) The substances which are stronger reducing agents than hydrogen are placed above hydrogen in the series and have negative values of standard reduction potentials. All those substances which have positive values of reduction potentials and placed below hydrogen in the series are weaker reducing agents than hydrogen.

(iii) The substances which are stronger oxidising agents than H^+ ion are placed below hydrogen in the series.

(iv) The metals on the top (having high negative values of standard reduction potentials) have the tendency to lose electrons readily. These are active metals. The activity of metals decreases from top to bottom. The non-metals on the bottom (having high positive values of standard reduction potentials) have the tendency to accept electrons readily. These are active non-metals. The activity of non-metals increases from top to bottom.

Applications of Electrochemical series

(i) Reactivity of metals: The activity of the metal depends on its tendency to lose electron or electrons, i.e., tendency to form cation (M''^+). This tendency depends on the magnitude of standard reduction potential. The metal which has high negative value (or smaller positive value) of standard reduction potential readily loses the electron or electrons and is converted into cation. Such a metal is said to be chemically active.

The chemical reactivity of metals decreases from top to bottom in the series. The metal higher in the series is more active than the metal lower in the series. For example,

(a) Alkali metals and alkaline earth metals having high negative values of standard reduction potentials are chemically active. These react with cold water and evolve hydrogen. These readily dissolve in acids forming corresponding salts and combine with those substances which accept electrons.

(b) Metals like Fe, Pb, Sn, Ni, Co, etc., which lie a little down in the series do not react with cold water but react with steam to evolve hydrogen.

(c) Metals like Cu, Ag and Au which lie below hydrogen are less reactive and do not evolve hydrogen from water.

(ii) **Electropositive character of metals:** The electropositive character also depends on the tendency to lose electron or electrons. Like reactivity, the electropositive character of metals decreases from top to bottom in the electrochemical series. On the basis of standard reduction potential values, metals are divided into three groups:

(a) Strongly electropositive metals: Metals having standard reduction potential near about -2.0 volt or more negative like alkali metals, alkaline earth metals are strongly electropositive in nature.

(b) Moderately electropositive metals: Metals having values of reduction potentials between 0.0 and about -2.0 volt are moderately electropositive. Al, Zn, Fe, Ni, Co, etc., belong to this group.

(c) Weakly electropositive metals: The metals which are below hydrogen and possess positive values of reduction potentials are weakly electropositive metals. Cu, Hg, Ag, etc., belong to this group.

(iii) **Displacement reactions:**

(a) To predict whether a given metal will displace another, from its salt solution. A metal higher in the series will displace the metal from its solution which is lower in the series, i.e., the metal having low standard reduction poten-tial will displace the metal from its salt's solution which has higher value of standard reduction potential. A metal higher in the series has greater tendency to provide electrons to the cations of the metal to be precipitated.

(b) Displacement of one nonmetal from its salt solution by another nonmetal: A nonmetal higher in the series (towards bottom side), i.e., having high value of reduction potential will displace another nonmetal with lower reduction potential i.e., occupying position above in the series. The nonmetal's which possess high positive reduction potentials have the tendency to accept electrons readily. These electrons are provided by the ions of the nonmetal having low value of reduction potential. Thus, Cl_2 can displace bromine and iodine from bromides and iodides.

$$Cl_2 + 2KI \rightarrow 2KCl + I_2$$

$$2I^- \rightarrow I_2 + 2e^- \qquad \text{(Oxidation)}$$

$$Cl_2 + 2e^- \rightarrow 2Cl^- \qquad \text{(Reduction)}$$

[The activity or electronegative character or oxidising nature of the nonmetal increases as the value of reduction potential increases.]

(c) Displacement of hydrogen from dilute acids by metals: The metal which can provide electrons to H^+ ions present in dilute acids for reduction, evolve hydrogen from dilute acids.

$$Mn \rightarrow Mn^+ + ne^- \qquad \text{(Oxidation)}$$
$$2H^+ + 2e^- \rightarrow H_2 \qquad \text{(Reduction)}$$

The metal having negative values of reduction potential possess the property of losing electron or electrons.

Thus, the metals occupying top positions in the electrochemical series readily liberate hydrogen from dilute acids and on descending in the series tendency to liberate hydrogen gas from dilute acids decreases.

The metals which are below hydrogen in electrochemical series like Cu, Hg, Au, Pt, etc., do not evolve hydrogen from dilute acids.

(d) Displacement of hydrogen from water: Iron and the metals above iron are capable of liberating hydrogen from water. The tendency decreases from top to bottom in electrochemical series.

Alkali and alkaline earth metals liberate hydrogen from cold water but Mg, Zn and Fe liberate hydrogen from hot water or steam.

(iv) Reducing power of metals: Reducing nature depends on the tendency of losing electron or electrons. More the negative reduction potential, more is the tendency to lose electron or electrons. Thus, reducing nature decreases from top to bottom in the electrochemical series. The power of the reducing agent increases as the standard reduction potential becomes more and more negative.

Sodium is a stronger reducing agent than zinc and zinc is a stronger reducing agent than iron.

Element	Na	Zn	Fe
Reduction potential	−2.71	−0.76	−0.44

Reducing nature decreases

Alkali and alkaline earth metals are strong reducing agents.

(v) Oxidising nature of nonmetals: Oxidising nature depends on the tendency to accept electron or electrons. More the value of reduction potential, higher is the tendency to accept electron or electrons. **Thus, oxidising nature increases from top to bottom in the electrochemical series.** The strength of an oxidising agent increases as the value of reduction potential becomes more and more positive.

F_2 (Fluorine) is a stronger oxidant than Cl_2, Br_2 and I_2.

Cl_2 (Chlorine) is a stronger oxidant than Br_2 and I_2.

Element	I_2	Br_2	Cl_2	F_2
Reduction potential	+0.53	+1.06	+1.36	+2.85

Oxidising nature increases

Thus, in electrochemical series

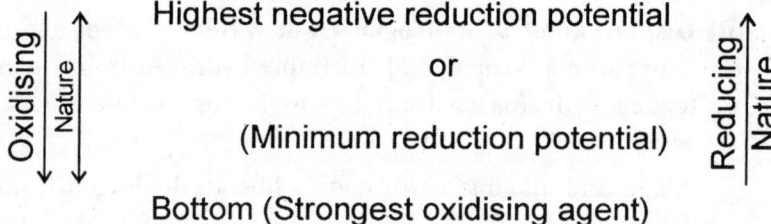

Top (Strongest reducing agent)

Oxidising Nature ↑

Highest negative reduction potential

or

(Minimum reduction potential)

Reducing Nature ↑

Bottom (Strongest oxidising agent)

Highest positive value of reduction potential

Fig. 5.14

(vi) Thermal stability of metallic oxides: The thermal stability of the metal oxide depends on its electropositive nature. As the electropositivity decreases from top to bottom, the thermal stability of the oxide also decreases from top to bottom. The oxides of metals having high positive reduction potentials are not stable towards heat. The metals which come below copper form unstable oxides, i.e., these are decomposed on heating.

$$Ag_2O \xrightarrow[2\,Ag]{Heat} \frac{1}{2}O_2$$

$$2H_gO \xrightarrow[2Hg]{Heat} \frac{1}{2}O_2$$

(vii) Products of electrolysis: In case two or more types of positive and negative ions are present in solution, during electrolysis certain ions are discharged or liberated at the electrodes in preference to others. **In general, in such com-petition the ion which is stronger oxidising agent (high value of standard reduction potential) is discharged first at the cathode.** The increasing order of deposition of few cations is:

$$K^+, Ca^{2+}, Na^+, Mg^{2+}, Al^{3+}, Zn^{2+}, Fe^{2+}, H^+, Cu^{2+}, Ag^+, Au^{3+}$$

Increasing order of deposition

Similarly, the anion which is stronger reducing agent (low value of standard reduction potential) is liberated first at the anode.

The increasing order of discharge of few anions is:

$$SO_4^{2-}, NO_3^-, OH^-, Cl^-, Br^-, I^-$$

Increasing order of discharge

Thus, when an aqueous solution of NaCl containing Na^+, Cl^-, H^+ and OH^- ions is electrolysed, H^+ ions are discharged at cathode and CF ions at the anode, i.e., H_2 is liberated at cathode and chlorine at anode.

When an aqueous solution of $CuSO_4$ containing Cu^{2+}, H^+ and OH^- ions is electrolysed, Cu^{2+} ions are dis-charged at cathode and OH^- ions at the anode.

$$Cu^{2+} + 2e^- \rightarrow Cu \qquad \text{(Cathodic reaction)}$$
$$4OH^- \rightarrow O_2 + 2H_2O + 4e^- \qquad \text{(Anodic reaction)}$$

Cu is deposited on cathode while O_2 is liberated at anode.

(viii) Corrosion of metals: Corrosion is defined as the deterioration of a substance because of its reaction with its environment. This is also defined as the process by which metals have the tendency to go back to their combined state, i.e., reverse of extraction of metals.

Ordinary corrosion is a redox reaction by which metals are oxidised by oxygen in presence of moisture. Oxidation of metals occurs more readily at points of strain. Thus, a steel nail first corrodes at the tip and head. The end of a steel nail acts as an anode where iron is oxidised to Fe^{2+} ions.

$$Fe \rightarrow Fe^2 + 2e^- \qquad \text{(Anode reaction)}$$

The electrons flow along the nail to areas containing im-purities which act as cathodes where oxygen is reduced to hydroxyl ions.

$$O_2 + 2H_2O + 4e^- \rightarrow 4OH^- \qquad \text{(Cathode reaction)}$$

Overall the metal containing the more electronegative reduction potential, will be oxidised easily or corroded easily.

(ix) Extraction of metals: A more electropositive metal can displace a less electropositive metal from its salt's solution. This principle is applied for the extraction of Ag and Au by cyanide process. Silver from the solution containing sodium argento cyanide, $NaAg(CN)_2$, can be obtained by the addition of zinc as it is more electro-positive than Ag.

$$2NaAg(CN)_2 + Zn \rightarrow Na_2Zn(CN)_4 + 2Ag$$

Relation between Equilibrium constant, Gibbs free energy and EMF of the cell

Concept of equilibrium in electrochemical cell

In an electrochemical cell a reversible redox process takes place, e.g., in Daniell cell:

$$Zn(s) + Cu^{2+}(aq) \Leftrightarrow Zn^{2+}(aq) + Cu(s)$$

(1) At equilibrium mass action ratio becomes equal to equilibrium constant,

i.e., $\qquad Q = K_e$

(2) Oxidation potential of anode = – Reaction potential of cathode

i.e., $\qquad$ emf = oxidation potential of anode

$\qquad\qquad\qquad\qquad$ + Reduction potential of cathode

$\qquad\qquad = 0$

Cell is fully discharged

According to Nernst equation:

$$E = E^\circ - 0.0591/n \ \log_{10} Q \text{ at } 25^\circ C$$

At equilibrium, $\quad E = 0, Q = K$

$$0 = E^\circ \ 0.0591/n \ \log_{10} K$$

$$K = \text{Antilog} \ [(nE^\circ)/0.0591]$$

Work done by the cell

Let n faraday charge be taken out of a cell of emf E; then work done by the cell will be calculated as:

$$\text{Work} = \text{Charge} \times \text{Potential}$$
$$= nFE$$

Work done by the cell is equal to decrease in free energy.

$$-\Delta G = nFE$$

Similarly, maximum obtainable work from the cell will be

$$W_{max} = nFE°$$

where, E_o = standard emf or standard cell potential.

$$-\Delta G = nFE$$

The relationship among K, $\Delta G°$ and $E°$ cell

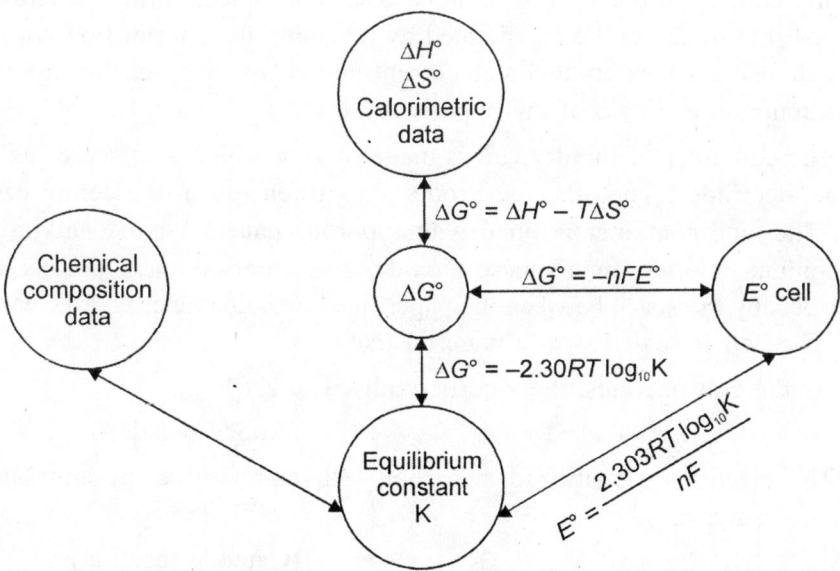

Fig. 5.15

Heat of reaction in an electrochemical cell

Let n Faraday charge flows out of a cell of emf E,

Then $-\Delta G = nFE$ ... (i)

Gibbs-Helmholtz equation from thermodynamics may be given as

$$\Delta G = \Delta H + T\ (\partial \Delta G/\partial T)_P \qquad \text{... (ii)}$$

From equation (i) and (ii) we get

$$-nFE = \Delta H + T\left(\partial(-nFE)/\partial T\right)_P = \Delta H - nFT(\partial E/\partial T)_P$$

$$\Delta H = -nFE + nFT(\partial E/\partial T)_P$$

Here $(\partial E/\partial T)_P$ = Temperature coefficient of cell

Case I: When $(\partial E/\partial T)_P = 0$, then $\Delta H = -nFE$

Case II: When $(\partial E/\partial T) > 0$, then $nFE > \Delta H$, i.e., process inside the cell is endothermic.

Case III: When $(\partial E/\partial T) < 0$, then $nFE < \Delta H$, i.e., process inside the cell is exothermic.

PRIMARY VOLTAIC CELL (THE DRY CELL)

In this cell, once the chemicals have been consumed, further reaction is not possible. It cannot be regenerated by reversing the current flow through the cell using an external direct current source of electrical energy. The most common example of this type is dry cell.

The container of the dry cell is made of zinc which also serves as one of the electrodes. The other electrode is a carbon rod in the centre of the cell. The zinc container is lined with a porous paper. A moist mixture of ammonium chloride, man-ganese dioxide, zinc chloride and a porous inert filler occupy the space between the paper lined zinc container and the carbon rod. The cell is sealed with a material like wax.

As the cell operates, the zinc is oxidised to Zn^{2+}

$$Zn \rightarrow Zn^{2+} + 2e^- \qquad \text{(Anode reaction)}$$

The electrons are utilized at carbon rod (cathode) as the ammonium ions are reduced.

$$2NH_4^+ + 2e^- \rightarrow 2NH_3 + H_2 \qquad \text{(Cathode reaction)}$$

The cell reaction is

$$Zn + 2\ NH_4^+ \rightarrow Zn^{2+} + 2NH_3 + H_2$$

Hydrogen is oxidized by MnO_2 in the cell.

$$2MnO_2 + H_2 \rightarrow 2MnO(OH)$$

Ammonia produced at cathode combines with zinc ions to form complex ion.

$$Zn^{2+} + 4NH_3 \rightarrow [Zn(NH_3)_4]_{2+}$$

E_{cell} is 1.6 volt

Alkaline dry cell is similar to ordinary dry cell. It contains potassium hydroxide. The reaction in alkaline dry cell are:

$$Zn + 2OH^- \rightarrow Zn(OH)_2 + 2e^- \qquad \text{(Anode reaction)}$$

$$2MnO_2 + 2H_2O + 2e^- \rightarrow 2MnO(OH) + 2OH^- \qquad \text{(Cathode reaction)}$$

$$Zn + 2MnO_2 + 2H_2O \rightarrow Zn(OH)_2 + 2MnO(OH) \qquad \text{(Overall)}$$

E_{cell} is 1.5 volt.

SECODARY VOLTAIC CELL (LEAD STORAGE BATTERY)

The cell in which original reactants are regenerated by passing direct current from external source, i.e., it is re-charged, is called secondary cell. Lead storage battery is the example of this type.

It consists of a group of lead plates bearing compressed spongy lead, alternating with a group of lead plates bearing leaf dioxide, PbO_2. These plates are immersed in a solution of about 30% H2SO4. When the cell discharge; it operates as a voltaic cell. The spongy lead is oxidized to Pb2+ ions and lead plates acquire a negative charge.

$$Pb \rightarrow Pb^{2+} + 2e^- \qquad \text{(Anode reaction)}$$

Pb^{2+} ions combine with sulphate ions to form insoluble lead sulphate, $PbSO_4$, which begins to coat lead electrode.

$$Pb^{2+} + SO_4^{2-} \rightarrow PbSO_4 \qquad \text{(Precipitation)}$$

The electrons are utilized at PbO_2 electrode.

$$PbO_2 + 4H^+ + 2e^- \rightarrow Pb^{2+}\, 2H_2O \qquad \text{(Cathode reaction)}$$

$$Pb^{2+} + SO_4^{2-} \rightarrow PbSO_4 \qquad \text{(Precipitation)}$$

Overall cell reaction is:

$$Pb + PbO_2 + 4H^+ + 2\ SO_4^2 \rightarrow 2PbSO_4 + 2H_2O$$

Ecell is 2.041 volt.

When a potential slightly greater than the potential of battery is applied, the battery can be re-charged.

$$2PbSO_4 + 2H_2O \rightarrow Pb + PbO_2 + 2H_2SO_4$$

After many repeated charge-discharge cycles, some of the lead sulphate falls to the bottom of the container, the sulphuric acid concentration remains low and the battery cannot be recharged fully.

FUEL CELL

Fuel cells are another means by which chemical energy may be converted into electrical energy. The main disadvantage of a primary cell is that it can deliver current for a short period only. This is due to the fact that the quantity of oxidising agent and reducing agent is limited. But the energy can be obtained indefinitely from a fuel cell as long as the outside supply of fuel is maintained. One of the examples is the hydrogen-oxygen fuel cell. The cell consists of three compartments separated by a porous electrode. Hydrogen gas is introduced into one compartment and oxygen gas is fed into another compartment. These gases then diffuse slowly through the electrodes and react with an electrolyte that is in the central compartment. The electrodes are made of porous carbon and the electrolyte is a resin containing concentrated aqueous sodium hydroxide solu-tion. Hydrogen is oxidised at anode and oxygen is reduced at cathode. The overall cell reaction produces water. The reactions which occur are:

Anode $[H_2(g) + 2OH^-(aq) \rightarrow 2H_2O(l) + 2e^-] \times 2$

Cathode $O_2(g) + 2H_2O(l) + 4e^- \rightarrow 4OH^-(aq)$

Overall $2H_2(g) + O_2(g) \rightarrow 2H_2O(l)$

This type of cells are used in space-crafts. Fuel cells are efficient and pollution free.

COMMERCIAL PRODUCTION OF CHEMICALS

The wide applications of electrolysis have been listed in section 12.4 of this chapter. A large number of chemicals are produced by electrolysis. A few of these are described below:

1. Manufacture of sodium: Sodium is obtained on large scale by two processes:

(i) **Castner's process:** In this process, electrolysis of fused sodium hydroxide is carried out at 330°C using iron as cathode and nickel as anode.

$$2NaOH \Leftrightarrow 2Na^+ + 2OH$$

At cathode $2Na^+ + 2e \rightarrow 2Na$

At anode $4OH^- \rightarrow 2H_2O + O_2 + 4e$

During electrolysis, oxygen and water are produced. Water formed at the anode gets partly evaporated and is partly broken down and hydrogen is discharged at cathode.

$$H_2O \Leftrightarrow H^+ OH^-$$

At cathode $2H^+ + 2e \rightarrow 2H \; H_2$

(ii) **Down's process:** Now-a-days sodium metal is manu-factured by this process. It involves the electrolysis of fused sodium chloride containing calcium chloride and potassium fluoride using iron as cathode and graphite as anode at about **600°C** (Fig. 5.16)

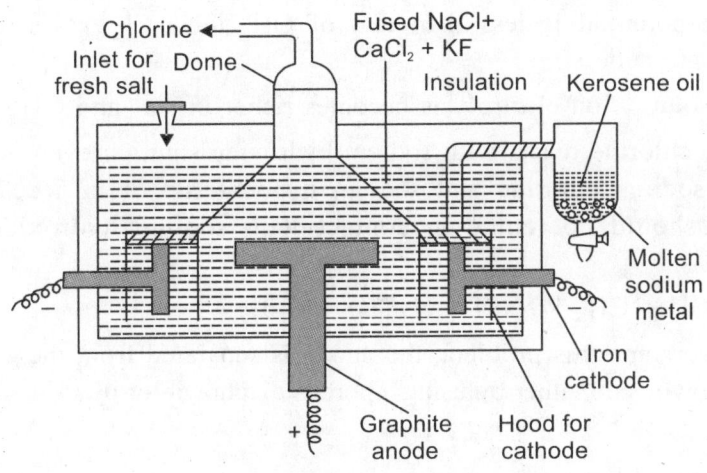

Fig. 5.16

$$NaCl \Leftrightarrow Na^+ + Cl^-$$

At cathode $Na^+ + e \rightarrow Na$

At anode $2Cl^- \rightarrow Cl_2 + 2e$

The electrolysis of pure NaCl presents the following difficulties:

(a) The fusion temperature of NaCl is high, *i.e.,* 803°C. At this temperature both sodium and chlorine are corrosive.

(b) Sodium forms a metallic fog at this temperature.

To remove above difficulties, the fusion temperature is reduced to 600°C by adding $CaCl_2$ and KF. This is a cheaper method and **chlorine is obtained as a by-product.** The sodium obtained is of high purity (about 99.5%).

2. Sodium hydroxide (Caustic soda), NaOH: Caustic soda is manu-factured by the electrolysis of aqueous solution of sodium chloride in an electrolytic cell.

Principle: A sodium chloride solution contains Na^+, H^+, Cl^- and OH^- ions.

$$NaCl \Leftrightarrow Na^+ + Cl^-$$
$$H_2O \Leftrightarrow H^+ + OH^-$$

On passing electricity, Na$^+$ and IF ions move towards cathode and Cl$^-$ and OH" ions move towards anode. The discharge potential of H$^+$ ions is less than Na$^+$ ions, thus hydrogen ions get discharged easily and hydrogen is liberated. Similarly, at anode Cl$^-$ ions are easily discharges as their discharge potential is less than that of OH$^-$ ions. Cl$_2$ gas is, therefore, liberated at anode.

The solution on electrolysis becomes richer in Na$^+$ and OH$^-$ ions.

Since chlorine reacts with sodium hydroxide solution even in the cold forming sodium chloride and sodium hypochlorite, it is necessary that chlorine should not come in contact with sodium hydroxide during electrolysis.

$$2NaOH + Cl_2 \rightarrow NaCl + NaCIO + H_2O$$

To overcome this problem, the anode is separated from the cathode in the electrolytic cell either by using a porous diaphragm or by using a mercury cathode.

Kellner-Solvay cell

This is the modified cell. This cell has no compartments. The flowing mercury as shown in Fig. 5.17 acts as cathode. A number of graphite rods dipping in sodium chloride solution acts as anode. A constant level of sodium chloride solution is maintained in the cell. On electrolysis chlorine gas is librated and Na+ ions are discharged ay cathode (mercury). Sodium discharged dissolves in Hg and forms amalgam. This amalgam flows out in a vessel containing water. sodium hydroxide is formed with evolution of hydrogen.

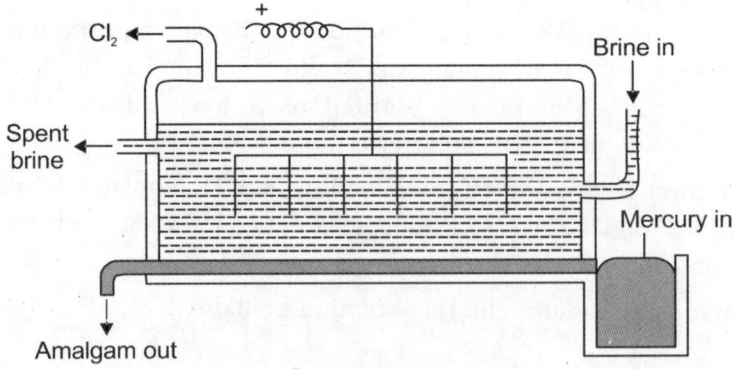

Fig. 5.17: Kellner -Solvay cell

Preparation of Pure Sodium Hydroxide:

Commercial sodium hydroxide is purified with the help of alcohol. Sodium hydroxide dissolves in alcohol while impurities like $NaCl$, Na_2CO_3, Na_2SO_4, etc., remain insoluble. The alcoholic filtrate is distilled. The alcohol distills off while pure solid sodium hydroxide is left behind.

3. Manufacture of Aluminium: Aluminium is manufactured from pure bauxite ore by electrolysis. The bauxite ore usually contains impurities such as iron oxide, silica, etc. These impurities are first removed by the application of the following methods in order to get pure alumina, *i.e.,* pure bauxite ore.

(a) Hall's process

(b) Baeyer's process

(c) Serpeck's process.

Electrolytic Reduction of Pure Alumina: The electrolysis of pure alumina faces two difficulties: (i) Pure alumina is a bad conductor of electricity, (ii) The fusion temperature of pure alumina is about 2000°C and at this temperature when the electrolysis is carried of the fused mass, the metal formed vapourises as the boiling point of aluminium is 1800°C.

The above difficulties are overcome by using a mixture containing alumina, cryolite (Na_3AlF_6) and fluorspar (CaF_2) in the ratio of 20 : 60 : 20. The fusion temperature of this mixture is 900°C and it is a good conductor of electricity.

The electrolysis is carried out in an iron box lined inside with gas carbon which acts as cathode. The anode consists of carbon rods which dip

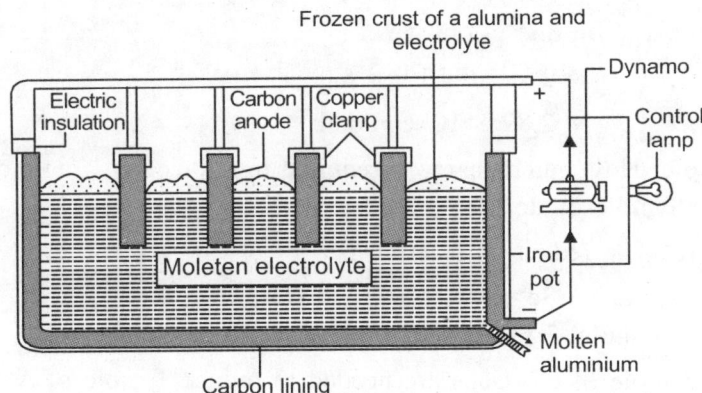

Fig. 5.18

in the fused mixture of the electrolyte from above. The fused electrolyte is covered with a layer of coke (Fig. 5.18).

The current passed through the cell serves two purposes: (i) Heating of the electrolyte: The temperature of the cell is automatically maintained at 900 – 950°C. (ii) Electrolysis: On passing current, aluminium is discharged at cathode.

Aluminium being heavier than the electrolyte sinks to the bottom and is tapped out periodically from a tapping hole. Oxygen is liberated at anode. It attacks the carbon rods forming CO and CO_2. The process is continuous. When the concentra-tion of the electrolyte decreases, the resistance of the cell increases. This is indicated by the glowing of a lamp placed in parallel. At this stage more of alumina is added.

One concept: Alumina (Al_2O_3) ionizes as

$$Al_2O_3 \rightarrow Al^{3+} + AlO_3^{3-}$$

Cathode   Anode

$$Al^{3+} + 3e \; Al \text{ (at cathode)}$$

At anode $AlO_3^- \rightarrow 2Al_2O_3 + 3O_2 + 12e$ (at anode)

Thus, the overall chemical reaction taking place during electrolysis is

$$2Al_2O_3 \rightarrow 4Al + 3O_2$$

Aluminum of 99.8% purity is obtained from this process.

Some More Problems

Example: Find the charge in coulomb on 1 g-ion of N^{3-}.

Solution: Charge on one ion of N^{3-}

$$= 3 \times 1.6 \times 10^{-19} \text{ coulomb}$$

Thus, charge on one g-ion of N^{3-}

$$= 3 \times 1.6 \; 10^{-19} \times 6.02 \times 10^{23}$$
$$= 2.89 \times 10^5 \text{ coulomb}$$

Example: How much charge is required to reduce (a) 1 mole of Al^{3+} to Al and (b) 1 mole of to Mn^{2+}?

Solution: (a) The reduction reaction is

$$Al^{3+} + 3e^- \rightarrow Al$$

1 mole 3 mole

Thus, 3 mole of electrons are needed to reduce 1 mole of Al^{3+}.

$$Q = 3 \times F$$
$$= 3 \times 96500 = 289500 \text{ coulomb}$$

(b) The reduction is

$$Mn_4^- + 8H + 5e^- \rightarrow MN^{2+} + 4H_2O$$

1 mole   5 mole

$$Q = 5 \times F$$

$$= 5 \times 96500 = 48500 \text{ coulomb}$$

Example . How much electric charge is required to oxidise (a) 1 mole of H_2O to O_2 and (b)1 mole of FeO to Fe_2O_3?

Solution: (a) The oxidation reaction is

$$H_2O \rightarrow 1/2\, O_2 + 2H^+ + 2e^-$$

1 mole   2 mole

$$Q = 2 \times F$$

$$= 2 \times 96500 = 193000 \text{ coulomb}$$

(b) The oxidation reaction is

$$FeO + 1/2\, H_2O \rightarrow 1/2\, Fe_2O_3 + H^+ + e^-$$

$$Q = F = 96500 \text{ coulomb}$$

Electrolyte Concentration Cells

In these cells, electrodes are identical but these are immersed in solutions of the same electrolyte of different concentrations. The source of electrical energy in the cell is the tendency of the electrolyte to diffuse from a solution of higher concentration to that of lower concentration. With the expiry of time, the two concentrations tend to become equal. Thus, at the start the emf of the cell is maximum and it gradually falls to zero. Such a cell is repre-sented in the following manner:

(C_2 is greater than C_1).

$$M|Mn^+(C_1) \| M^{n+}(C_2)|M$$

or $(Zn|Zn^{2+}\,(C_1))$/Anode $\|$ $(Zn^{2+}\,(C_2\,)|Zn)$/Cathode

The emf of the cell is given by the following expression:

$Ecell = 0.0591/n \log C_{(2(R.H.S.))}/C_{(1(L.H.S.))}$ at 25°C

The concentration cells are used to determine the solubility of sparingly soluble salts, valency of the cation of the electrolyte and transition point of the two allotropic forms of a metal used as electrodes, etc.

Example: A cell contains two hydrogen electrodes. The negative electrode is in contact with a solution of 10^{-6} M hydrogen ions. The emf of the cell is 0.118 volt at 25°C. Calculate the concentration of hydrogen ions at the positive electrode.

Solution: The cell may be represented as

$$Pt|H_2(1atm)|H^+ \, \| H^+|H_2(1 \, atm)|Pt$$

$$10^{-6} M \, CM$$

Anode	Cathode
(–ve)	(+ve)

$$H_2 \rightarrow 2H^+ + 2e^- \quad 2H^+ + 2 \rightarrow H_2$$

$$E_{cell} = 0.0591/2 \, \log([H^+]_{cathode}^2)/[10^{-6}]^2$$

$$0.081 = (0.0591) \, \log ([H^+])/10^{-6}$$

$$\log[H^+]_{cathode}/10^{-6} = 0.118/0.0591 = 2$$

$$[H^+]_{cathode}/10^{-6} = 10^2$$

$$[H^+]_{cathode} = 10\text{-}6 = 10\text{-}4 \, M$$

Example. The emf of the cell Ag|AgI in 0.05 M KI solution. NH_4NO_3| 0.05 M $AgNO_3$\Ag is 0.788 volt at 25°C. The activity coefficient of KI and silver nitrate in the above solution is 0.90 each. Calculate (i) the solubility product of AgI, and (ii) the solubility of AgI in pure water at 25°C.

Solution: Ag^+ ion concentration on $AgNO_3$ side

$$= 0.9 \times 0.5 = 0.045 \, M$$

Similarly I^- ion concentration in 0.05 M KI solution

$$= 0.05 \times 0.9 - 0.045 \, M$$

$$E_{cell} = 0.0591/1 \, \log[Ag^+]_{(R.H.S.)}/[Ag^+]_{(L.H.S.)}$$

$$= 0.0591 \, \log 0.045/[Ag^+]_{(L.H.S.)}$$

or $\log 0.045/[Ag^+]_{(L.H.S.)} = 0.788/0.0591 = 13.33$

$$[Ag^+]_{L.H.S.} = 0.045/(2.138 \times 10^{13})$$

$$= 2.105 \times 10^{-15} \, M$$

Solubility product of AgI $= [Ag^+][I^-]$

$$= 2.105 \times 10^{-15} \times 0.045$$

$$= 9.427 \times 10^{-17}$$

Solubility of   AgI $= \checkmark$(Solubility product of AgI)

$$= \checkmark(9.472 \times 0100^{\wedge}(-17) \,)$$

$$= 9.732 \times 10^{-9} \, g \, mol \, L^{-1}$$

$$= 9.732 \times 10^{-9} \times 143.5 \, g \, L^{-1}$$

$$= 1.396 \times 10^{-6} \, gL^{-1}$$

Example: The observed emf of the cell

$$Pt|H_2(1\,atm)|H^+(3 \times 10^{-4}\ M)\|H^+(M_1)|H_2(1\ atm)|Pt$$

is 0.154 V. Calculate the value of M_1 and pH of cathodic solution.

Solution: $E_{cell} = 0.0591 \log M_1/(3\times10^{-4})$

or $\qquad \log M_1/(3\times10^{-4}) = 0.0154/0.0591 = 2.6058$

$$M_1/(3\times10^{-4}) = 4.034 \times 10^2$$

$$M_1 = 4.034 \times 10^2 \times 3 \times 10^{-4}\ M$$

$$= 0.121\ M$$

$$pH = -\log [H^+] = -\log 0.121 = 0.917$$

Example: Calculate the emf of the following cell at 25°C.

$$\text{Pt } H_2|HCl|H_2 \text{ Pt}$$

$$2 \text{ atm} \qquad 10 \text{ atm}$$

Solution: $\qquad E_{cell} = 0.0591/2 \log P_1/P_2$

$$= 0.0591/2 \log 2/10$$

$$= -0.0206 \text{ volt}$$

Buffer Solution

Buffer solutions are those solutions which resist the change in the pH of the solution.

A **buffer solution** is an aqueous solution consisting of a mixture of a weak acid and its conjugate base or a weak base and its conjugate acid. It has the property that the pH of the solution changes very little when a small amount of strong acid or base is added to it. Buffer solutions are used as a means of keeping pH at a nearly constant value in a wide variety of chemical applications. Many life forms thrive only in a relatively small pH range; an example of a buffer solution is blood.

Principles of Buffering

Buffer solutions achieve their resistance to pH due to the presence of a 'reservoir' of both acid HA and conjugate base A^-. In contrast to a buffer, strong acids in solution will be almost entirely in the form of the conjugate base A^-, while weak acids will be predominantly HA. Because the buffering effect depends on the presence of both species, buffer solutions are most effective at pH values near to the pK_a of the acid, where the concentrations are equal.

Adding H^+ to the solution will result in the reaction $H^+ + A^- \rightarrow HA$. Because HA is a weak acid, it will remain mostly in its protonated state, so the increase in free H^+ concentration will be lower than the amount of H^+ added to the solution.

Adding OH^- to the solution will decrease the H^+ concentration by combining with H^+ to form H_2O. However, this will perturb the dissociation equilibrium of HA: $HA \rightleftharpoons H^+ + A^-$, so that more H^+ dissociates from HA to counteract the change.

Calculating Buffer pH

The acid dissociation constant for a weak acid, HA, is defined as

$$K_a = \frac{\left[H^+\right]\left[A^-\right]}{[HA]}.$$

Simple manipulation with logarithms gives the Henderson-Hasselbalch equation, which describes pH in terms of pK_a

$$pH = pK_a + \log_{10}\frac{\left[A^-\right]}{[HA]}.$$

In this equation $[A^-]$ is the concentration of the conjugate base and $[HA]$ is the concentration of the acid. By manipulating this equation, it is possible either to calculate the pH of a buffer solution of known composition, or to calculate the relative concentrations of acid and conjugate base required to achieve a specific pH value. An ICE table can also be used for this purpose. When the concentrations of acid and conjugate base are equal, often described as half-neutralization, $pH = pK_a$.

The *calculated* pH may be different from *measured* pH. Glass electrodes found in common pH meters respond not to the concentration of hydrogen ions ($[H^+]$), but to their activity, which depends on several factors, primarily on the ionic strength of the media. For example, calculation of pH of phosphate-buffered saline would give the value of 7.96, whereas the actual pH is 7.4.

The same considerations apply to a mixture of a weak base, B and its conjugate acid BH^+.

$$B + H_2O\ BH^+ + OH^-.$$

The pK_a value to be used is that of the acid conjugate to the base.

In general a buffer solution may be made up of more than one weak acid and its conjugate base

Applications

Buffer solutions are necessary to keep the correct pH for enzymes in many organisms to work. Many enzymes work only under very precise conditions; if the pH strays too far out of the margin, the enzymes slow or stop working and can denature, thus permanently disabling their catalytic activity.[1] A buffer of carbonic acid (H_2CO_3) and bicarbonate (HCO_3^-) is present in blood plasma, to maintain a pH between 7.35 and 7.45.

Industrially, buffer solutions are used in fermentation processes and in setting the correct conditions for dyes used in colouring fabrics. They are also used in chemical analysis[2] and calibration of pH meters.

The majority of biological samples that are used in research are made in buffers, especially phosphate buffered saline (PBS) at pH 7.4.

Solubility and Solubility product

Solubility product constants are used to describe saturated solutions of ionic compounds of relatively low solubility. A saturated solution is in a state of dynamic equilibrium between the dissolved, dissociated, ionic compound and the undissolved solid.

$$M_xA_y(s) \rightarrow x\ M^{y+}(aq) + y\ A^{x-}(aq)$$

The general equilibrium constant for such processes can be written as:

$$K_c = [M^{y+}]^x[A^{x-}]^y$$

Since the equilibrium constant refers to the product of the concentration of the ions that are present in a saturated solution of an ionic compound, it is given the name *solubility product constant*, and given the symbol K_{sp}. Solubility product constants can be calculated, and used in a variety of applications.

Relation between solubility s (mole/litre) and solubility product (K_{sp})

For binary salt (AB type-NaCl, AgCl, KBr), if solubility is s mole/litre then solubility product(K_{sp})

$$K_{sp} = s.s = s^2\ mole^2/litre^2$$

Similarly for ternary salt like AB_2 or A_2B type ($MgCl_2$, Na_2SO_4)

$$MgCl_2 = Mg^{++} + 2Cl^-\ (if\ solubility\ is\ s\ mole/litre)\ then$$

$$S = s + 2s$$

$$K_{sp} = (Mg^{++})\ (2Cl^-)^2$$

$$= s.(2s)^2 = 4s^3$$

Similarly for salts like

$$Ca_3(PO4)_2 K_{sp} = 108s^5$$

Example: Calculate the solubility product constant for lead (II) chloride, if 50.0 mL of a saturated solution of lead (II) chloride was found to contain 0.2207 g of lead(II) chloride dissolved in it.

- First, write the equation for the dissolving of lead(II) chloride and the equilibrium expression for the dissolving process.

$$PbCl_2(s) \rightarrow Pb^{2+}(aq) + 2\ Cl^-(aq)$$
$$K_{sp} = [Pb^{2+}][Cl^-]^2$$

- Second, convert the amount of dissolved lead(II) chloride into moles per liter.

(0.2207 g $PbCl_2$)(1/50.0 mL solution)(1000 mL/1 L)(1 mol $PbCl_2$/278.1 g $PbCl_2$) = 0.0159 M $PbCl_2$

$$K_{sp} = [0.0159][0.0318]^2 = 1.61 \times 10^{-5}$$

Determining Whether a Precipitate will, or will not Form When Two Solutions are Combined

When two electrolytic solutions are combined, a precipitate may, or may not form. In order to determine whether or not a precipitate will form or not, one must examine two factors. First, determine the possible combinations of ions that could result when the two solutions are combined to see if any of them are deemed "insoluble" base on solubility tables (K_{sp} tables will also do). Second, determine if the concentrations of the ions are great enough so that the reaction quotient Q exceeds the K_{sp} value. One important factor to remember is there is a dilution of all species present and must be taken into account.

Example: 25.0 mL of 0.0020 M potassium chromate are mixed with 75.0 mL of 0.000125 M lead (II) nitrate. Will a precipitate of lead(II) chromate form K_{sp} of lead(II) chromate is 1.8×10^{-14}.

- First, determine the overall and the net-ionic equations for the reaction that occurs when the two solutions are mixed.

$$K_2CrO_4(aq) + Pb(NO_3)_2(aq) \rightarrow 2\ KNO_3(aq) + PbCrO_4(s)$$

$$Pb^{2+}(aq) + CrO_4^{2-}(aq) \rightarrow PbCrO_4(s)$$

The latter reaction can be written in terms of K_{sp} as:

$$PbCrO_4(s) \rightarrow Pb^{2+}(aq) + CrO_4^{2-}(aq)$$
$$Ksp = [Pb^{2+}][CrO_4^{2-}]$$

- Using the dilution equation, $C_1V_1 = C_2V_2$, determine the initial concentration of each species once mixed (before any reaction takes place).

(0.0020 M K_2CrO_4)(25.0 mL) = (C_2)(100.0 mL)

C_2 for K_2CrO_4 = 0.00050 M

Similar calculation for the lead(II) nitrate yields:

C_2 for $Pb(NO_3)_2$ = 0.0000938 M

- Using the initial concentrations, calculate the reaction quotient Q, and compare to the value of the equilibrium constant, K_{sp}.

$Q = (0.0000938 \text{ M } Pb^{2+})(0.00050 \text{ M } CrO_4^{2-}) = 4.69 \times 10^{-8}$

Q is greater than K_{sp} so a precipitate of lead(II) chromate will form.

PRACTICE PROBLEMS: EQUILIBRIUM CONCENTRATIONS

Q. The K_{sp} for AgCl is 1.8×10^{-10}. If Ag^+ and Cl^- are both in solution and in equilibrium with AgCl. What is $[Ag^+]$ if $[Cl^-]$ = .020 M? If Na^+ and Cl^- were both present at 0.0001 $\underline{M}$, would a precipitate occur?

What concentration of Ag^+ would be necessary to bring the concentration of Cl^- to 1.0×10^{-6} M or lower?

Answers: Equilibrium Concentrations

Here are the answers to the questions above.

The K_{sp} for AgCl is 1.8×10^{-10}. If Ag^+ and Cl^- are both in solution and in equilibrium with AgCl. What is $[Ag^+]$ if $[Cl^-]$ = .020 M?

$[Ag^+] = 9.0 - 10^{-9}M$

If Ag^+ and Cl^- were both present at 0.0001 M, would a precipitate occur?

Yes, a precipitate would occur because these concentrations together are higher than what the K_{sp} allows.

What concentration of Ag^+ would be necessary to bring the concentration of Cl^- to 1.0×10^{-6} M or lower?

$[Ag^+] = 9.0 \times 10^{-9}$ M or higher

Using K_{sp}. As A Measure Of the Solubility of a Salt

The value of K_a for an acid is proportional to the strength of the acid.

$$K_a = \frac{[H_3O^+][A^*]}{[HA]}$$

If we find the following K_a values in a table, we can immediately conclude that formic acid is a stronger acid than acetic acid.

Formic acid (HCO$_2$H):

$K_a = 1.8 \times 10^{-4}$

Acetic acid (CH$_3$CO$_2$H):

$$K_a = 1.8 \times 10^{-5}$$

Nernst Distribution Law: [After Walther Hermann Nernst (1864–1941), German physical chemist.] when, at a constant temperature, a solute distributes itself between two immiscible phases, then the ratio of its concentrations in the two phases is constant, and is described by the relation $C_1/C_2 = K$, where C_1 and C_2 are, respectively, the amount of substance concentrations of the solute in phases 1 and 2 at equilibrium, and K is the distribution constant. The law only applies in dilute solution. The Nernst distribution law permits us to determine the most favorable conditions for the extraction of substances from solutions.

Chapter 6
CORROSION

➤ **Definition**
➤ **Types and Mechanism**
➤ **Protection**

GENERAL

Corrosion can be defined as the deterioration of a material, due to its interaction with the surroundings, usually a metal surface is deteriorated due to presence of air and moisture present in the environment. Rusting of iron or steel, blistering of steel, etc. are the examples of corrosion.

Corrosion can be due to gases like oxygen, chlorine sulphur oxides present in the atmosphere, this is known as dry corrosion and it takes place in the absence of moisture while other type of corrosion is wet corrosion which takes place in the presence of moisture. We have all seen corrosion and know that the process produces a new and less desirable material from the original metal and can result in a loss of function of the component or system.

DRY CORROSION

This is decay of metal surface due to generally metal oxide layer formation in the absence of moisture. In this type of corrosion , first electrons are lost from the metal surface and metal cation is formed then in the second step corrosive gaseous atoms accept the electron and form anions. Finally metal cations combine with anions and form metal oxide or halide.

$$M \Rightarrow M^{n+} + ne \qquad \text{... (1)}$$

Like
$$Mg \Rightarrow Mg^{++} + 2e$$

$$O + 2e \Rightarrow O^- \qquad \text{... (2)}$$

or
$$Cl + e \Rightarrow Cl^-$$

finally
$$Mg^{++} + O^- \Rightarrow MgO \text{ (oxide layer formation)}$$

Wet Corrosion

The corrosion product we see most commonly is the rust which forms on the surface of iron or steel. For this to happen the major component of steel, iron (Fe) at the surface of a component undergoes a number of simple changes. Firstly,

$$Fe \Rightarrow Fe^{n+} + n \text{ electrons}$$

the iron atom can lose some electrons and become a positively charged ion. This allows it to bond to other groups of atoms that are negatively charged.

Most common is

$$Fe \Rightarrow Fe^{2+} + 2e$$

Wet iron or steel rusts to give a variant of iron oxide so the other half of the reaction must involve water (H_2O) and oxygen (O_2) something like this

$$O_2 + 2H_2O + 4e^- \Rightarrow 4OH^-$$

This makes sense as we have a negatively charged material that can combine with the iron and electrons, which are produced in the first reaction are used up.

$$Fe^{2+} + 2OH^- \Rightarrow Fe(OH)_2$$

or we can, for clarity, ignore the electrons and write

$$2Fe + O_2 + 2H_2O \Rightarrow 2Fe(OH)_2$$

Iron + Water with oxygen

$\Rightarrow$ Iron Hydroxide, which is dissolved as given in next step

Oxygen dissolves quite readily in water and because there is usually an excess of it, reacts with the iron hydroxide.

$$4Fe(OH)_2 + O_2 \Rightarrow 2H_2O + 2Fe_2O_3.H_2O$$

Iron hydroxide + oxygen $\Rightarrow$ water + Hydrated iron oxide (brown rust)

Electrochemical Corrosion Theory

Electrochemical corrosion involves two half-cell reactions; an oxidation reaction at the **anode** and a reduction reaction at the **cathode**. For iron corroding in water with a near neutral pH, these half cell reactions can be represented as:

Anode reaction: $2Fe \Rightarrow 2Fe^{2+} + 4e^-$

Cathode reaction: $O_2 + 2H_2O + 4e^- \Rightarrow 4OH^-$

There are obviously different anodic and cathodic reactions for different alloys exposed to various environments. These half cell reactions are thought to occur (at least initially) at microscopic anodes and cathodes covering a corroding surface (Fig. 6.1). Macroscopic anodes and cathodes can develop as corrosion damage progresses with time.

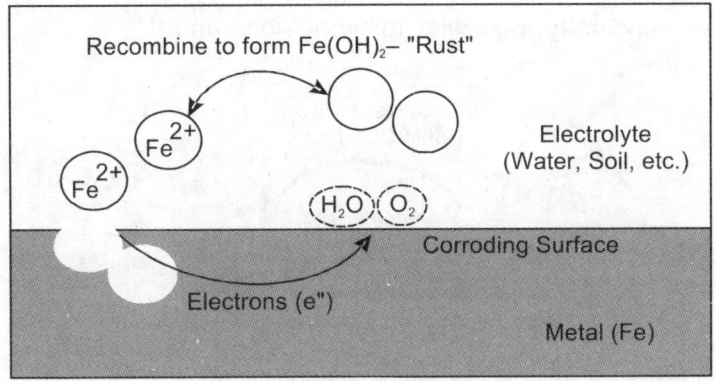

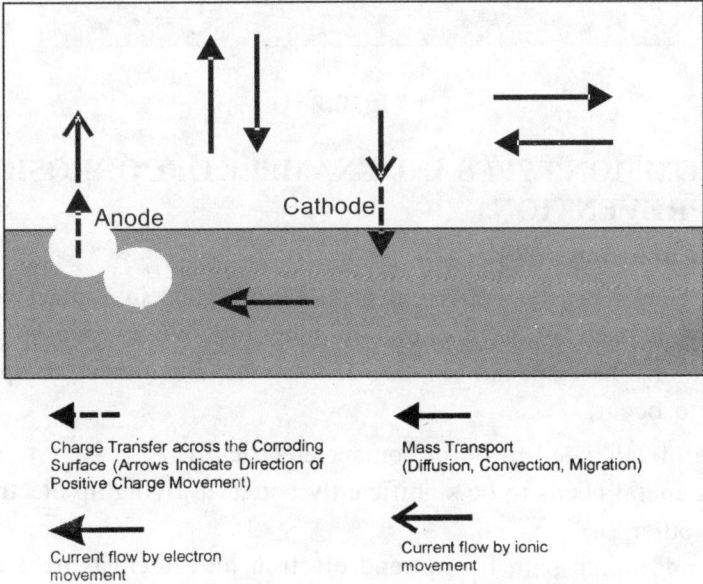

Fig. 6.1

From the above theory it should be apparent that there are four fundamental components in an electrochemical corrosion cell:

- An anode.
- A cathode.
- A conducting environment for ionic movement (electrolyte).

- An electrical connection between the anode and cathode for the flow of electron current

If any of the above components is missing or disabled, the electrochemical corrosion process will be stopped. Clearly, these elements are thus fundamentally important for corrosion control.

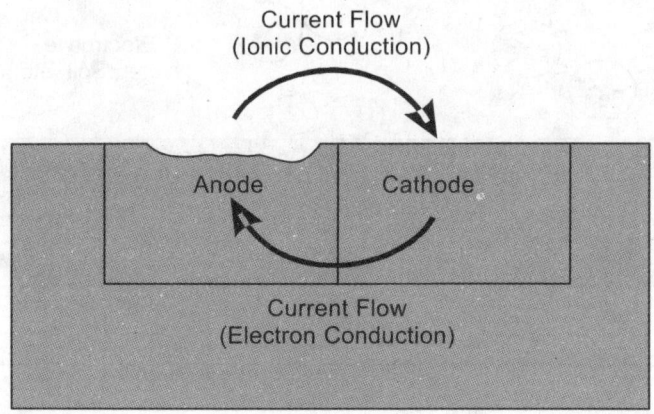

Fig. 6.2

SOME COMMON TYPES AND EXAMPLE OF CORROSION AND THEIR PREVENTION

Galvanic Corrosion

This can occur when two different metals are placed in contact with each other and is caused by the greater willingness of one to give up electrons than the other. Three special features of this mechanism need to operate for corrosion to occur:

* The metals need to be in contact electrically
* One metal needs to be significantly better at giving up electrons than the other
* An additional path for ion and electron movement is necessary.

Prevention of this problem is based on ensuring that one or more of the three features do not exist. Break the electrical contact using plastic insulators or coatings between the metals.

Select metals close together in the galvanic series.Prevent ion movement by coating the junction with an impermeable material, or ensure environment is dry and liquids cannot be trapped.

Pitting Corrosion

Pitting corrosion occurs in materials that have a protective film such as a corrosion product or when a coating breaks down. The exposed metal gives up electrons easily and the reaction initiates tiny pits with localised chemistry supporting rapid attack. Control can be ensured by:

* Selecting a resistant material
* Ensuring a high enough flow velocity of fluids in contact with the material or frequent washing
* Control of the chemistry of fluids and use of inhibitors
* Use of a protective coating
* Maintaining the material's own protective film.

Selective Attack

This occurs in alloys such as brass when one component or phase is more susceptible to attacke than another and corrodes preferentially leaving a porous material that crumbles. It is best avoided by selection of a resistant material but other means can be effective such as:

* Coating the material
* Reducing the aggressiveness of the environment
* Use of cathodic protection

Stray Current Corrosion

When a direct current flows through an unintended path and the flow of electrons supports corrosion. This can occur in soils and flowing or stationary fluids. The most effective remedies involve controlling the current by:

* Insulating the structure to be protected or the source of current
* Earthing sources and/or the structure to be protected.
* Applying cathodic protection
* Using sacrificial targets.

Stress Corrosion Cracking

The combined action of a static tensile stress and corrosion which forms cracks and eventually catastrophic failure of the component. This is specific to a metal material paired with a specific environment. Prevention can be achieved by:

* Reducing the overall stress level and designing out stress concentrations
* Selection of a suitable material not susceptible to the environment
* Design to minimise thermal and residual stresses

    * Developing compressive stresses in the surface the material
    * Use of a suitable protective coating

Microbial Corrosion

This general class covers the degradation of materials by bacteria, moulds and fungi or their by-products. It can occur by a range of actions such as:

Attack of the metal or protective coating by acid by-products, sulphur, hydrogen sulphide or ammonia.Direct interaction between the microbes and metal which sustains attack.

Prevention can be achieved by:

* Selection of resistant materials
* Frequent cleaning
* Control of chemistry of surrounding media and removal of nutrients
* Use of biocides
* Cathodic protection.

GENERAL METHODS OF CONTROL OF CORROSION

Corrosion can be mitigated or prevented by basic methods like coating, cathodic protection, material selection or change of environment. Some important basic methods are described here.

Protection by Coatings

Galvanization: Plating, painting, and the application of enamel are the most common anti-corrosion treatments. They work by providing a barrier of corrosion-resistant material between the damaging environment and the (often cheaper, tougher, and/or easier-to-process) structural material. Aside from cosmetic and manufacturing issues, there are tradeoffs in mechanical flexibility versus resistance to abrasion and high temperature. Platings usually fail only in small sections, and if the plating is more noble than the substrate (for example, chromium on steel), a galvanic couple will cause any exposed area to corrode much more rapidly than an unplated surface would. For this reason, it is often wise to plate with a more active metal such as zinc or cadmium. Painting either by roller or brush is more desirable for tight spaces; spray would be better for larger coating areas such as steel decks and waterfront applications. Flexible polyurethane coating can provide an anti-corrosive seal with a highly durable slip resistant membrane. Painted coatings are relatively easy to apply and have fast drying times although temperature and humidity may cause dry times to vary.

Organic Coatings

The coatings covered are limited to organic paint materials, with the exception of inorganic zinc coatings which are included, because they are most commonly used in conjunction with organic coatings and are applied by spray, like organic coatings. Powder coatings are also described, although their application is somewhat different from typical brush, roller, or spray application.

METHODS BY WHICH COATINGS PROTECT METALS FROM CORROSION

Coatings have three basic mechanisms for protecting metals from corrosion, although more than one of these mechanisms may be used by a coating.

These mechanisms are:

* Cathodic protection
* Corrosion inhibitors.

Barrier Protection

Most coatings provide corrosion protection by forming a barrier relatively impermeable to moisture and electrolytes necessary for corrosion. Obviously, for optimum protection, the barrier should be as impermeable, thick, and continuous as practical.

Cathodic Protection of Steel

Some protective coatings have a high loading of fine zinc particles, so the particles in the cured film are in electrical contact with each other and with the underlying steel. This permits a type of cathodic protection. Presently, two basic types of zinc-rich coatings are used on steel: organic and inorganic products.

Inhibitive Pigments

Some pigments are added to primers to inhibit corrosion at the coating/metal interface. Red lead is the most common example of an inhibitive pigment.

COMPOSITIONS AND PROPERTIES OF COATINGS

Components of Coatings and Their Functions

All ingredients used to formulate a coating can be placed in one of three basic categories: solvent, resin, and pigment. Each of these categories has a special function in the coating's formulation.

Solvent

The solvent is used to dissolve the resin material that actually forms the coating film. It also reduces the viscosity of the product to permit easier application, as well as affecting its leveling, drying, durability, and adhesion. Because the different organic polymers in different resins greatly differ in their solubilities, some resins require much stronger than others to dissolve them. In water-based coatings, the water is a dispersing rather than a dissolving agent.

The emission of virtually all organic solvents in coatings gives rise to photochemical smog. Thus, there is a great pressure to reduce the amount of solvent in coatings or to use water-based coatings.

Resin

The resin is the binder or film-forming part of the coating that is responsible for most of the properties of the coating. Thus, coatings are identified by the generic types of their resins. The resin and the solvent portions of coatings are sometimes called the nonvolatile and the volatile vehicle, respectively, and are sometimes referred to collectively as the vehicle.

Pigment

The pigment constitutes the solid portion of a coating. It is generally heavier than the liquid vehicle portion and may settle out on prolonged standing. Pigments are usually modified or unmodified natural earth materials, although less stable organic pigments are occasionally used. The chief function of the pigment is to provide opacity (hiding) to protect the organic vehicle from degradation by sunlight. Titanium is the pigment most frequently used to give opacity to white paints and light tints. Pigments also provide color, improve adhesion and weather resistance, decrease moisture permeability, and control gloss. Leafing pigments, such as aluminum, tend to form parallel plates in the film to effectively increase its thickness by increasing the path moisture must penetrate. Other things being equal, the finer the pigment particle size and the less the pigment/resin ratio, the glossier will be the coating.

The pigment and the resin portions are sometimes called the solids portion, since they remain after all the solvent has evaporated. Obviously, the greater the coating solids, the greater will be the dry film thickness received from a given wet film thickness. There are also many additives or extenders added to coatings to modify gloss or consistency, emulsify components, improve weathering, or obtain some other desirable

Reactive coatings

If the environment is controlled (especially in recirculating systems), corrosion inhibitors can often be added to it. These form an electrically insulating and/or chemically impermeable coating on exposed metal surfaces, to suppress electrochemical reactions. Such methods obviously make the system less sensitive to scratches or defects in the coating, since extra inhibitors can be made available wherever metal becomes exposed. Chemicals that inhibit corrosion include some of the salts in hard water (Roman water systems are famous for their mineral deposits), chromates, phosphates, polyaniline, other conducting polymers and a wide range of specially-designed chemicals that resemble surfactants (i.e. long-chain organic molecules with ionic end groups)..

Anodization-Aluminium alloys often undergo a surface treatment. Electrochemical conditions in the bath are carefully adjusted so that uniform pores several nanometers wide appear in the metal's oxide film. These pores allow the oxide to grow much thicker than passivating conditions would allow. At the end of the treatment, the pores are allowed to seal, forming a harder-than-usual surface layer. If this coating is scratched, normal passivation processes take over to protect the damaged area. Anodizing is very resilient to weathering and corrosion, so it is commonly used for building facades and other areas that the surface will come into regular contact with the elements. Whilst being resilient, it must be cleaned frequently. If left without cleaning Panel Edge Staining will naturally occur.

Electroplating

The process of coating an inferior metal with a superior metal by electrolysis is known as electroplating.

The aims of electroplating are:

(i) To prevent the inferior metal from corrosion.

(ii) To make it more attractive in appearance.

The object to be electroplated is made the cathode and block of the metal to be deposited is made the anode in an electrolytic bath containing a solution of a salt of the anodic metal. On passing electric current in the cell, the metal of the anode dissolves out and is deposited on the cathode-article in the form of a thin film. The following are the requirements for fine coating:

(i) The surface of the article should be free from greasy matter and its oxide layer. The surface is cleaned with chromic acid or detergents.

(ii) The surface of the article should be rough so that the metal deposited sticks permanently.

(iii) The concentration of the electrolyte should be so adjusted as to get smooth coating.

(iv) Current density must be the same throughout.

Table is given below for suistable selection of cathode/anaode and electrolyte for electroplating.

For electroplating	Anode	Cathode	Electrolyte
With copper	Cu	Object	$CuSo_4$ + dilute H_2So_4
With silver	Ag	Object	$KAg(CN)_2$
With nickel	Ni	Object	Nickel ammonium sulphate
With gold	Au	Object	$KAu(CN)_2$
With zinc	Zn	Object	$ZnSO_4$
With thin	Sn	Iron objects	$SnSO_4$

Cathodic protection

Cathodic protection (CP) is a technique to control the corrosion of a metal surface by making that surface the cathode of an electrochemical cell. Cathodic protection systems are most commonly used to protect steel, water, and fuel pipelines and tanks; steel pier piles, ships, and offshore oil platforms.

Sacrificial anode protection

A sacrificial anode is a block of metal that is more reactive than the metal of material to be protected like for the protection of ship material Zinc is used as sacrificial anode. Metal having more negative standard reduction potential is used as a sacrificial anode, since it is more susceptible for oxidation i.e. easily oxidised. Samemethod is used for the protection of pipe lines in sea/underground. Generally Mg metal hollow sphere or cylinder is used as sacrificial anode. This metal is replaced after definite time intervals for continuous protection of pipe lines. If we wrap zinc around an iron nail the nail is protected from rusting. Notice that the iron docs not have to be completely covered in order to be fully protected. This is a real advantage to using a sacrificial anode. iron. The more reactive a metal is the easier it gives away electrons. This reactive block of metal acts as a source of electrons for the iron. When oxygen takes electrons from the iron during the process of rusting iron atoms simply take electrons from the reactive metal.

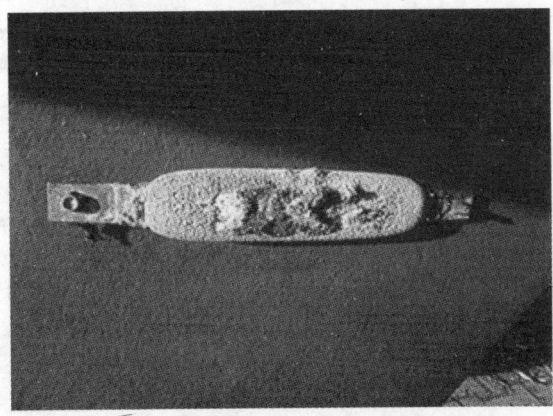

Fig. 6.3: Sacrificial anode in the hull of a ship

The hulls of large sea vessels use small zinc blocks placed at regular intervals to prevent rust. Periodically these zinc blocks have to be replaced as they corrode away.

Impressed Current Cathodic Protection

For larger structures, galvanic anodes cannot economically deliver enough current to provide complete protection. Impressed Current Cathodic Protection (ICCP) systems use anodes connected to a DC power source (such as a cathodic protection rectifier). Anodes for ICCP systems are tubular and solid rod shapes of various specialized materials. These include high silicon cast iron, graphite, mixed metal oxide or platinum coated titanium or niobium coated rod and wires.

Anodic protection

Anodic protection (AP) is a technique to control the corrosion of a metal surface by making it the anode of an electrochemical cell and controlling the electrode potential in a zone where the metal is passive.

AP is used to protect metals that exhibit passivation in environments whereby the current density in the freely corroding state is significantly higher than the current density in the passive state over a wide range of potentials.

Anodic protection is used for carbon steel storage tanks containing extreme pH environments including concentrated sulfuric acid and 50 percent caustic soda where cathodic protection is not suitable due to very high current requirements.

An anodic protection system includes an external power supply connected to auxiliary cathodes and controlled by a feedback from reference electrode. Careful design and control is required when using anodic protection for several reasons, including excessive current when passivation is lost or unstable, leading to possible accelerated corrosion.

Anodic protection impresses anodic current on the structure to be protected (opposite to the cathodic protection). It is appropriate for metals that exhibit passivity (e.g., stainless steel) and suitably small passive current over a wide range of potentials. It is used in aggressive environments, e.g., solutions of sulfuric acid.

Chapter 7
WATER CHEMISTRY

➢ **Water**
➢ **Hardness as Impurities**
➢ **Determination of Hardness**
➢ **Types of hardness,**
➢ **External Treatment of Water:**
  ● **Lime Soda Method**
  ● **Ion Exchange Method**
  ● **Zeolite Method**
  ● **Reverse Osmosis**
➢ **Internal Treatment of Water:**
  ● **Calgon Method**
➢ **Numerical Problems**

WATER

Life cannot be imagine without water. For the existence of all living beings (humans, animals or plants) water is essential. Without water we cannot survive. Almost all human activities- domestic, agricultural and industrial demand use of water. Although water is nature's most wonderful and abundant compound but only less than 1% of the world's water resources are available for drinking purpose.Drinking water should be free from impurities and microbial contamination. Any thing present in the water sample other than H_2O is termed as impurity.

There are various sources of water like Surface water, Underground water, rain water, sea water tec. Surface water includes flowing water (streams and rivers) and still water (lakes, ponds and reservoirs) while underground water includes wells and springs.

Any water sample taken from any source contains dissolved minerals like chlorides, sulphates, bicarbonates of sodium, magnesium and iron. It also contains suspended impurities of sand and rock and organic matter.

Impurities in Water

The following types of impurities are present in water:

1. **Suspended Impurities:** These impurities are in the form of suspended material which impart turbidity, colour and odour to water. It may be clay or silica, oily matter, vegetable and animal matter. These are termed as total suspended solids, which can be removed by proper filtration.

2. **Dissolved Impurities:** These impurities are in the soluble form. It may be due to the presence of dissolved salts like carbonates, bicarbonates, chlorides and sulphates of calcium, magnicium, iron and sodium. This is termed as total dissolved solids (TDS). Hardness in water is due to the presence of these salts. Dissolved gases like O_2, CO_2 etc, also come under this category.

3. **Microorganisms:** They include bacterias, fungi and algae.

HARDNESS OF WATER

Hardness in water is the characteristic, "which prevents the lathering of soap". It may be defined as the soap consuming capacity of water sample, since more the hardness, more soap will be consumed. Hardness is due to the presence of certain salts of Ca, Mg and other heavy metal ions like Al^{3+}, Fe^{3+} and Mn^{2+}. A sample of hard water, when treated with soap (sodium or potassium salt of higher fatty acid like $C_{17}H_{35}COONa$) does not produce lather, but forms insoluble white precipitate which do not posssess any detergent action. Typical reactions of sodium stearate with calcium chloride and magnesium sulphate (hardness producing salt present in the water) are shown below:

$2C_{17}H_{35}COONa$ $+$ $CaCl_2$ $\rightarrow$ $(C_{17}H_{35}COO)_2Ca \downarrow + 2NaCl$
Soap (sodium stearate)   (Hardness)   Calcium stearate   (Insoluble)

$2C_{17}H_{35}COONa$ $+$ $MgSO_4$ $\rightarrow$ $(C_{17}H_{35}COO)_2Mg + Na_2SO_4$
Soap   (Hardness)   Magnesium stearate (Insoluble)

In fact, any cation which produces insoluble matter with soap solution will contribute to hardness. Thus, on this basis water can be classified into two types: viz., Hard and Soft water. Generally soft water contains less than 100 ppm TDS and hardness while hardwater has more TDS.

Types of Hardness

Hardness is of two types, temporary and permanent.

(1) Temporary hardness is caused due to the presence of dissolved bicarbonates of calcium, magnesium and other heavy metals. Thus main salts responsible for temporary hardness are $Ca(HCO_3)_2$ and $Mg(HCO_3)_2$. This type of hardness can be removed by boiling the water, when bicarbonates are decomposed, yielding insoluble carbonates and hydroxides, which are deposited as precipitate in the bottom of container. Since this is alkaline hardness hence can be determined by titration with HCl using methyl orange as indicator.

$$Ca(HCO_3)_2 = {}^{boiling}CaCO_3 + CO_2$$
$$Mg(HCO_3)_2 = {}^{boiling} Mg(OH)_2 + 2CO_2$$

(2) **Permanent Hardness**—It is due to the presence of dissolved chlorides, sulphates and nitrates of calcium, magnesium, iron and other heavy metals. Hence, the main salts responsible for permanent hardness are: $CaCl_2$, $MgCl_2$, $CaSO_4$, $MgSO_4$, $FeSO_2$, $Al_2(SO_4)_3$. Unlike temporary hardness, permanent hardness is not destroyed on boiling. It is also known as non-carbonate or non-alkaline hardness.

Advantages of Hard Water

The taste of hard water is usually better than soft water. The label on the bottle of mineral water shows that it contains Mg^{2+} and Ca^{2+} ions and it tastes good. The dissolved calcium in hard water can help to produce strong teeth and healthy bones.

Disadvantages of Hard Water

Hard water produce scum with soap. Thus, the washed clothes look dull. Efficiency of soap decreases in hard water so economy decreases. Boiler feed water should be free from hardness otherwise even explosion can occur.

Degree of Hardness

Although hardness of water is never present in the form of calcium carbonate because it is insoluble in water, hardness of water is conveniently expressed in terms of equivalent amount (equivalents) of $CaCO_3$ as its molecular weight is perfect 100 (eq.wt-50). Moreover, it is the most insoluble salt that can be precipitated in water treatment.

CaCO equivalent of hardness =

$$\text{Wt. of substance producing hardness} \times \frac{\text{Mol. wt. of } CaCO_3(100)}{\text{Mol. wt. of substance}}$$

$$\text{Or} = \text{Wt. of substance producing hardness} \times \frac{\text{Eq. wt. of CaCO}_3 (50)}{\text{Eq. wt. of substance}}$$

Problem: What are the parameters for checking water quality for domestic use.

Ans. The parameters for checking water quality for domestic use follows as:

   (i) Water should not contain hardness (not more than 300 ppm)

   (ii) Turbidity should not be more than 10 ppm.

   (iii) pH of domestic water should be around 7.5 – 8.0.

   (iv) Coloured impurities should not be more than 20 ppm.

   (v) It should not contain dissolved solids more than 500 ppm any how, desirable is less than 100 ppm.

Problem: Given atomic weights of elements as H = 1, C = 12, N = 14, O = 16, Na = 23, Mg = 24, Al = 27, S = 32, Cl = 35.5, Ca = 40, Fe = 56. Find multiplication factor for converting into equivalents of $CaCO_3$.

For $Ca(HCO_3)_2$, $Mg(HCO_3)_2$, $CaSO_4$, $CaCl_2$, $MgSO_4$, $MgCl_2$, $MgCO_3$, CO_2, $Mg(NO_3)_2$, HCO^-_3, OH^-, $NaAlO_2$, $Al_2(SO_4)_3$ and $FeSO_4. 7H_2O$

Table 7.1

Constituent salt/ion	Molar Mass	n-factor	Chemical equivalent Molar mass = n-factor	Multiplication factor for converting into equivalent of $CaCO_3$
$Ca(HCO_3)_2$,	162	2	162/2 = 81	100/(2 × 81) = 100/162
$Mg(HCO_3)_2$,	146	2	146/2 = 73	100/(2 × 73) = 100/146
$CaSO_4$,	136	2	136/2 = 68	100/(2 × 68) = 100/136
$CaCl_2$,	120	2	120/2 = 60	100/(2 × 60) = 100/120
$MgSO_4$,	111	2	111/2 = 55.5	100/(2 × 55.5) = 100/111
$MgCl_2$,	95	2	95/2 = 417.5	100/(2 × 47.5) = 95100/
$MgCO_3$,	84	2	84/2 = 42	100/(2 × 4842) = 100/
CO_2,	44	2	44/2 = 22	100/(2 × 2244) = 100/
$Mg(NO_3)_2$,	148	2	148/2 = 74	100/(2 × 74)148 = 100/
HCO^-_3,	61	1	61/1 = 61	100/(2 × 61) = 122100/
OH^-,	17	1	17/1 = 17	100/(2 × 17) = 13400/
CO_3^{-2},	60	2	60/2 = 30	100/(2 × 30) = 10600/
$NaAlO_2$,	82	1	82/1 = 82	100/(2 × 82) = 100164/
$Al_2(SO_4)_3$,	342	6	342/6 = 57	100/(2 × 57) = 100/114
$FeSO_4, 7H_2O$,	278	2	278/2 = 139	100/(2 × 139) = 100/278

(i) **Parts per million (ppm):** It is defined as the number of parts by weight of calcium carbonate present per million (10^6) parts by weight of water,

i.e., 1 ppm = 1 part of $CaCO_3$ equivalents hardness in (10^6) parts of water.

(ii) **Milligrams per litre (mg/L):** It is defined as the number of milligrams of $CaCO_3$ present in one litre of water,

i.e, 1 mg/L = 1 mg of $CaCO_3$ equivalent per liter of water. It can be easily proved that 1 mg/L = 1 ppm for water

As for water, 1L = 1kg = 10^6mg

∴ 1mg of $CaCO_3$ eq-hardness per L of water

= 1mg of $CaCO_3$ eq-hardness per 10^6mg of water

= 1 part of $CaCO_3$ per 10^6 parts of water = 1 ppm

Hence, 1mg/L = 1 ppm

(iii) Degree clarke (^0Cl) : It is defined as the parts of $CaCO_3$ equivalent per 70,000 parts of water.

Or It is number of grains of $CaCO_3$ equivalent hardness per gallon of water

i.e., 1^0Cl = 1 part of $CaCO_3$ per 70,000 parts of water.

(iv) Degree French (^0Fr) : It is defined as the parts of $CaCO_3$ equivalent hardness per 10^5 parts of water.

i.e., ^0Fr = 1 part of $CaCO_3$ equivalent hardness per 10^5 parts of water.

Relationship between various units of hardness :

As 1 ppm = 1 part per 10^6 parts of water.

1 ^0Fr = 1 part per 10^5 parts of water.

1 ^0Cl = 1 part per 70,000 parts of water.

and

∴ 10^6 ppm = 10^5 ^0Fr = 70,000 ^0Cl

Hence, 1ppm = 0.1 ^0Fr = 0.07 ^0Cl = 1mg/L.

↘ / ↓	ppm	mg/l	^0Fr	^0Cl
ppm	1	1	0.1	0.07
mg/l	1	1	0.1	0.07
^0Fr	10	10	1	0.7
^0Cl	0.07	0.07	0.7	1

Examples based on Determination of Hardness of Water

Example –

A water sample contains 200 mg of $CaSO_4$ per liter. Calculate the hardness in terms of $CaCO_3$ equivalents.

Solution:

$$\text{Hardness} = (\text{strength of } CaSO_4 \text{ in mg/L}) \times \text{multiplication factor}$$

$$= (\text{strength of } CaSO_4 \text{ in mg/L}) \times [\text{chemical equivalent}$$

$$\text{of } CaCO_3/ \text{ chemical equivalent of } CaSO_4]$$

$$= (200 \text{ mg/L}) \times \frac{[50]}{68} = 147 \text{ mg/L} = 147 \text{ ppm}$$

Expample –

How many gram of $MgCO_3$ dissolved per liter gives 44 ppm of hardness?

Solution:

$$\text{Hardness} = (\text{strength of } MgCO_3 \text{ in mg/L}) \times [\text{Chemical equivalents}$$

$$\text{of } CaCO_3/\text{Chemical equivalents of } MgCO_3]$$

Hence, strength of

$$MgCO_3 = \text{Hardness} \times \text{Chemical equivalents of } MgCO_3$$

Chemical equivalents of $CaCO_3$

$$= (44 \text{ ppm}) \times \frac{[42]}{50} = 36.96 \text{ ppm} = 30.96 \text{ mg/L}$$

Thus, 30.96×10^{-3} gms of $MgCO_3$ dissolved per litre gives 84ppm of hardness.

Example:

A sample of water on analysis was found to contain the following impurities:

Impurity	$Ca(HCO_3)_2$	$Mg(HCO_3)_2$	$CaSO_4$	$MgSO_4$
Quantity (mg/L)	24	20	16	10
Mol. Wt.	162	146	136	120

Calculate the temporary, permanent and total hardness of water, in ppm, ^0Fr and ^0Cl.

Solution: Step (i) Conversion into $CaCO_3$ equivalents.

Constituent	Amount mg/L [A]	Multiplication factor [M]	CaCO₃ equivalent = [A] × [M]
$Ca(HCO_3)_2$	24	100/162	$24 \times \dfrac{100}{162} = 14.81$ mg/L
$Mg(HCO_3)_2$	20	100/146	$20 \times \dfrac{100}{146} = 13.69$ mg/L
$CaSO_4$	16	100/136	$16 \times \dfrac{100}{136} = 11.76$ mg/L
$MgSO_4$	10	100/120	$10 \times \dfrac{100}{120} = 8.33$ mg/L

Step (ii) Determination for Temporary Hardness :

As Temporary hardness is due to bicarbonates of Calcium and Magnesium

$\therefore$ Temporary hardness = 14.81 + 13.69 = 28.5 mg/L

As $\qquad$ 1 mg/L = 1 ppm = 0.1 ^{0}Fr = 0.07 ^{0}Cl

Hence,

$\qquad$ Temporary hardness = 28.5ppm or

$$= 28.5 \times 0.1 = 2.85^0 Fr$$
$$28.5 \times 0.07 = 1.995 \ ^0Cl$$

Step (ii) Determination for Permanent Hardness:

As permanent hardness is this case is due to $CaSO_4$ and $MgSO_4$

$\therefore$ Permanent hardness = 11.76 + 8.33 = 20.09 mg/L

$$= 20.09 \text{ ppm} = 20.09 \times 0.1 = 2.009 \ ^0Fr$$
$$= 20.09 \times 0.07 = 01.4063 \ ^0Cl$$

BOILER FEED WATER (WATER FOR STEAM GENERATION)

Water is mainly used in boilers for the generation of steam (for industries and power houses). For such water all the impurities are not necessarily eliminated, and only those impurities which lead to operational troubles in boilers are eliminated or kept within the tolerable limits.

Boiler water specification:

(i) Its hardness should be below 0.2 ppm.

(ii) Its caustic alkalinity (due to OH⁻) should lie in between 0.15 and 0.45 ppm.

(iii) Its soda alkalinity (due to Na_2CO_3) should be 0.45 − 1 ppm.

Excess of impurities, if present, in boiler feed water generally cause the following problems : Scale and sludge formation, corrosion, priming and foaming, caustic embitterment.

BOILER PROBLEMS

Sludge and Scale Formation in Boilers

In a boiler, water is continuously evaporated to form steam. This increases the concentration of dissolved salts. Finally a stage is reached when the ionic product of these salts exceeds their solubility product and hence they are thrown out as precipitates.

If the precipitates formed are soft loose and slimy, these are known as sludges; while if the precipitate is hard and adhering on the inner walls, it is called as scale.

The essential differences are given:

Differences between Sludges and Scales

S.No.	Sludges	Scales
1.	Sludges are soft, loose and slimy precipitate.	Scales are hard deposits.
2.	They are non-adherent deposits and can be easily removed to remove.	They stick very firmly to the inner surface of boiler and are very difficult
3.	Formed by substances like $CaCl_2$, $MgCl_2$, $MgSO_4$, $MgCO_3$	Formed by substance like $CaSO_4$, $Mg(OH)_2$ etc.
4.	Formed at comparatively colder portions of the boiler	Formed generally at heated portions of the boiler
5.	They decrease the efficiency of boiler but are less dangerous	Decrease the efficiency of boiler and chances of explosions are also there.
6.	Can be removed by blow-drawn operation	Cannot be removed by blows-down operation.

Priming and Foaming

When steam is produced rapidly in the boilers, some droplets of the liquid water are carried along with the steam. This process of 'wet-steam' formation, is called priming. **Priming** refers to the propulsion of water into the steam drum by extremely rapid, almost explosive boiling of the water at the heating surfaces.

Foaming is the formation of small but persistent foam or bubbles at the water surface in boilers, which do not break easily. Foaming is caused by the presence of an oil and alkails in boiler –feed water. Actually oils and alkalis react to form soaps which greatly lowers the surfaces tension of water and thus increase the foaming tendency of the liquid.

Boiler Corrosion

Boiler corrosion is "decay" or "disintegration" of boiler body material due to chemical or electrochemical reaction with its environment having O_2, CO_2 and mineral acids.

The disadvantages of corrosion are :

   (i) Shortening of boiler life

  (ii) leakages of the joints and rivets;

 (iii) increased cost of repairs and maintenance.

Corrosion in boilers is due to following reasons.

Caustic Embritlement

Caustic embrittlement is the phenomenon during which the boiler material becomes brittle due to the accumulation of caustic substances. This type of boiler corrosion is caused by the use of highly alkaline water in the high pressure boiler.

TREATMENT OF WATER OR SOFTENING OF WATER:

The process whereby we remove or reduce the hardness of water, irrespective of whether it is temporary or permanent is termed as 'softening' of water. It is very essential process since hard water is unsuitable for domestic as well as industrial use. One of the most important applications of water is in steam production for the generation of electricity. For this water need to be fed to industrial boilers. We just cannot feed any water into the industrial boilers because it has been identified that hard water creates large numbers of problems like scale and sludge formation, priming and foaming etc.

The hardness causing salts can be removed from water broadly by following two ways :

  (a) External treatment, and

  (b) Internal treatment

The External treatment of water is carried out before its entry into the boiler. This treatment prevents boiler problems. It can be done by lime-soda, zeolite, RO or ion-exchange processes.While Internal treatment is done in the boiler by the addition of chemicals known as conditioning of water. This is essentially a corrective method of remove those salts which are not completely removed by external treatment of water softening. Colloidal, Phosphate, Calgon and Carbonate conditioning methods are used in the Internal treatment .

Internal Treatment of Water

Internal treatment can constitute the unique treatment when boilers operate at low or moderate pressure, when large amounts of condensed steam are used for feed water, or when good quality raw water is available. The purpose of an internal treatment is to

(1) react with any feed-water hardness and prevent it from precipitating on the boiler metal as scale;

(2) condition any suspended matter such as hardness sludge or iron oxide in the boiler and make it non-adherent to the boiler metal;

(3) provide anti-foam protection to allow a reasonable concentration of dissolved and suspended solids in the boiler water without foam carry-over;

(4) eliminate oxygen from the water and provide enough alkalinity to prevent boiler corrosion.

In addition, as supplementary measures an internal treatment should prevent corrosion and scaling of the feed-water system and protect against corrosion in the steam condensate systems. During the conditioning process, which is an essential complement to the water treatment program, specific doses of conditioning products are added to the water.

The commonly used products include:

- **Phosphates-dispersants, polyphosphates-dispersants (softening chemicals):** Reacting with the alkalinity of boiler water, these products neutralize the hardness of water by forming tricalcium phosphate, and insoluble compound that can be disposed and blow down on a continuous basis or periodically through the bottom of the boiler.

- **Natural and synthetic dispersants (Anti-scaling agents):** increase the dispersive properties of the conditioning products. They can be:
  - o Natural polymers: lignosulphonates, tannins
  - o Synthetic polymers: polyacrilates, maleic acrylate copolymer, maleic styrene copolymer, polystyrene sulphonates etc.

- **Sequestering agents**: such as inorganic phosphates, which act as inhibitors and implement a threshold effect.
- **Oxygen scavengers**: sodium sulphite, tannis, hydrazine, hydroquinone/progallol-based derivatives, hydroxylamine derivatives, hydroxylamine derivatives, ascorbic acid derivatives, etc. These scavengers, catalyzed or not, reduce the oxides and dissolved oxygen. Most also passivate metal surfaces. The choice of product and the dose required will depend on whether a deaerating heater is used.
- **Anti-foaming or anti-priming agents**: mixture of surface-active agents that modify the surface tension of a liquid, remove foam and prevent the carry over of fine water particles in the steam.
- **Softening** chemicals used include soda ash, caustic and various types of sodium phosphates, calgon(SHMP). These chemicals react with calcium and magnesium compounds in the feed water to separate Softening chemicals may be added continuously or intermittently depending on feed-water hardiness and other factors. Chemicals added to react with dissolved oxygen (sulphate, hydrazine, etc.) and chemicals used to prevent scale and corrosion in the feed-water system (polyphosphates, organics, etc.) should be fed in the feed-water system as continuously as possible.
- Internal treatment involves addition of chemical to the boiler water either to precipitate the scale forming impurities in the form of sludges, which can be easily removed or convert the impurities to soluble compounds, so that scale formation can be avoided. Important internal treatments involve.
- *Colloidal Conditioning:* Organic substances like kerosene, tannin, agar-agar are addedto form gels and form loose non-sticky deposits with scale-forming precipitates, whichcan be easily removed by blow-down operations in low pressure boilers.Different sodium phosphates like NaH_2PO_4, $Na_2HPO_4$and Na_3PO_4
- are added to high pressure boilers to react with the hardness forming impurities to form soft sludge of calcium and magnesium phosphates and finally this can be removed by blow down operation.
- $3CaCl_2 + 2Na_3PO_4 \rightarrow Ca_3(PO4)_2 + 6NaCl$
- *Carbonate conditioning:*
- Sodium carbonate is added to the water of low pressure boiler whereby the scale forming $CaSO_4$ gets converted to loose sludge of $CaCO_3$,which can be easily removed by blow-down operation.
- $CaSO_4 + Na_2CO_3 = CaCO_3 + Na_2SO_4$

- *Calgon conditioning:*
- Calgon conditioning–"Calgon" the original product consisted of powdered sodium hexametaphosphate (amorphous sodium poly-phospate), its name was derived from the phrase "calcium gone", originally promoted for general use in bathing and cleaning, it gave rise to derivative products which have diverged from the original composition. It forms complex with ambient calcium ion and certain other cations, preventing formation of unwanted salts and interference by those cations with the actions of soap or other detergents.
- In calgon conditioning, sodium hexa metaphosphate (SHMP) is added in boiler water to prevent the formation of scale and sludge. Calgon removes scale forming Ca^{+2} i.e. it converts insoluble sludge into soluble complex. This treatment can be done in both hot and cold conditions.
- $Na_2 [Na_4(PO_3)_6] \rightleftharpoons 2Na^+ + [Na_4)PO_3)_6]^{-2}$
- $[Na_4 (PO_3)_6]^{-2} + 2CaSO_4 \rightleftharpoons [Ca_2(PO_3)_6]^{-2} + 4Na^+$
- Or $2CaSO_4 + [Na_4P_6O_{18}]^{2-} \rightleftharpoons [Ca_2P_6O_{18}]^{2-} + 2Na_2SO_4$
- Calgon *i.e.*, sodium hexa meta phosphate when added to very hot boilerwater then SHMP is converted into sodium orthophosphate which reacts with Calcium salts to form calcium orthophosphate (CaP_2O_7) which is loose sludge, then it can be removed by blow down of boiler.
- $CaSO_4 + Na_2P_2O_7 \rightleftharpoons CaP_2O_7 + Na_2SO_4$
  Picture of boiler is shown in figure 7.1.

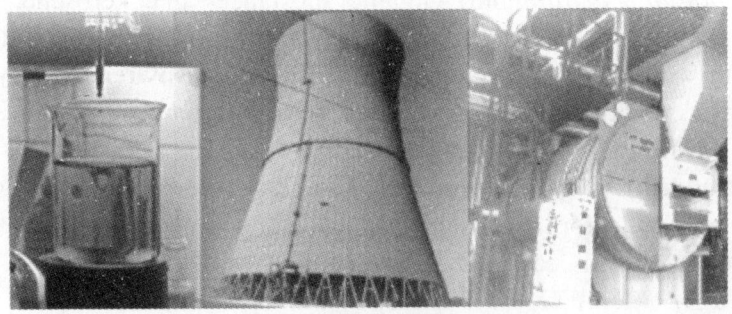

Fig. 7.1: Boiler

EXTERNAL TREATMENT

It can be done by the following methods :

(i) Lime-soda process

    (ii) Zeolite process

  (iii) Ion Exchange process

  (iv) Reverse Osmosis

Lime Soda Process (L-S Process)

The basic principle of this process is to add Lime($Ca(OH)_2$ and Soda (Na_2CO_3) to convert all the soluble hardness into insoluble precipitates which then may be removed by settling and filtration. A calculated amount of Lime ($Ca(OH)_2$ and sodium carbonate, Na_2CO_3, (soda) is added in the hard water. Proper mixing of the chemicals and water is carried out. Calcium carbonate, $CaCO_3$; magnesium hydroxide, $Mg(OH_2)$; ferric hydroxide, $Fe(OH_3)$ and aluminum hydroxide, $Al(OH)_3$ are precipitated, which are filtered off.

    Calcium hardness is precipitated as calcium carbonate. Magnesium hardness is precipitated as magnesium hydroxide ($Mg(OH)_2$). These precipitates are then removed by conventional processes of coagulation/flocculation, sedimentation, and filtration. Because precipitates are very slightly soluble, some hardness remains in the water—usually about 50 to 85 mg/l (as $CaCO_3$). This hardness level is desirable to prevent corrosion problems associated with water being too soft and having little or no hardness. At room temperature, the precipitates formed are very fine. They do not settle down easily and cause difficulty in filtration. If small amount of coagulants like Alum [K_2SO_4. $Al_2(SO_4)_3$. $24H_2O$]; Aluminum sulphate [$Al_2(SO_4)_3$] or Sodium aluminate [$NaAlO_2$] are added, they hydrolyse to precipitate of aluminum hydroxide which entraps the fine precipitate of $CaCO_3$ and $Mg(OH)_2$. Thus coagulant helps in the formation of coarse precipitates.

Lime Addition

Hardness Lime Precipitate

    $CO_2 + Ca(OH)_2 \rightarrow CaCO_3 + H_2O$

    $Ca(HCO_3)_2 + Ca(OH)_2 \rightarrow 2CaCO_3 + 2H_2O$

    $Mg(HCO_3)_2 + Ca(OH)_2 \rightarrow CaCO_3 + MgCO_3 + 2H_2O$

    $MgCO_3 + Ca(OH)_2 \rightarrow CaCO_3 + Mg(OH)_2$

    CO_2 does not contribute to the hardness, but it reacts with the lime, and therefore uses up some lime before the lime can start removing the hardness.

Lime and Soda Ash Addition

$$MgSO_4 + Ca(OH)_2 \rightarrow Mg(OH)_2 \text{ (ppt)} + CaSO_4$$

$$CaSO_4 + Na_2CO_3 \text{ (Soda ash)} \rightarrow CaCO_3 \text{ (ppt)} + Na_2SO_4$$

For each molecule of calcium bicarbonate hardness removed, one molecule of lime is used. For each molecule of magnesium bicarbonate hardness removed, two molecules of lime are used. For each molecule of non-carbonate calcium hardness removed, one molecule of soda ash is used. For each molecule of non-carbonate magnesium hardness removed one molecule of lime plus one molecule of soda ash is used.

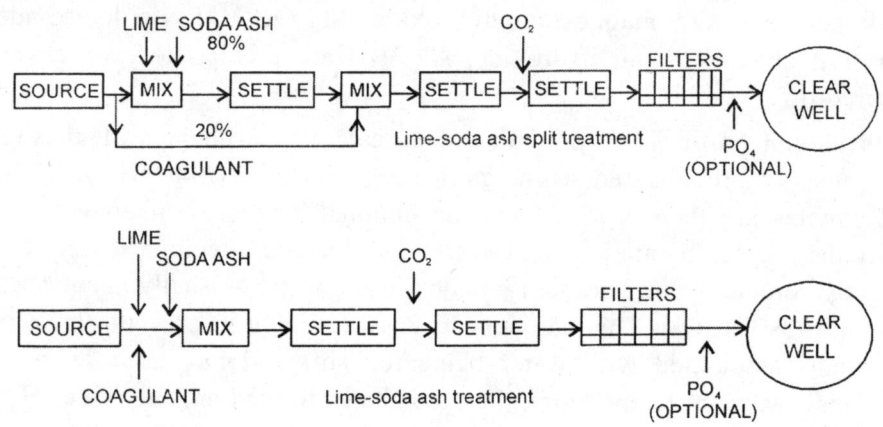

Fig. 7.2

Hot and Cold Process

If L-S Process is used at 3o-40°C temperature, then it is normally termed as Cold process, if at 60-70°C, then it is known as hot process. In cold process requirement of Lime and soda is more and efficiency may be low while in hot process, some steam may by supplied in the water and requirement of chemical is low, efficiency is high .

CALCULATIONS OF THE REQUIREMENT OF LIME AND SODA

Rules for solving numerical problems on lime-soda requirements for softening of hard water:

1. The units in which the impurities are analyzed and expressed are to be noted.

2. Substances which do not contribute towards hardness (KCl, NaCl, SiO_2, Na_2SO_4 etc.) should be ignored and explicitly stated.

3. A substances causing "hardness should be converted into their respective $CaCO_3$ equivalents.

   $CaCO_3$ equivalent of hardness causing impurity .

   = 100 × wt. of the impurity/2 × chemical equivalent of impurity

   = Multiplication factor × wt. of impurity

Salt	Molecular weight	Chemicale quivalent	Multiplication Factor
$Ca(HCO_3)_2$	162	81	100/162
$Mg(HCO_3)_2$	146	73	100/146
$CaSO_4$	136	68	100/136
$CaCl_2$	111	55·5	100/111
$MgSO_4$	120	60	100/120
$MgCl_2$	95	47·5	100/95
$CaCO_3$	100	50	100/100
$MgCO_3$	84	42	100/84
CO_2	44	22	100/44
$Mg(NO_3)_2$	148	74	100/148
HCO_3	61	61	100/122
OII	41	17	100/34
CO^2_3	60	30	100/60
$NaAlO_2$	82	82	100/164
$Al_2(SO_4)_3$	342	57	100/114
$FeSO_4.7H_2O$	278	139	100/278
H^+	1	1	100/2
HCl	36·5	36·5	100/73

4. If the impurities are given as $CaCO_3$ or $MgCO_3$, these should be considered due to $Ca(HCO_3)_2$ and $Mg(HCO_3)_2$ respectively and they must only be expressed in terms of $CaCO_3$ and $MgCO_3$

5. The amount expressed as $CaCO_3$ does not require any further conversion. However, the amount expressed as $MgCO_3$ should be converted into its $CaCO_3$ equivalents by multiplying with 100/84

6. The amount of lime and soda required are calculated as follows.

   Lime = (74/100) {temporary calcium hardness + (2 × temporary magnesium hardness) + Perm Mg hardness + CO_2 + HCl + H_2SO_4 + HCO^-_3 + salts of Fe^{2+}, Al^{3+} − $NaAlO_2$)

   Soda = (106/100) {Perm Ca hardness + Perm Mg hardness + salts of Fe^{2+}, Al^{3+} + HCl + H_2SO_4 + HCO^-_3 + −$NaAlO_2$}

7. If Ca^{2+} and Mg^{2+} is given, 1 equivalent of lime and 1 equivalent of soda is required for Mg^{2+} whereas 1 equivalent of soda is required for Ca^{2+}. The ions Ca^{2+} and Mg^{2+} are treated as permanent hardness due to Ca and Mg.

8. If the lime and soda used are impure and if the percentage purity is given, then the actual requirements of the chemicals should be calculated accordingly. Thus, if lime is 90% pure, then the value obtained in step (6) must be multiplied by 100/90 to get actual lime requirement. Similarly, if the soda is 95% pure then the value obtained in step (6) is multiplied by 100/95 to get actual soda requirement.

9. The value obtained in step (6) is also multiplied by the volume of water which has to be purified.

Thus the final complete formula for calculating the amount of lime or soda required is given as

Lime requirement = (74/100) {temporary calcium hardness + (2 × temporary magnesium hardness) + Perm Mg hardness + CO_2 + HCl + H_2SO_4 + HCO^-_3 + salts of 100 Fe^{2+}, Al^{3+} − $NaAlO_2$} × 100/% purity × volume of water

Soda requirement = (106/100) {Perm Ca hardness + Perm Mg hardness + salts of Fe^{2+}, Al^{3+} + HCl + H_2SO_4 − HCO^-_3 − $NaAlO_2$} × 100/% purity × volume of water.

And the most general formulae for calculating the amount of lime or soda required are

Lime requirement = (74/100) {temporary calcium hardness + (2 × temporary magnesium hardness) + Perm Mg hardness} × 100/% purity × volume of water

Soda requirement = (106/100) {Perm Ca hardness + Perm Mg hardness + salts of Fe^{2+}, Al^{3+} +} × 100/% purity × volume of water.

Zeolite or Permutit Process

It is a process by which ions held on a porous, essentially insoluble solids are exchanged for ions in solution that is brought in contact with it; Let us take the details of zeolite or permutite process for removal of permanent hardness of water. Permutite-is the trade name given to sodium zeolites.

These are hydrated sodium alumino silicate minerals i.e.

$Na_2O. Al_2O_3. xSiO_2. yH_2O.$ (where x = 2-10 & y = 2-6)When y = 2, we get $Na_2O. Al_2O_3. 2SiO_2. yH_2O$ For simplicity, we can write zeolites as Na_2Z. Where $Z = O. Al_2O_3. 2SiO_2. yH_2O$.

In this method, hard water is passed' through a bed of permutite contained in a cylindrical vessel. The water percolates at a specified rate through the bed. The loose sodium ions are exchanged for Ca^{2+} and Mg^2 ions. Thus calcium and magnesium salts get removed in the form of the insoluble zeolites and soft water is collected.

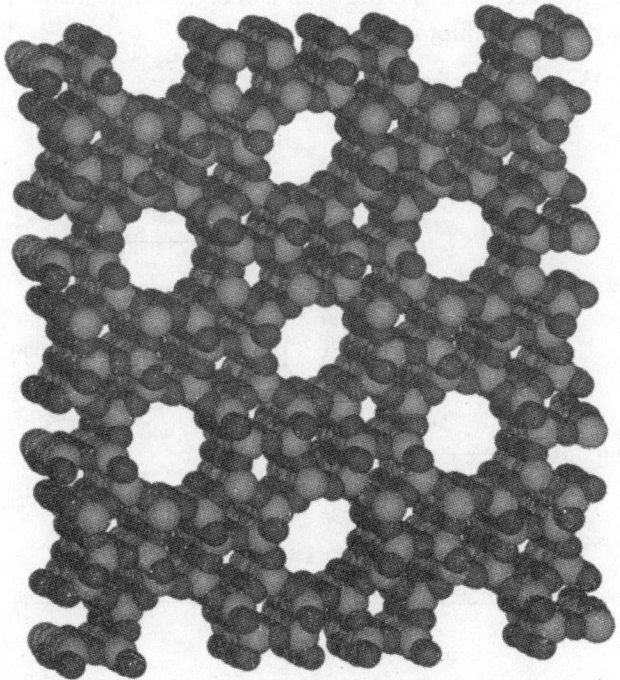

Fig. 7.3: Zeolite and Zeolite Softener

This process involves treatment of water by using zeolites.Zeolites may be natural or synthetic. Natural occurring Zeolite is hydrated sodium alumino silicate minerals (like $Na_2O. Al_2O_3. xSiO_2. yH_2O$) which is capable of exchanging its sodium ions reversibly for hardness-producing ions in water. Synthetic zeolites are prepared from sodium silicates and sodium aluminate. Durability is more for natural zeolites while synthetic has higher exchange capacity. Zeolites are also known as permutits and in Greek it means 'boiling stone.' A zeolite crystal structure consists of f several SiO_4 tetrahedrally, each oxygen of a tetrahedron being shared with an adjacent one. The empirical formula is thus $(SiO_2)_n$. However, some of the Si^{4+} ions may be isomorphostly replaced by Al^{3+} ions and in order to balance the charges an extra positive-ion such as Na^+ and K^+ must also be incorporated for every Al^{3+} introduced. The linking of these results in an open structure with cavities. The porous nature of the structure permits free movement of water molecules and ions. Zeolite holds sodium ions loosely and can be simply represented as Na_2Z where Z represents remaining part of the zeolite other than Na. The hardness-causing ions (Ca^{2+}, Mg^{2+}, Fe^{++} etc) are retained by the zeolite as CaZ and MgZ respectively, while the outgoing water contains salts. In the process, the water becomes free from Ca^{2+} and Mg^{2+}, the main hardness producing cations.

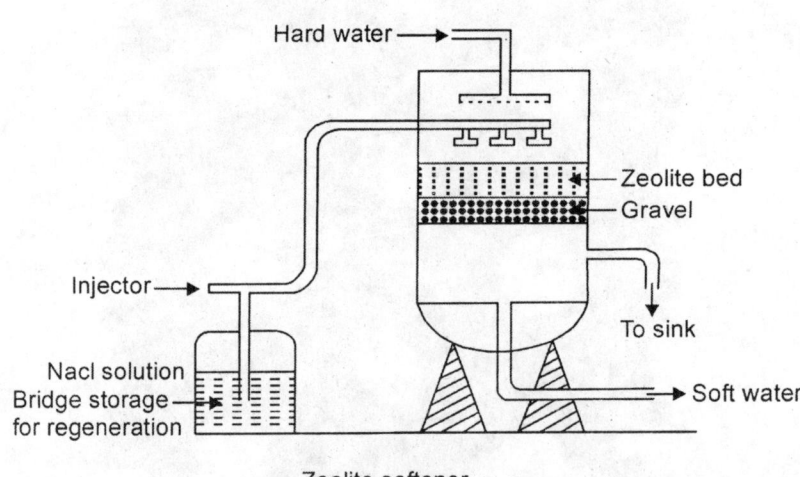

Zeolite softener

General reactions taking place during the softening process are :

$$Na_2Z + Ca(HCO_3)_2 \longrightarrow CaZ + 2NaHCO_3$$
$$Na_2Z + Mg(HCO_3)_2 \longrightarrow MgZ + 2NaHCO_3$$
$$CaSO_4 + Na_2Z \longrightarrow CaZ \downarrow + Na_2SO_4$$
$$MgSO_4 + Na_2Z \longrightarrow MgZ \downarrow + Na_2SO_4$$
$$CaCl_2 + Na_2Z \longrightarrow CaZ \downarrow + 2NaCl$$

Regeneration of Zeolites

This process removes both temporary and permanent hardness. After long use, the zeolite bed gets exhausted. CaZ or MgZ are exhausted zeolites. After some time, the zeolite is completely converted into calcium and magnesium zeolites by replacement of Na+ ions with Ca++ and Mg++ ions. At this stage, the supply of hard water is stopped and exhausted zeolite is regenerated by using chemicals, such as brine solution, NaCI or sodium nitrate or sodium sulphate. However, NaCI is preferred on account of its cheapness, easy availability and low molecular weight. The products 'calcium chloride and magnesium chloride are highly soluble in water and can be easily washed out. Following reactions take place during regeneration.

$$CaZ \ + 2 \ NaCl \longrightarrow Na_2Z + CaCl_2$$

$$MgZ + 2 \ NaCl \longrightarrow Na_2Z + MgCl_2$$

The softening and regeneration process can be represented as follows:

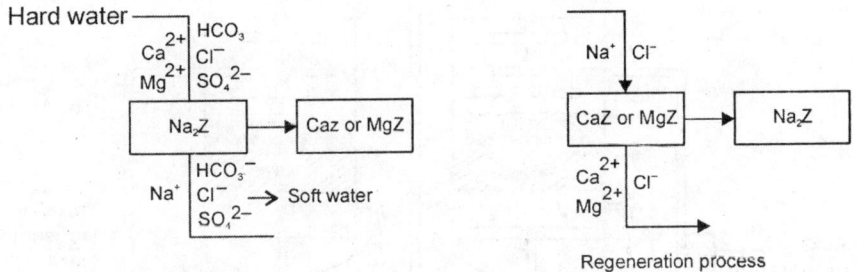

Regeneration process

Limitation of Zeolite Process

when the supplied water is having high amount of the the suspended matter then it must be removed by coagulation or filtration, before the water is fed to the zeolite bed. Otherwise the pores of the zeolite bed will get clogged by the turbidity and soon process will become inactive. Mineral acids, if present in water, destroy the zeolite bed and hence they must be neutralized with soda in advance, before feeding the water into the zeolite bed. The feed water should not be hot as the zeolite tends to dissolve in it. Anions are not removed by this process, only harder cations are replaced by softer (Sodium ions) ions hence the bicarbonates present in hard water get converted $NaHCO_3$ which goes into soft water effluent. If it is used as boiler feed, under the boiler conditions $NaHCO_3$ dissociated as:

$$NaHCO_3 \longrightarrow NaOH + CO_2,$$

Both the products are not desirable. Since NaOH may lead to caustic embrittlement and CO_2 makes the condensed water acidic and corrosive. Thus it is desirable to remove temporary hardness before feeding to zeolite softener. compared to ion-exchange process, water treated by the zeolite process contains20- 25% more dissolved solids. Moreover, cost of the plant and materials are also limiting factors.

Advantages of Zeolite Process

The hardness is nearly completely removed (about 10-15 ppm hardness). The Plant set up is compact and occupies less space with cleanliness. Impurities are not precipitated, so there is no danger of sludge formation.It is rapid process which required less time for softening and maintenance as well as operations are simple.

Ion-exchange process

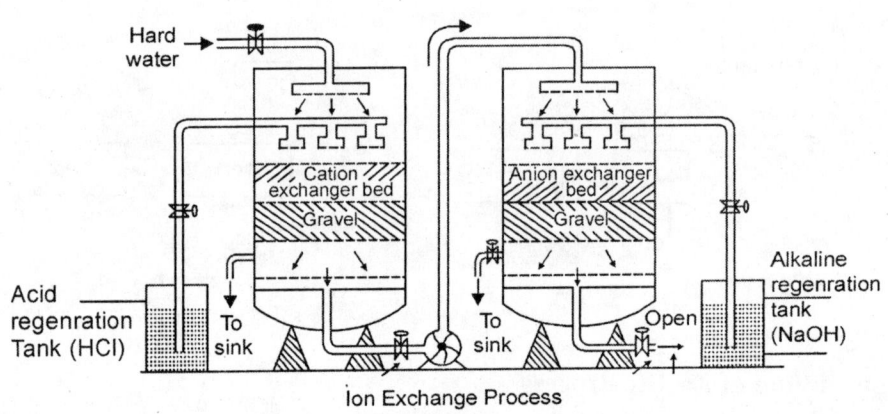

Ion Exchange Process

Fig. 7.4

Ion Exchange process

In this process, the ions present in solution are exchanged by ion-exchange resin. Ion-exchange resins are insoluble, high molecular mass polymers with a porous structure. These are further of two types:

  (i) Cation exchange resins

  (ii) Anion exchange resins.

  (i) Cations exchange resins have acidic functional groups like— COOH, $-SO_3H$ etc. Which exchange cations with the H^+ ions.

  (ii) Anion exchange resins contain basic functional groups like $-NH_2$, ammonium ions or quaternary phosphonium ions. These are capable of exchanging OH^- ions with anion exchangers.

The schematic diagram of this process is shown in fig. Hard water is first passed through first column containing cation exchange resins where all cations of hard water get exchanged with H^+ ions as:

$$2RH + Ca^{+2} \rightarrow R_2Ca + 2H^+$$
$$2RH + Mg^{+2} \rightarrow R_2Mg + 2H^+$$

After this, water is passed through second column containing ion exchange resins. All anions of hard water get removed with the OH^- ions as:

$$R'OH + Cl^- \rightarrow RCl + OH^-$$
$$2R'OH + SO_4^{-2} \rightarrow R'_2SO_4 + 2OH^-$$

H^+ and OH' ions combine to form water—

$$H^+ + OH^- \rightarrow H_2O$$

Finally, water is made free from dissolved gases like CO_2 by passing through degasifier.

The tower is heated from sides by steam and it is connected to vacuum pump. The water coming is free from all type of ions.

During process, the resins get exhausted. These resins can be generated by passing solution of dil. HCl or H_2SO_4 through first column or acid regeneration tank.

The regeneration reactions are:

$$R_2Ca + 2H^+ \rightarrow 2RH + Ca^{+2}$$
$$R_2Mg + 2H^+ \rightarrow 2RH + Mg^{+2}$$

Similarly the anion exchange resins can be regenerated by passing solution of dil. NaOH through alkaline (NaOH solution) storage tank second and reaction is shown below.

$$R'Cl + OH^- \rightarrow R'OH + Cl^-$$
$$R'_2 SO_4 + 2OH^- \rightarrow 2R'OH + SO_4^2$$

Ion-exchange resins are insoluble, cross linked, high molecular weight, organic polymers with a porous structure, and the "functional group" attached to the chains are responsible for the ion-exchange properties.

The ion-exchange resins may be classified as :

(i) **Cation exchange resins (R^-H^+):** They are mainly styrene-divinyl benzene copolymers, which on sulphonation or carboxylation, become capable to exchange their hydrogen ions with the cations in the water.

Such resins have acidic functional groups like $-SO_3H$, $-COOH$ or $-OH$ (phenolic) capable of exchanging the cationic portion of minerals by their hydrogen ion, and hence they are termed as cation exchangers.

(ii) **Anion exchange resins (R^+OH^-):** They are styrene-divinyl benzene or amine formaldehyde copolymers, which contain basic functional groups such as amino or quaternary ammonium ($-N^+R_3$) or quaternary phosphonium or tertiary sulphonium group as an integral part of the resin matrix. These after treatment with dil. NaOH solution, become capable to exchange their OH^- anions with anions in water and therefore they are known as anion exchangers.

Treatment of Water by Reverse Osmosis Method

Reverse Osmosis

Reverse osmosis (RO) is a membrane-technology filtration method that removes many types of large molecules and ions from solutions by applying pressure to the solution when it is on one side of a selective membrane. The result is that the solute is retained on the pressurized side of the membrane and the pure solvent is allowed to pass to the other side. To be "selective," this membrane should not allow large molecules or ions through the pores (holes), but should allow smaller components of the solution (such as the solvent) to pass freely.

In the normal osmosis process, the solvent naturally moves from an area of low solute or dissolved solids concentration (High Water Potential), through a membrane (semi permeable membrane), to an area of high solute concentration (Low Water Potential). The movement of a pure solvent to equalize solute concentrations on each side of a membrane generates osmotic pressure. Applying an external pressure to reverse the natural flow of pure solvent, thus, is **reverse osmosis**.

Reverse osmosis i.e basic principle is the reverse of osmosis,when the pressure higher than osmotic pressure is applied on the solution side, then the solvent flows from the region of higher conc. to the lower conc. through semipermeable membrane is known as reverse osmosis.

The process is similar to other membrane technology applications. Reverse osmosis, however, involves a diffusive mechanism so that separation efficiency is dependent on solute concentration, pressure, and water flux rate. Reverse osmosis is most commonly known for its use in drinking water purification from seawater, removing the salt and other substances from the water molecules.

In. this process of reverse osmosis, the pure water is separated from brackish water or saline water. Pressure of the order of $20 - 40$ kg/cm$_2$.

The phenomenon of reverse osmosis, as shown in the Fig. 7.5.

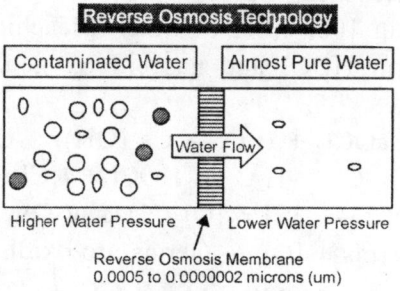

Fig. 7.5

OTHER IMPORTANT QUESTIONS

Q.1. What are disinfectants? What are the main requirements in a good disinfectant? Name few disinfectants (at least three) used in our daily life with use and principle of working.

Ans. The substances used for killing the pathogenic bacteria's, micro-organisms etc. from the water to make it safe for drinking purposes.

Main requirements:

  (i) It should kill the disease producing micro-organisms quickly at room temperature,

 (ii) It should be inexpensive,

(iii) It should not be toxic to human beings

(iv) It should provide protection against any contamination in water during storage.

The three disinfectants with their use and principle of working are as follows:

 (a) By using chlorine gas: Chlorine can be used directly as a gas or chlorine water r sterilization in municipal water supply. It reacts with water to form hypochiorous acid and nascent oxygen both of which are powerful germicides.

$$Cl_2 + H_2O \rightarrow HOCl + HCl$$
$$\text{(Hypochlorous acid)}$$
$$HOCl \rightarrow HCl + [O] \text{ (Nascent Oxygen)}$$
$$\text{Germs} + [O] \rightarrow \text{Germs are Oxidised}$$

Excess of chlorine cannot be used because it produces unpleasant, odour taste and irritating effect on mucous membrane.

(b) **By adding bleaching powder:** About 1kg of bleaching powder is added to about 1000 litres of water. Bleaching powder reacts with water to form HOCl and nascent oxygen which are powerful germicides i.e.

$$CaOCl_2 + H_2O \rightarrow Ca(OH)_2 + Cl_2$$
$$Cl_2 + H_2O \rightarrow HOCl + HCl$$
$$HOCl \rightarrow HCl + [O] \text{ (Nascent Oxygen)}$$
$$\text{Germs} + [O] \rightarrow \text{Germs are oxidised.}$$

Disadvantages of adding bleaching powder:

1. Bleaching powder introduces calcium in water therefore making it more hard.

2. Bleaching powder undergoes decomposition continuously, therefore it should be analysed for its effective chlorine contents.

(c) **By using chloramine:** Chlorine and ammonia are mixed in the ratio of 2 : 1 by volume to produce a compound known as given below:

$$Cl_2 + NH_3 \rightarrow ClNH_2 + HCl$$
$$\text{(Chloramine)}$$

This process is known as chloramination

Chloramine reacts with water to form HOCl and [0] which are powerful germicides.

$$ClNH_2 + 2H_2O \rightarrow HOCl + NH_4OH$$
$$HOCl \rightarrow HCl + [O] \text{ (Nascent oxygen)}$$
$$\text{Germs} + [O] \rightarrow \text{Germs are oxidised}$$

This method has following advantages

1. It removes irritating smell due to excess of chlorine.

2. It imparts good taste to water.

Break Point Chlorination: The disinfecting action of chlorine is not so simple. Being an oxidising agent, it first oxidises organic matter and other reducing agents such s NH_3, H_2S etc. For example NH_3-reacts with hypochiorous acid (HOCI) (produced from reaction of chlorine with water) in the following way.

$$NH_3 + HOCI \rightarrow NH_2CI + H_2O$$

$$NHCI_2 + HOCI \rightarrow NHCI_2 + H_2O$$

$$NHCI_2 + HOCI \rightarrow NCI_3 + H_2O$$

Similarly chlorine reacts with other reducing agents. After completely oxidising the organic matter and reducing agents the chlorine left behind is now available for disinfecting action against bacteria and other micro-organisms. The chlorine is called free residual chlorine or break point chlorination. Therefore Break point chlorination is the addition of sufficient amount of chlorine to oxidise organic matter and reducing substances leaving behind mainly free chlorine which possesses disinfecting action against pathogenic bacteria's.

Q.2. What is demineralised water? How is it different from soft water?

Ans. Water of zero hardness is obtained. Water can be used in high pressure boilers. It gives best quality water similar to distilled water. Soft water can not be used in boilers. It contains total dissolved solids lesser than the raw water.

Differences between soft water and demineralized water:

Soft Water	Demineralized Water
1. Soft water has hardness ← 85 ppm ($CaCO_3$ eq.). Thus, soft water has more hardness than demineralized water.	Demineralized water does not have any salt (or cations and anions) present in it. So, hardness ≤ 2 ppm.
2. It is fit for domestic use.	It is not recommended as such for drinking purposes.
3. It can be made by using either Lime-Soda process or Zeolite process.	It can be made either by distillation or by suing cation and anion exchangers.
4. Soft water is unfit for feeding into boilers.	It is very good for use in high pressure boilers.

Q.3. How scales are formed in boilers?

Ans. Scales are formed in boilers as follows:

    (i) Decomposition of bicarbonates: At high temperature, bicarbonates decompose into sticky water insoluble material.

    (ii) Hydrolysis of magnesium salts.

(iii) **Presence of silica:** Silica may be in the form of colloidal particles and it can deposit as calcium silicate or magnesium silicate as firmly adhering material.

(iv) **Decreased solubility of Ca SO₄:** $CaSO_4$ has lesser solubility at higher temperatures. Hence at high temperatures $CaSO_4$ present dissolved in boiler feed water will precipitate out as hard scale forming material.

SOLVED NUMERICAL

Example

The hardness of 20,000 liters of a sample of water removed by passing it through a zeolite softener. The zeolite softener then required 150 litres of sodium chloride solution containing 200 gm/litre of NaCl for generation. Find the hardness of water sample.

Solution.

NaCl contained in 150 L of NaCl solution

$$= 200 \text{ gm/L} \times 150 \text{ L}$$

$$= 30,000 \text{ gm of NaCl}$$

Let hardness be H ppm (or mg/l), then total hardnessin the water = 20000 litreX mg/litre = 20,000 XH (mg) = 20 X H gm

Now **number of gm equivalents of NaCl= number of gm equivalents of hardness** as $CaCO_3$ water,

or remember simple formula is

[Wt of NaCl in gm/58.5 = V(volume of water in litre)X H(Hardness in mg/l)/50,000]

i.e. $30,000 \dfrac{1}{58.5} = 20XH \times \dfrac{1}{50}$

then H =1282 ppm hence hardness of water is 1282 ppm

Example:

An exhausted zeolite softener was regenerated by passing 200 liters of NaCl solution, having a strength of 0.25 gm/L of NaCl. Find the total volume of water that can be softened by this zeolite softener, if the hardness of water is 600 ppm.

Solution. 200 L of NaCl solution contains

$$= 200 \text{ L} \times (0.25 \text{ g/L}) \text{ of NaCl}$$
$$= 50 \text{ gm of NaCl}$$

Now by using direct simple formula

[Wt of NaCl in gm/58.5 = V(volume of water in litre)

$$\times \text{ H(Hardness in mg/l)/50,000]}$$

$$50/58.5 = V \times 600/50,000$$

Then $\qquad$ V = 71.22 litre.

Chapter 8
POLYMER CHEMISTRY

- ➤ **Introduction**
- ➤ **Classification of Polymers**
- ➤ **Mechanism**
- ➤ **Polymerization Techniques**
- ➤ **Elastomer**
- ➤ **Synthetic Fibre**
- ➤ **Biodegradable Polymer**

INTRODUCTION

Humans have taken advantage of the versitility of polymers for centuries in the form of oils, tars, resins, and gums. However, it was not until the industrial revolution that the modern polymer industry began to develop. In the late 1830s, Charles Goodyear succeeded in producing a useful form of natural rubber through a process known as "vulcanization". Some 40 years later, Celluloid (a hard plastic formed from nitrocellulose) was successfully commercialized. Despite these advances, progress in polymer science was slow until the 1930s, when materials such as vinyl, neoprene, polystyrene, and nylon were developed. The introduction of these revolutionary materials began an explosion in polymer research that is still going on today.

Prior to the early 1920's, chemists doubted the existence of molecules having molecular weights greater than a few thousand. This limiting view was challenged by Hermann Staudinger, a German chemist with experience in studying natural compounds such as rubber and cellulose. In contrast to the prevailing rationalization of these substances as aggregates of small molecules, Staudinger proposed they were made up of macromolecules composed of 10,000 or more atoms. He formulated a polymeric structure for rubber, based on a repeating isoprene unit (referred to as a monomer). For his contributions to chemistry, Staudinger received the 1953 Nobel Prize. The terms polymer and monomer were derived from the Greek roots poly (many), mono (one) and meros (part).

Polymer: *Polymers* are a large class of materials consisting of many small molecules (called *monomers*) that can be linked together to form long chains, thus they are known as *macromolecules*. A typical polymer may include thousands to millions of monomers. Although the term polymer is sometimes taken to refer to plastics, it actually encompasses a large class of compounds comprising both natural and synthetic materials with a wide variety of properties.

Like, A is the monomer unit and $(A)_n$ is polymer, where nmolecules of A are joint together in head to tail arrangement to give a giant molecule or macromolecule $(A)_n$ where n is degree of polymerization.

CLASSIFICATION OF POLYMERS

Polymers may be classified in many ways depending upon their availability or occurance, or thermal effect or structure.

On the basis of occurance or availability, polymers can be classified as natural polymer and synthetic polymer.

Natural Polymers

The polymers which are available naturally or they are obtained from the nature directly like cellulose, starch, wood, natural rubber,amber etc. They are easily biodegradable.

Synthetic Polymer

The polymers which can not be obtained from nature,but they are prepared by synthetic methods, like Bakelite, PVC, PMMA, Teflon etc.

According to the thermal effect or mechanical response at elevated temperatures, polymers are classified in two categories;

(a) Thermoplasts, and

(b) Thermosets

(a) Thermoplasts

- Thermoset polymers soften when heated and harden when cooled i.e they are reversible. Simultaneous application of heat and pressure is required to fabricate these materials.
- On the molecular level, when the temperature is raised, secondary bonding forces are diminished so that the relative movement of adjacent chains is facilitated when a stress is applied.

- Most Linear polymers and those having branched structures with flexible chains are thermoplastics.
- Thermoplastics are very soft and ductile.
- The commercial available thermoplasts are, Polyvinyl Chloride (PVC) and Polystyrene, Polymethyl methacrylate, Polystyrene etc.

(b) Thermosets

- Thermosetting polymers become soft during their first heating and become permanently hard when cooled. They do not soften during subsequent heating. Hence, they cannot be remolded/reshaped by subsequent heating i.e. they are irreversible.
- In thermosets, during the initial heating, covalent cross-links are formed between adjacent molecular chain. These bonds anchor the chains together to resist the vibration and rotational chain motions at high temperatures. Cross linking is usually extensive in that 10 to 15% of the chain mer units are cross linked. Only heating to excessive temperatures will cause severance of these crosslink bonds and polymer degradation.
- Thermoset polymers are harder, stronger, more brittle than thermoplastics and have better dimensional stability. Thermosets cannot be recycle, do not melt, are usable at higher temperatures than thermoplastics, and are more chemically inert.
- They are more usable in processes requiring high temperatures
    - o Most of the cross linked and network polymers which include, Vulcanized rubbers, Epoxies,Phenolic resins,Polyester resins are thermosetting.

On the basis of type of monomer unit, polymers can be termed as homopolymer or copolymer.

Homopolymer

The polymer which is formed by using one kind of monomer unit is known as homopolymer, like PVC is the polymer of vinyl chloride.

$$A\text{-}A\text{-}A\text{-}A\text{-}A\text{-}A \text{———}n \text{ units} = (A)n$$

Copolymer

The polymer which is formed by using more than one type of monomer units is known as copolymer. In this respect, it is useful to distinguish several ways in which different monomeric units might be incorporated in a polymeric molecule. The following examples refer to a two component system, in which one monomer is designated A and the other B.

Random or Statistical Copolymers

Also called random copolymers. Here the monomeric units are distributed randomly, and sometimes unevenly, in the polymer chain:

~**ABBAAABAABBBABAABA**~.

Alternating Copolymers

Here the monomeric units are distributed in a regular alternating fashion, with nearly equimolar amounts of each in the chain:

~**ABABABABABABABAB**~.

Block Copolymers

Instead of a mixed distribution of monomeric units, a long sequence or block of one monomer is joined to a block of the second monomer:

~**AAAAA-BBBBBBB~AAAAAAA~BBB**~.

Graft Copolymers

As the name suggests, side chains of a given monomer are attached to the main chain of the second monomer:

~**AAAAAAA(BBBBBBB~)AAAAAAA(BBBB~)AAA**~.

```
Alternating
—R—B—R—B—R—B—R—B—R—B—
Random
—R—R—R—B—R—B—B—R—B—R—
Block
—R—R—R—R—R—B—B—B—B—B—
Graft
—R—R—R—R—R—R—R—R—R—R—
       |         |
       B         B
       |         |
       B         B
       |         |
       B         B
       |         |
```

Some Useful Copolymers

Monomer A	Monomer B	Copolymer	Uses
$H_2C=CHCl$	$H_2C=CCl_2$	Saran	films and fibers
$H_2C=CHC_6H_5$	$H_2C=C-CH=CH_2$	SBR styrene butadiene rubber	tires
$H_2C=CHCN$	$H_2C=C-CH=CH_2$	Nitrile Rubber	adhesives, hoses

$H_2C=C(CH_3)_2$ $H_2C=C\text{-}CH=CH_2$ Butyl Rubber   inner tubes

$F_2C=CF(CF_3)$ $H_2C=CHF$ Viton   gaskets

On the basis of structure, polymers can be classified as:

(a) LinearPolymer: In this type of polymer,monomer units are attached linearly forming a continuous chain. Like polythene

$$n(CH_2 = CH_2) \Rightarrow -CH_2\text{--}CH_2\text{--}CH_2\text{--}CH_2\text{--}CH_2\text{--}CH_2- \;\text{------}\; \text{or}\; (-CH_2\text{--}CH_2-)_n$$

(b) Branched Polymer: In this type of polymer, some groups are attached to the main chain of polymer. For example LDPE (low dense polyethene).

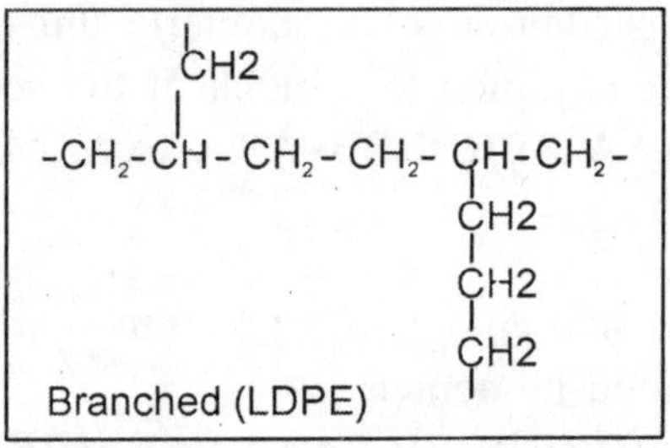

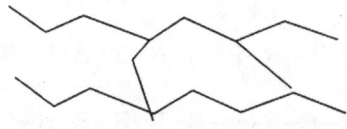

$$\begin{array}{c} \overset{|}{C}H2 \\ | \\ -CH_2\text{-}\overset{|}{C}H\text{-}CH_2\text{-}CH_2\text{-}\underset{|}{C}H\text{-}CH_2\text{-} \\ CH2 \\ | \\ CH2 \\ | \\ CH2 \end{array}$$

Branched (LDPE)

(c) Crosslinked Polymer: This is the 3-dimensional interlinked polymer. During the polymerization, many linear or branched polymer chains are interlinked by the functional group of same compound or another different compound.

Crosslinked polymer

On the basis of tacticity i.e configuration or orientation of side groups, polymers may be classified as isotactic,atactic and syndiotactic polymer. Tacticity describes the relative stereochemistry of chiral centers in neighboring structural units within a macromolecule.

Isotactic: If all substituents are present on the same side about the main chain.e.g Natural rubber

Atactic: If all substituents or side groups are present randomely about the main chain, that is known as atactic polymer e.g. polypropylene

Syndiotactic: If all substituents or side groups are present in alternating fashion, it is called Syndiotactic polymer, e.g. gutta percha

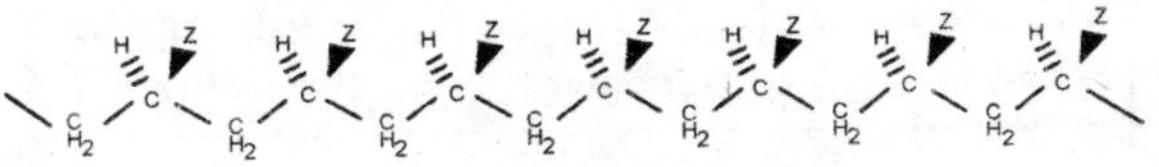

isotactic

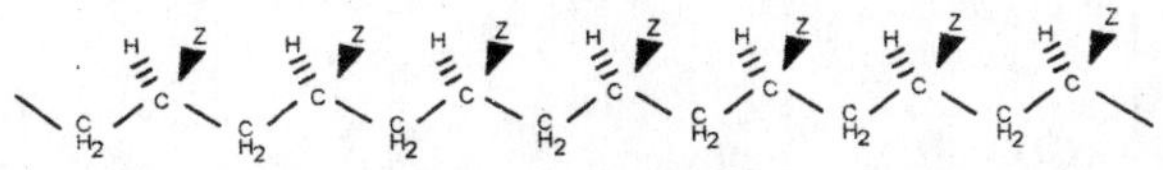

Syndiotactic

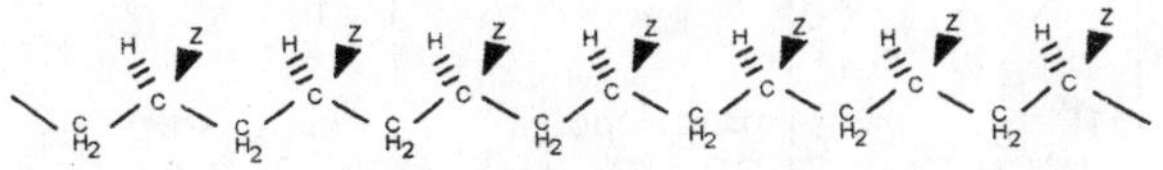

atactic

Many common and useful polymers, such as polystyrene, polyacrylonitrile and poly(vinyl chloride) are atactic as normally prepared. Customized catalysts that effect stereoregular polymerization of polypropylene and some other monomers have been developed, and the improved properties associated with the increased crystallinity of these products has made this an important field of investigation. The following values of T_g have been reported.

Polymer	T_g atactic	T_g isotactic	T_g syndiotactic
PP	–20°C	0°C	–8°C
PMMA	100°C	130°C	120°C

The properties of a given polymer will vary considerably with its tacticity. Thus, atactic polypropylene is useless as a solid construction material, and is employed mainly as a component of adhesives or as a soft matrix for composite materials. In contrast, isotactic polypropylene is a high-melting solid (ca. 170°C) which can be molded or machined into structural components.

Polymers on the basis of polymerisation process (addition and condensation polymerisation) can be divided in two types, addition and condensation polymers.

Many polymeric materials having chain-like structures similar to polyethylene are known. Polymers formed by a straightforward linking together of monomer units, with no loss or gain of material, are called **addition polymers** or **chain-growth polymers**. A listing of some important addition polymers and their monomer precursors is presented in the following table.

Some Common Addition Polymers

Name(s)	Formula	Monomer	Properties	Uses
Polyethylene low density (LDPE)	$-(CH_2-CH_2)_n-$	ethylene $CH_2=CH_2$	soft, waxy solid	film wrap, plastic bags
Polyethylene high density (HDPE)	$-(CH_2-CH_2)_n-$	ethylene $CH_2=CH_2$	rigid, translucent solid	electrical insulation bottles, toys
Polypropylene (PP) different grades	$-[CH_2-CH(CH_3)]_n-$	propylene $CH_2=CHCH_3$	atactic: soft, elastic solid isotactic: hard, strong solid	similar to LDP Ecarpet, upholstery
Poly (vinyl chloride) (PVC)	$-(CH_2-CHCl)_n-$	vinyl chloride $CH_2=CHCl$	strong rigid solid	pipes, siding, flooring
Poly (vinylidene chloride) (Saran A)	$-(CH_2-CCl_2)_n-$	vinylidene chloride $CH_2=CCl_2$	dense, high-melting solid	seat covers, films
Polystyrene(PS)	$-[CH_2-CH(C_6H_5)]_n-$	styrene $CH_2=CHC_6H_5$	hard, rigid, clear solid soluble in organic solvents	toys, cabinet spackaging (foamed)
Polyacrylonitrile (PAN, Orlon, Acrilan)	$-(CH_2-CHCN)_n-$	acrylonitrile $CH_2=CHCN$	high-melting solidsoluble in organic solvents	rugs, blankets clothing
Polytetrafluoroethylene (PTFE, Teflon)	$-(CF_2-CF_2)_n-$	tetrafluoroethylene $CF_2=CF_2$	resistant, smooth solid	non-stick surface selectrical insulation
Poly(methyl methacrylate) (PMMA, Lucite, Plexiglas)	$-[CH_2-C(CH_3)CO_2CH_3]_n-$	methyl methacrylate $CH_2=C(CH_3)CO_2CH_3$	hard, transparent solid	lighting covers, signsskylights
Poly(vinyl acetate)(PVAc)	$-(CH_2-CHOCOCH_3)_n-$	vinyl acetate $CH_2=CHOCOCH_3$	soft, sticky solid	latex paints, adhesives
cis-Polyisoprene natural rubber	$-[CH_2-CH=C(CH_3)-CH_2]_n-$	isoprene $CH_2=CH-C(CH_3)=CH_2$	soft, sticky solid	requires vulcanization for practical use
Polychloroprene (cis + trans) (Neoprene)	$-[CH_2-CH=CCl-CH_2]_n-$	chloroprene $CH_2=CH-CCl=CH_2$	tough, rubbery solid	synthetic rubber, oil resistant

2. Condensation Polymers

Condensation polymers are generally formed by step growth process. They are formed more slowly than addition polymers, often requiring heat, and they are generally lower in molecular weight. The terminal functional groups on a chain remain active, so that groups of shorter chains combine into longer chains in the late stages of polymerization. The presence of polar functional groups on the chains often enhances chain-chain attractions, particularly if these involve hydrogen bonding, and thereby crystallinity and tensile strength. The following examples of condensation polymers are illustrative.

Note that for commercial synthesis the carboxylic acid components may actually be employed in the form of derivatives such as simple esters. Also, the polymerization reactions for Nylon 6 and Spandex do not proceed by elimination of water or other small molecules. Nevertheless, the polymer clearly forms by a step-growth process.

Some Condensation Polymers

Formula	Type	Monomers	$T_g \degree C$	$T_m \degree C$
~[CO(CH$_2$)$_4$CO-OCH$_2$CH$_2$O]$_n$~	polyester	HO$_2$C-(CH$_2$)$_4$-CO$_2$H HO-CH$_2$CH$_2$-OH	< 0	50
[para-terephthalate ester structure] ─O–(CH$_2$)$_2$–O─$_n$	polyester Dacron Mylar	para HO$_2$C-C$_6$H$_4$-CO$_2$H HO-CH$_2$CH$_2$-OH	70	265
[meta-isophthalate ester structure] ─O–(CH$_2$)$_2$–O─$_n$	polyester	meta HO$_2$C-C$_6$H$_4$-CO$_2$H HO-CH$_2$CH$_2$-OH	50	240
[Bisphenol A carbonate structure with C(CH$_3$)$_2$ and -O-C(=O)-]$_n$	poly-carbonate Lexan	(HO-C$_6$H$_4$-)$_2$C(CH$_3$)$_2$ (Bisphenol A) X$_2$C=O (X = OCH$_3$ or Cl)	150	267
~[CO(CH$_2$)$_4$CO-NH(CH$_2$)$_6$NH]$_n$~	polyamide Nylon 66	HO$_2$C-(CH$_2$)$_4$-CO$_2$H H$_2$N-(CH$_2$)$_6$-NH$_2$	45	265
~[CO(CH$_2$)$_5$NH]$_n$~	polyamide Nylon 6 Perlon	[caprolactam ring structure, N-H, =O]	53	223

polyamide Kevlar	para $HO_2C-C_6H_4-CO_2H$ para $H_2N-C_6H_4-NH_2$	—	500	
polyamide Nomex	meta $HO_2C-C_6H_4-CO_2H$ meta $H_2N-C_6H_4-NH_2$	273	390	

POLYMERIZATION MECHANISM

Addition or Chain-growth polymerization

Chain-growth polymerization (or addition polymerization) involves the linking together of molecules incorporating double or triple carbon-carbon bonds. These unsaturated *monomers* (the identical molecules that make up the polymers) have extra internal bonds that are able to break and link up with other monomers to form the repeating chain. Chain-growth polymerization is involved in the manufacture of polymers such as polyethylene, polypropylene, and polyvinyl chloride (PVC). A special case of chain-growth polymerization leads to living polymerization.

In the radical polymerization of ethylene, its Å bond is broken, and the two electrons rearrange to create a new propagating center like the one that attacked it. The form this propagating center takes depends on the specific type of addition mechanism. There are several mechanisms through which this can be initiated. The free radical mechanism is one of the first methods to be used. Free radicals are very reactive atoms or molecules that have unpaired electrons. Taking the polymerization of ethylene as an example, the free radical mechanism can be divided in to three stages: chain initiation, chain propagation, and chain termination.

Polymerization of Ethene

Free radical addition polymerization of ethylene must take place at high temperatures and pressures, approximately 300 °C and 2000 atm. While most other free radical polymerizations do not require such extreme temperatures and pressures, they do tend to lack control. One effect of this lack of control is a high degree of branching. Also, as termination occurs randomly, when two chains collide, it is impossible to control the length of individual chains. A newer method of polymerization similar to free radical, but allowing more control involves the Ziegler-Natta catalyst, especially with respect to polymer branching.

Other forms of chain growth polymerization include cationic addition polymerization and anionic addition polymerization. While not used to a large extent in industry yet due to stringent reaction conditions such as lack of water and oxygen, these methods provide ways to polymerize some monomers that cannot be polymerized by free radical methods such as polypropylene. Cationic and anionic mechanisms are also more ideally suited for living polymerizations, although free radical living polymerizations have also been developed.

Esters of acrylic acid contain a carbon-carbon double bond which is conjugated to an ester group. This allows the possibility of both types of polymerization mechanism. An acrylic ester by itself can undergo chain-growth polymerization to form a homopolymer with a carbon-carbon backbone, such as poly (methyl methacrylate). Also, however, certain acrylic esters can react with diaminemonomers by nucleophilic conjugate addition of amine groups to acrylic C = C bonds. In this case the polymerization proceeds by step-growth and the products are poly (beta-amino ester) copolymers, with backbones containing nitrogen (as amine) and oxygen (as ester) as well as carbon.

All the monomers from which addition polymers are made are alkenes or functionally substituted alkenes. The most common and thermodynamically favored chemical transformations of alkenes are addition reactions. Many of these addition reactions are known to proceed in a stepwise fashion by way of reactive intermediates, and this is the mechanism followed by most polymerizations. A general diagram illustrating this assembly of linear macromolecules, which supports the name **chain growth polymers**, is presented here. Since a pi-bond in the monomer is converted to a sigma-bond in the polymer, the polymerization reaction is usually exothermic by 8 to 20 kcal/mol. If heat is not controlled properly, explosion may occur.

Z∗ is an initiating species   ∗ may be a radical, a cation or an anion

Mechanism: Polymerization procedures involve following mechanism.

- **Radical Polymerization** The initiator is a radical, and the propagating site of reactivity is a carbon radical.
- **Cationic Polymerization** The initiator is an acid, and the propagating site of reactivity is a carbocation.

- **Anionic Polymerization** The initiator is a nucleophile, and the propagating site of reactivity is a carbanion.
- **Coordination Catalytic Polymerization** The initiator is a transition metal complex, and the propagating site of reactivity is a terminal catalytic complex.

1. Radical Chain-Growth Polymerization

Since this can be initiated by traces of oxygen or other minor impurities, pure samples of these compounds are often "stabilized" by small amounts of radical inhibitors to avoid unwanted reaction. When radical polymerization is desired, it must be started by using a **radical initiator**, such as a peroxide or certain azo compounds. The formulas of some common initiators, and equations showing the formation of radical species from these initiators are presented below:

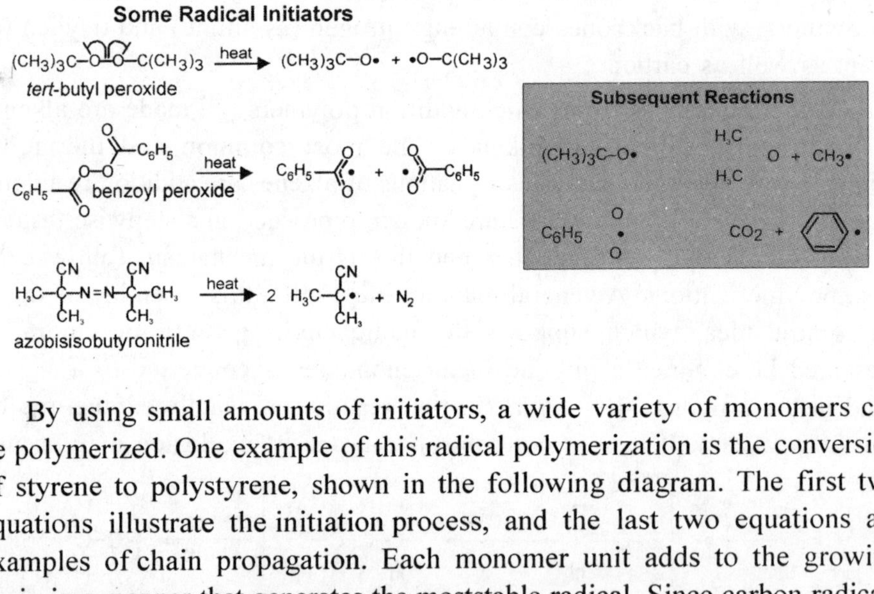

By using small amounts of initiators, a wide variety of monomers can be polymerized. One example of this radical polymerization is the conversion of styrene to polystyrene, shown in the following diagram. The first two equations illustrate the initiation process, and the last two equations are examples of chain propagation. Each monomer unit adds to the growing chain in a manner that generates the moststable radical. Since carbon radicals are stabilized by substituents of many kinds, the preference for head-to-tail regioselectivity in most addition polymerizations is understandable. Because radicals are tolerant of many functional groups and solvents (including water), radical polymerizations are widely used in the chemical industry.

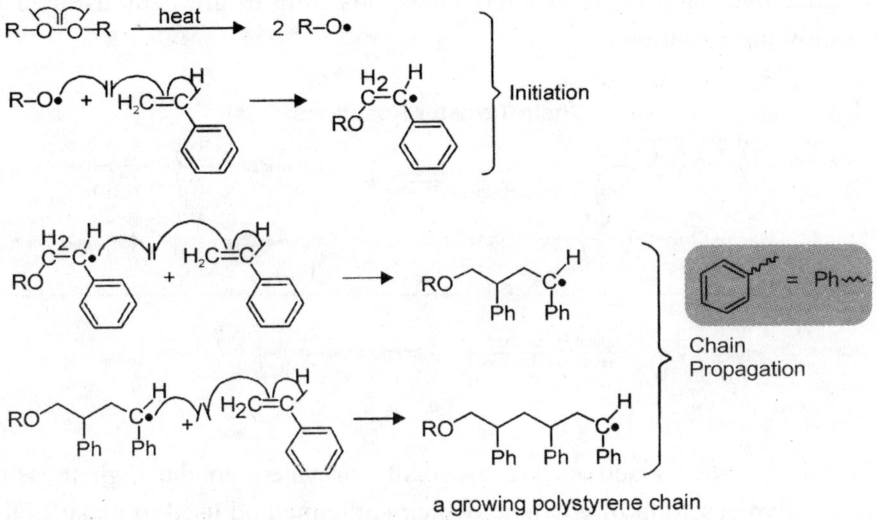

Initiation

Chain Propagation

a growing polystyrene chain

In principle, once started a radical polymerization might be expected to continue unchecked, producing a few extremely long chain polymers. In practice, larger numbers of moderately sized chains are formed, indicating that chain-terminating reactions must be taking place. The most common termination processes are Radical Combination and Disproportionation.

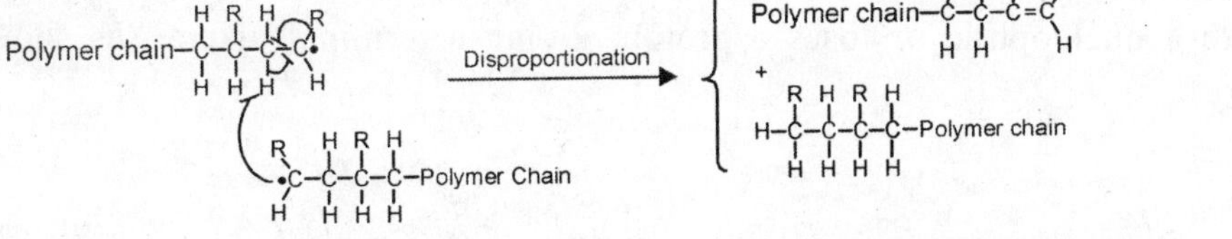

Chain Termination Reactions

The relative importance of these terminations varies with the nature of the monomer undergoing polymerization. For acrylonitrile and styrene combination is the major process. However, methyl methacrylate and vinyl acetate are terminated chiefly by disproportionation. Another reaction that diverts radical chain-growth polymerizations from producing linear macromolecules is called chain transfer. As the name implies, this reaction moves a carbon radical from one location to another by an intermolecular or intra-molecular hydrogen atom transfer. These possibilities are demonstrated by the following equations

Chain Transfer Reactions

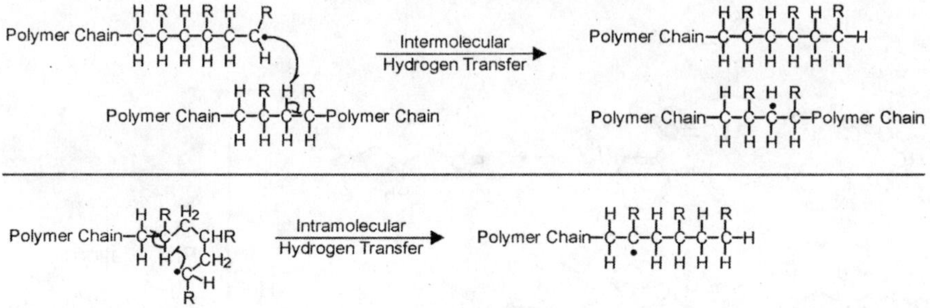

Chain transfer reactions are especially prevalent in the high pressure radical polymerization of ethylene, which is the method used to make LDPE (low density polyethylene). The 1°-radical at the end of a growing chain is converted to a more stable 2°-radical by hydrogen atom transfer. Further polymerization at the new radical site generates a side chain radical, and this may in turn lead to creation of other side chains by chain transfer reactions. As a result, the morphology of LDPE is an amorphous network of highly branched macromolecules.

2. Cationic Chain-Growth Polymerization

Polymerization of isobutylene (2-methylpropene) by traces of strong acids is an example of cationic polymerization. The polyisobutylene product is a soft rubbery solid, $T_g = -70°C$, which is used for inner tubes. This process is similar to radical polymerization, as demonstrated by the following equations. Chain growth ceases when the terminal carbocation combines with a nucleophile or loses a proton, giving a terminal alkene (as shown here).

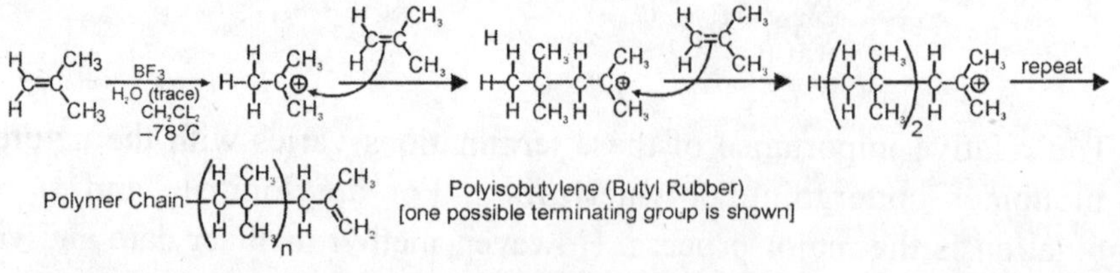

Polyisobutylene (Butyl Rubber)
[one possible terminating group is shown]

Monomers bearing cation stabilizing groups, such as alkyl, phenyl or vinyl can be polymerized by cationic processes. These are normally initiated at low temperature in methylene chloride solution. Strong acids, such as $HClO_4$, or Lewis acids containing traces of water (as shown above) serve as initiating reagents. At low temperatures, chain transfer reactions are rare in such polymerizations, so the resulting polymers are cleanly linear (unbranched).

3. Anionic Chain-Growth Polymerization

Treatment of a cold THF solution of styrene with 0.001 equivalents of n-butyllithium causes an immediate polymerization. This is an example of anionic polymerization, the course of which is described by the following equations. Chain growth may be terminated by water or carbon dioxide, and chain transfer seldom occurs. Only monomers having anion stabilizing substituents, such as phenyl, cyano or carbonyl are good substrates for this polymerization technique. Many of the resulting polymers are largely isotactic in configuration, and have high degrees of crystallinity.

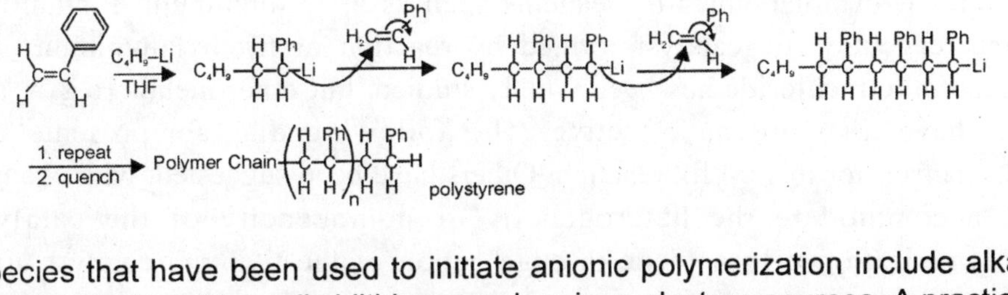

Species that have been used to initiate anionic polymerization include alkali metals, alkali amides, alkyl lithiums and various electron sources. A practical application of anionic polymerization occurs in the use of superglue. This material is methyl 2-cyanoacrylate, $CH_2=C(CN)CO_2CH_3$. When exposed to water, amines or other nucleophiles, a rapid polymerization of this monomer takes place.

4. Ziegler-Natta Catalytic Polymerization

An efficient and stereospecific catalytic polymerization procedure was developed by Karl Ziegler (Germany) and Giulio Natta (Italy) in the 1950's. Their findings permitted, for the first time, the synthesis of unbranched, high molecular weight polyethylene (HDPE), laboratory synthesis of natural rubber from isoprene, and configurational control of polymers from terminal alkenes like propene (e.g. pure isotactic and syndiotactic polymers). In the case of ethylene, rapid polymerization occurred at atmospheric pressure and moderate to low temperature, giving a stronger (more crystalline) product (HDPE) than that from radical polymerization (LDPE). For this important discovery these chemists received the 1963 Nobel Prize in chemistry.

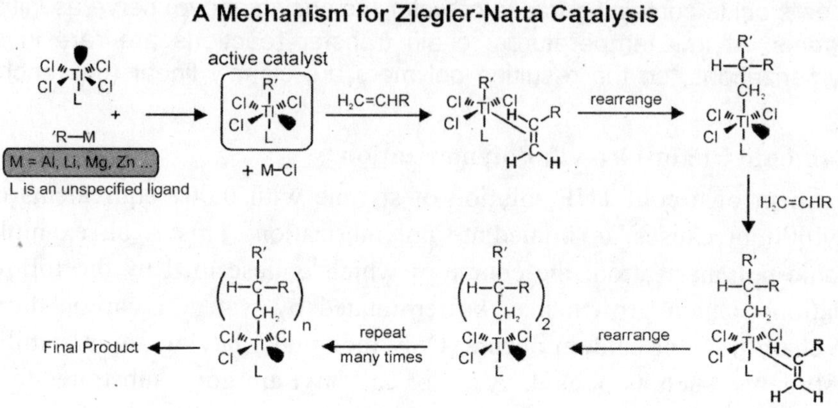

A Mechanism for Ziegler-Natta Catalysis

Ziegler-Natta catalysts are prepared by reacting certain transition metal halides with organometallic reagents such as alkyl aluminum, lithium and zinc reagents. The catalyst formed by reaction of triethylaluminum with titanium tetrachloride has been widely studied, but other metals (e.g. V and Zr) have also proven effective. The following diagram presents one mechanism for this useful reaction. Others have been suggested, with changes to accommodate the heterogeneity or homogeneity of the catalyst. Polymerization of propylene through action of the titanium catalyst gives an isotactic product; whereas, a vanadium based catalyst gives a syndiotactic product.

Polymerization Techniques

Broadly polymerisation techniques are of two types, Homogeneous and Heterogeneous polymerisation.

Homogeneous Polymerisation Systems

In this technique, reaction takes place in one homogenous system i.e. monomer, initiator and solvent form a single homogeneous phase after mixing. It is of two types

(a) Bulk Polymerization, and

(b) Solution Polymerization

(a) **Bulk polymerization:** Polymerization of the undiluted monomer is done for high conversion. Addition and condensation, both type of polymers can be synthesised by this technique. Polymerisation process is carried in two stages i.e. pre polymerisation and post polymerisation In the first stage (pre polymerisation), initiator is dissolved in monomer to get single phase, in this further solvent is not required. Till 10-12% conversion, reaction is slow but viscosity increases dramatically during further conversion. When polymerisation is completed by 25% then it becomes very viscous and high amount of heat is eveloved, then post polymerisation is carried out in another reactor, which is called main reactor, by transferring the material heat is also controlled.After completion of reaction, polymer is precipitated by adding suitable solvent like methanol. Styrene, vinyl chloride, methymethacrylate, Nylon-6 etc. monomers can be synthesised. Model for equipment is shown below:

Advantages	Disadvantages
• * Pure products	* heat control
• * Simple equipment	* dangerous
* No organic solvents	* molecular weights

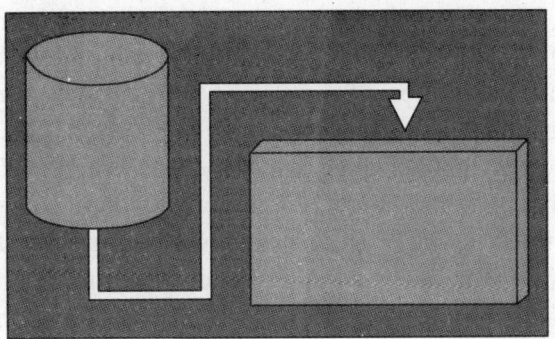

Fig. 8.1: Equipment for bulk polymerization

Solution polymerization

- In this polymerisation process,monomer is dissolved in solvent then initiator is dissolved to get homogeneous phase. Depending on concentration of monomer the solution does not increase in viscosity. When reaction is over, polymer is precipitatedby using solvent, then polyer filtered off and dried for use. Vinyl acetate, acronitrile, Acrylic coating, fibrespinning, film casting can ve synthesised by this method.In this heat is controlled due to proper solvent taken but very high molecular weight compound cannot be synthesied.

- **Heterogeneous systems**—In this technique, reaction takes place in more than one phase, i.e heterogeneous system. Mmonomer, initiator and solvent form heterogeneous phase, it may be emulsion or suspension form, hence it is also of two types: emulsion and suspension. **Suspension polymerization**—Water insoluble monomers are dispersed in water as large droplets about 0.1 to 1mm and kept suspended by mechanical agitator. Initiator is dissolved in monomer. Stabilization of droplets/polymer particles is done with non-micelle forming emulsifiers like gelatine or Na-carboxymethylcellulose. This is Equivalent to bulk polymerization, small droplets dispersed in water.Product can easily be separated. Pore sizes can be controlled by adding a combination of solvent (swelling agent) and non-solvent. Viscosity does not change much. Its advantages are that heat control is simple, product can be used directly and handling is easy, while disadvantages are that contamination may occur with stabilizing agent and coagulation is possible. Examples of polymer are Ion-exchange resins, polystyrene foam, PVC.

Emulsion polymerization

In this process, the monomer (organic) is dispersed in water, which forms fine droplets of 10^{-6} to 10^{-5} mm in size. Initiator is water soluble, addition of initiator leads to initiation of reaction in the micelles. A micelle forming emulsifier or surfactant like soap or detergent is used. The surfactant will form micelles when their concentration exceeds critical micelle size. Due to formation of polymer these micelles increase in size. The formed latex particles are much smaller than suspension particles. Kinetics differ considerable from other techniques. Polymer is formed within the micelles and not in the monomer droplets. Finally polymer is formed in the suspension form and polymer can be used as such in the suspension form. Advantages are that high Mwt polymer can be synthesized,easy control of temperature but cost of polymer may be high, some impurities may bepresent.Different types of paints, polystyrene, PVA can be synthesised by this technique.

SOME IMPORTANT EXAMPLES OF POLYMERS

Condensation Polymers

A large number of important and useful polymeric materials are not formed by chain-growth processes involving reactive species such as radicals, but proceed instead by conventional functional group transformations of polyfunctional reactants. These polymerizations often (but not always) occur with loss of a small byproduct, such as water, and generally (but not always) combine two different components in an alternating structure. The polyester Dacron and the polyamide Nylon 66, shown here, are two examples of synthetic condensation polymers, also known as **step-growth** polymers. In contrast to chain-growth polymers, most of which grow by carbon-carbon bond formation, step-growth polymers generally grow by carbon-heteroatom bond formation (C-O and C-N in Dacron and Nylon respectively). Although polymers of this kind might be considered to be alternating copolymers, the repeating monomeric unit is usually defined as a combined moiety.

Examples of naturally occurring condensation polymers are cellulose, the polypeptide chains of proteins, and poly (^{2}-hydroxybutyric acid), a polyester synthesized in large quantity by certain soil and water bacteria. Formulas for these will be displayed below by clicking on the diagram.

Many polymers, both addition and condensation, are used as fibers The chief methods of spinning synthetic polymers into fibers are from melts or viscous solutions. Polyesters, polyamides and polyolefins are usually spun from melts, provided the T_m is not too high. Polyacrylates suffer thermal degradation and are therefore spun from solution in a volatile solvent. **Cold-drawing** is an important physical treatment that improves the strength and appearance of these polymer fibers. At temperatures above T_g, a thicker than desired fiber can be forcibly stretched to many times its length; and in

Examples of Condensation Polymers

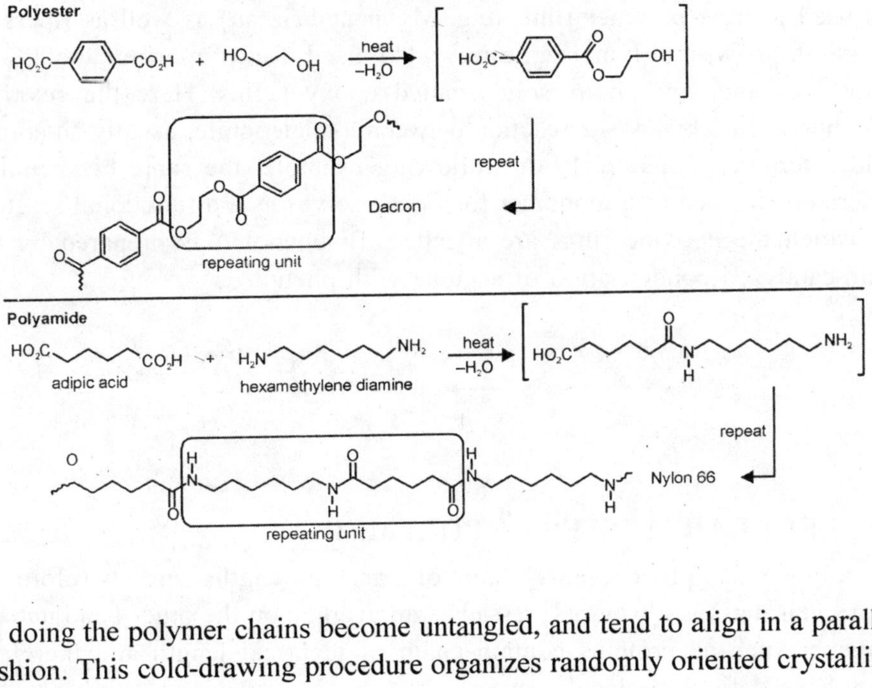

so doing the polymer chains become untangled, and tend to align in a parallel fashion. This cold-drawing procedure organizes randomly oriented crystalline domains (Fig. 8.2), and also aligns amorphous domains so they become more crystalline. In these cases, the physically oriented morphology is stabilized and retained in the final product. This contrasts with elastomeric polymers, for which the stretched or aligned morphology is unstable relative to the amorphous random coil morphology.

Random Crystalline Domains

Fig. 8.2

By clicking on the following diagram, a cartoon of these changes will toggle from one extreme to the other. This cold-drawing treatment may also be used to treat polymer films (e.g. Mylar and Saran) as well as fibers.

Step-growth polymerization is also used for preparing a class of adhesives and amorphous solids called epoxy resins. Here the covalent bonding occurs by an S_N2 reaction between a nucleophile, usually an amine, and a terminal epoxide. In the following example, the same bisphenol A intermediate used as a monomer for Lexan serves as a difunctional scaffold to which the epoxide rings are attached. Bisphenol A is prepared by the acid-catalyzed condensation of acetone with phenol.

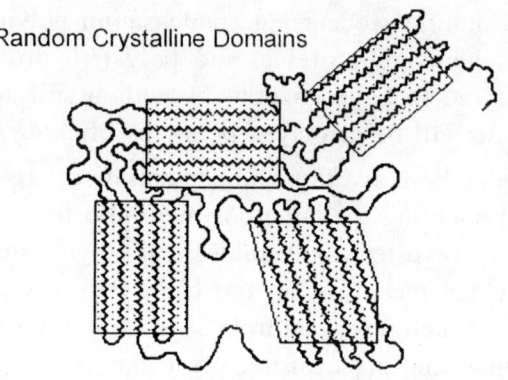

an epoxy resin

MOLECULAR MASSES OF POLYMERS

A polymer sample contains chain of varying lengths and therefore its molecular mass is always expressed as an average on the other hand natural polymer such as proteins contain chain of identical length and therefore they have definite molecular mass.

The molecular mass of a polymer can be expressed in two ways.

(1) Number average molecular mass (M_N)

(2) Weight average molecular mass (M_W).

(1) Number average molecular mass (M_N): If N_1, N_2, N_3..... are the number of molecules with molecular masses M_1, M_2, M_3...... respectively, then the number average molecular mass is

$$M_N = N_1M_1 + N_2M_2 + N_3M_3 +.../N_1 + N_2 + N_3...$$

This may be expressed as:

$$M_N = \Sigma N_iM_i/\Sigma N_i$$

Where N_i is the number of molecules of the ith type with molecular mass M_i.

(2) Weight average molecular mass (M_W): If m_1, m_2, m_3.... are the masses of species with molecular masses M_1, M_2, M_3... respectively, then the weight average molecular mass is

$$M_W = m_1M_1 + m_2M_2 + m_3M_3 .../m_1 + m_2 + m_3 +...$$
or
$$= \Sigma m_iM_i/\Sigma m_i$$

But $\quad m_i = N_iM_i$, so that $M_W = \Sigma N_iM_i^2/\Sigma N_iM_i$

where N_i is the number of molecules of mass M_i.

Another types of Polymer : Based upon molecular forces

Depending upon the intermolecular forces, the polymers have been classified into four type.

(i) Elastomers

(ii) Fibers

(iii) Thermoplastics

(iv) Thermosetting polymers

(i) *Elastomers* : The polymers that have elastic character like rubber (a material that can return to its original shape after stretching is said to be elastic) are called elastomers. In elastomers the polymers chains are held together by weak intermolecular forces. Because of the presence of weak forces, the polymers can be easily stretched by applying small stress and regains their original shape when the stress is removed. The most important example of elastomers is rubber.

(ii) *Fibers* : These are the polymers which have strong intermolecular forces between the chain. These forces are either hydrogen bonds or dipole-dipole interaction. Because of strong forces, the chains are closely packed giving them high tensil strength and less elasticity. Therefore, these polymers have sharp melting points. These polymers are long, thin and thread like and can be woven in fabric. Therefore, these are used for making fibers. Example: Nylon 66, dacron, silk etc.

(iii) *Thermoplastics* : These are the polymers which can be easily softened repeatedly when heated and hardened when cooled with little change in their properties. The intermolecular forces in these polymers are intermediate between those of elastomers and fibres. There is no cross linking between the chain. The softening occurs as the polymer chain move more and more freely because of absence of cross link. When heated, they melt and form a fluid which can be moulded into any desired shapes and then cooled to get the desired product. Polythene, polystyrene, PVC, teflon are the examples of this category.

(iv) *Thermosetting polymers* : These are the polymers which undergo permanent change on heating. They become hard and infusible on heating. They are generally prepared from low molecular mass semifluid substances. When heated they get highly cross linked to form hard infusible and insoluble products. The cross links hold the molecule in place so that heating does not allow them to move freely. Therefore a thermosetting plastic is cross linked and is permanently rigid. *Example* : Bakelite, melamine formaldehyde resin etc.

Details about Some Important Polymers

Polythene (PE)

Polyethylene (abbreviated PE) is the most common plastic. Its primary use is within packaging (plastic bag, plastic films, containers including bottles, etc.). Many kinds of polyethylene are known, but they almost always have the chemical formula $(C_2H_4)_nH_2$. Thus PE is usually a mixture of similar organic compound that differ in terms of the value of n.

Polyethylene is a thermoplastic polymer consisting of long hydrocarbon chains. Depending on the crystallinity and molecular weight, polythene may be Ultra-high-molecular-weight polyethylene, High-density polyethylene, Cross-linked polyethylene and Low-density polyethylene .The temperature at which these occur varies strongly with the type of polyethylene. For common commercial grades of medium- and high-density polyethylene the melting point is typically in the range 120 to 130°C. The melting point for average low-density polyethylene is typically 105 to 115°C.

Polyethylene is manufactured by the polymerization of ethylene (C_2H_4), which is the building block unit. Each molecule of ethylene consists of two methylene (CH_2) groups connected by a double bond.

Monomer

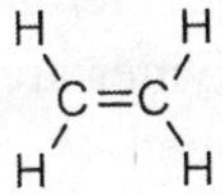

polythene-

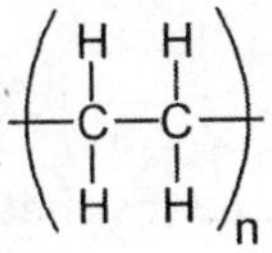

Polyethylene can be produced by various methods: Radical polymerization, anionic addition polymerization, cationic addition polymerization, or ion coordination polymerization. Each of these methods results in a different type of polyethylene. Some types of polyethylene like LDPE, HDPE, XDPE are discussed below.

Ultra-high-molecular-weight polyethylene (UHMWPE):

UHMWPE is polyethylene with a molecular weight numbering in the millions, usually between 3.1 and 5.67 million. The high molecular weight makes it a very tough material, but results in less efficient packing of the chains into the crystal structure as evidenced by densities of less than high density polyethylene (0.930–0.935 g/cm^3). UHMWPE can be made through Ziegler catalysts. Because of its outstanding toughness and its cut, wear and excellent chemical resistance, UHMWPE is used in a diverse range of applications. These include can and bottle handling machine parts, moving parts on weaving machines, bearings, gears, artificial joints, edge protection on ice rinks and butchers' chopping boards.

High-density polyethylene (HDPE)

HDPE is defined by a density of greater or equal to 0.941 g/cm^3. HDPE has a low degree of branching and thus stronger intermolecular forces and tensile strength. HDPE can be produced by chromium/silica catalysts, Ziegler-Natta catalysts or metallocene catalysts. The lack of branching is ensured by an appropriate choice of catalyst (for example, chromium catalysts or Ziegler-Natta catalysts) and reaction conditions. HDPE is used in products and packaging such as milk jugs, detergent bottles, margarine tubs, garbage containers and water pipes. One third of all toys are manufactured from HDPE.

Cross-linked polyethylene (PEX or XLPE)

PEX is a medium- to high-density polyethylene containing cross-link bonds introduced into the polymer structure, changing the thermoplast into an elastomer. The high-temperature properties of the polymer are improved, its flow is reduced and its chemical resistance is enhanced.

Low-density polyethylene (LDPE)

LDPE is defined by a density range of 0.910–0.940 g/cm^3. LDPE has a high degree of short and long chain branching, which means that the chains do not pack into the crystal structure as well. It has, therefore, less strong intermolecular forces as the instantaneous-dipole induced-dipole attraction is less. This results in a lower tensile strength and increased ductility. LDPE is created by free radical polymerization. The high degree of branching with long chains gives molten LDPE unique and desirable flow properties. LDPE is used for both rigid containers and plastic film applications such as plastic bags and film wrap.

PVC (Polyvinyl chloride)

Polyvinyl chloride, commonly abbreviated PVC, is the third-most widely produced plastic, after polyethylene and polypropylene.

Polyvinyl chloride is produced by polymerization of the monomer vinyl chloride (VCM), as shown.

About 80% of production involves suspension polymerization. Emulsion polymerization accounts for about 12 % and bulk polymerization is 8 %. Pure polyvinyl chloride without any plasticizer is a white, brittle solid. It is insoluble in alcohol, but slightly soluble in tetrahydrofuran The weight average molecular weights of PVC polymer range from 50,000 to 200,000.

PVC's relatively low cost, biological and chemical resistance and workability have resulted in it being used for a wide variety of applications. PVC is used in construction because it is cheaper than more durable longer lasting alternatives such as ductile iron. It can be made softer and more flexible by the addition of plasticizers, the most widely used being phthalates. In this form, it is used in clothing and upholstery, electrical cable insulation, inflatable products and many applications in which it replaces rubber. It is used for sewerage pipes and other pipe applications where cost or vulnerability to corrosion limit the use of metal. With the addition of impact modifiers and stabilizers, it has become a popular material for window and door frames. By adding plasticizers, it can become flexible enough to be used in cabling applications as a wire insulator.

Polystyrene

In chemical terms, polystyrene is a long chain hydrocarbon wherein alternating carbon centers are attached to phenyl groups . Polystyrene's chemical formula is $(C_8H_8)_n$; it contains the chemical elements carbon and hydrogen. The material's properties are determined by short-range van der Waals attractions between polymers chains. Since the molecules are long hydrocarbon chains that consist of thousands of atoms, the total attractive force between the molecules is large. When heated, the chains are able to take on a higher degree of conformation and slide past each other.

Polystyrene is formed by polymerization of styrene monomers. In the polymerization, one carbon-carbon double bond (in the vinyl group) is replaced by a much stronger carbon-carbon single bond, hence it is very difficult to depolymerize polystyrene. About a few thousand monomers typically comprise a chain of polystyrene, giving a molecular weight of 100,000–400,000..

styrene   polystyrene

Polystyrene can either be a thermoset or a thermoplastic. A thermoplastic polystyrene is in a solid (glassy) state at room temperature, but flows if heated above its glass transition temperature of about 100 °C (for molding or extrusion), and becomes solid again when cooled. Pure solid polystyrene is a colorless, hard plastic with limited flexibility. It can be cast into molds with fine detail. Polystyrene can be transparent or can be made to take on various colors. Solid polystyrene is used in disposable cutlery, plastic models, CD and DVD cases, and smoke detector housings. Products made from foamed polystyrene are nearly ubiquitous, for example packing materials, insulation, and foam drink cups.

Polypropylene (PP)

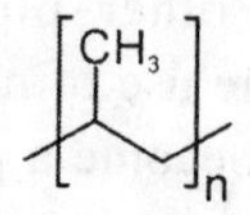

$$\left[\begin{array}{c} CH_3 \\ | \\ -CH-CH_2- \end{array} \right]_n$$

Polypropylene (PP), also known as **polypropene**, is a thermoplastic polymer, made from the monomer propylene, it is rugged and unusually resistant to many chemical solvents, bases and acids. It is used in a wide variety of applications including packaging and labeling, textiles (e.g., ropes, thermal underwear and carpets), stationery, plastic parts and reusable containers of various types, laboratory equipment, loudspeakers, automotive components, and polymer banknotes.

Short segments of polypropylene, showing isotactic (above) and syndiotactic tacticity (below).

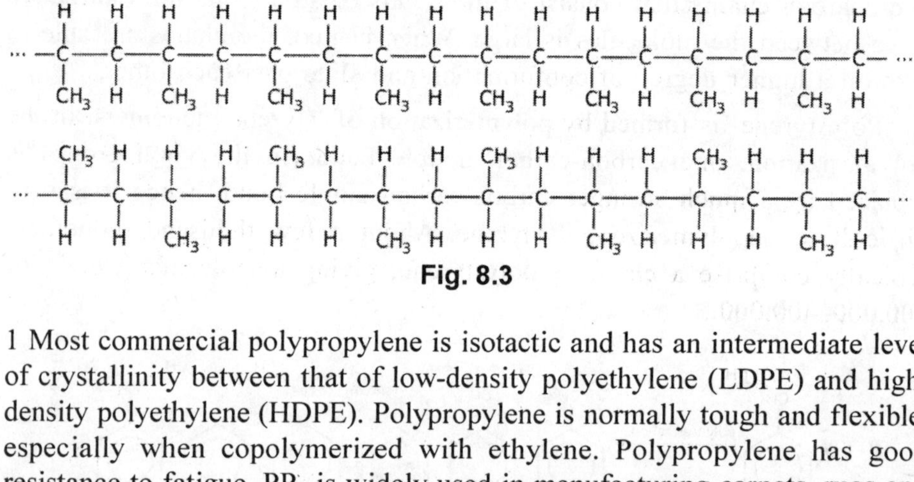

Fig. 8.3

1 Most commercial polypropylene is isotactic and has an intermediate level of crystallinity between that of low-density polyethylene (LDPE) and high-density polyethylene (HDPE). Polypropylene is normally tough and flexible, especially when copolymerized with ethylene. Polypropylene has good resistance to fatigue. PP is widely used in manufacturing carpets, rugs and mats to be used at home. Polypropylene is widely used in ropes, distinctive because they are light enough to float in water. For equal mass and construction, polypropylene rope is similar in strength to polyester rope. Polypropylene costs less than most other synthetic fibers.

TEFLON

Polytetrafluoroethylene

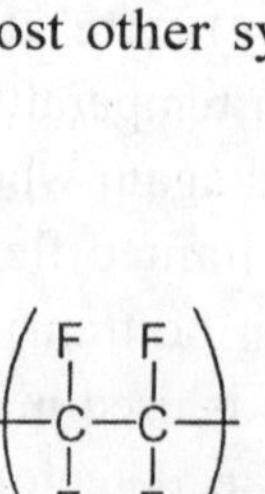

$$\left(\begin{array}{cc} F & F \\ | & | \\ -C - C- \\ | & | \\ F & F \end{array} \right)_n$$

Teflon is formed by polymerization of tetrafluoroethylene as reaction is shown below.

$$n(CF_2 = CF_2) \rightarrow -(CF_2 - CF_2)_{-n}$$

Polytetrafluoroethylene (PTFE) is a synthetic fluoropolymer of tetrafluoro-ethylene that finds numerous applications. The most well known brand name of PTFE is Teflon. PTFE is hydrophobic: neither water nor water-containing substances wet PTFE, as fluorocarbons demonstrate mitigated London dispersion forces due to the high electronegativity of fluorine. PTFE has one of the lowest coefficients of friction against any solid.

PTFE is used as a non-stick coating for pans and other cookware. It is very non-reactive, partly because of the strength of carbon–fluorine bonds, and so it is often used in containers and pipework for reactive and corrosive chemicals. Where used as a lubricant, PTFE reduces friction, wear, and energy consumption of machinery.

PMMA or plexi glass or lucite

Methacrylic acid, derived from acrylic acid, was formulated in 1865. The reaction between methacrylic acid and methanol results in the ester methyl methacrylate. The German chemists Fittig and Paul discovered in 1877 the polymerization process that turns methyl methacrylate into polymethyl methacrylate.

PMMA is also known for other names as Lucite, Plexiglas, Optix (Plaskolite), Perspex, and Altuglas

Synthesis

PMMA can be produced by emulsion polymerization or solution polymerization, or bulk polymerization. Generally radical or anionic polymerization of PMMA can also be performed..

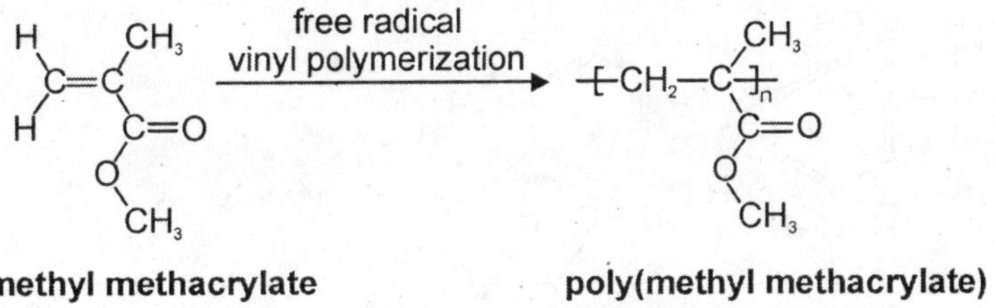

methyl methacrylate   poly(methyl methacrylate)

The glass transition temperature (T_g) of atactic PMMA is 105 °C.

Orlon

It is a Acrylic fiber. It is a polymer of acronitrile and the polymerization is carried out in aqueous phase. Acrylic fibers are synthetic fibers made from a polymer (polyacrylonitrile) with an average molecular weight of ~100,000, about 1900 monomer units. It can be blended with wool after dissolving in organic solvent like Dioxane or dimethyl formamide.

$$n(CH_2 = CHCN) \rightarrow -(CH_2 - CHCN)_{-n}$$

or

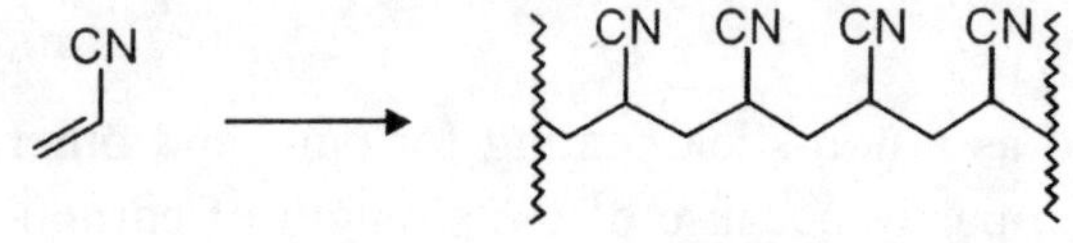

Orlon (Polyacrylonitrile)

Bakelite

It is a thermosetting phenol formaldehyde resin which is formed by condensation of phenol with formaldehyde.

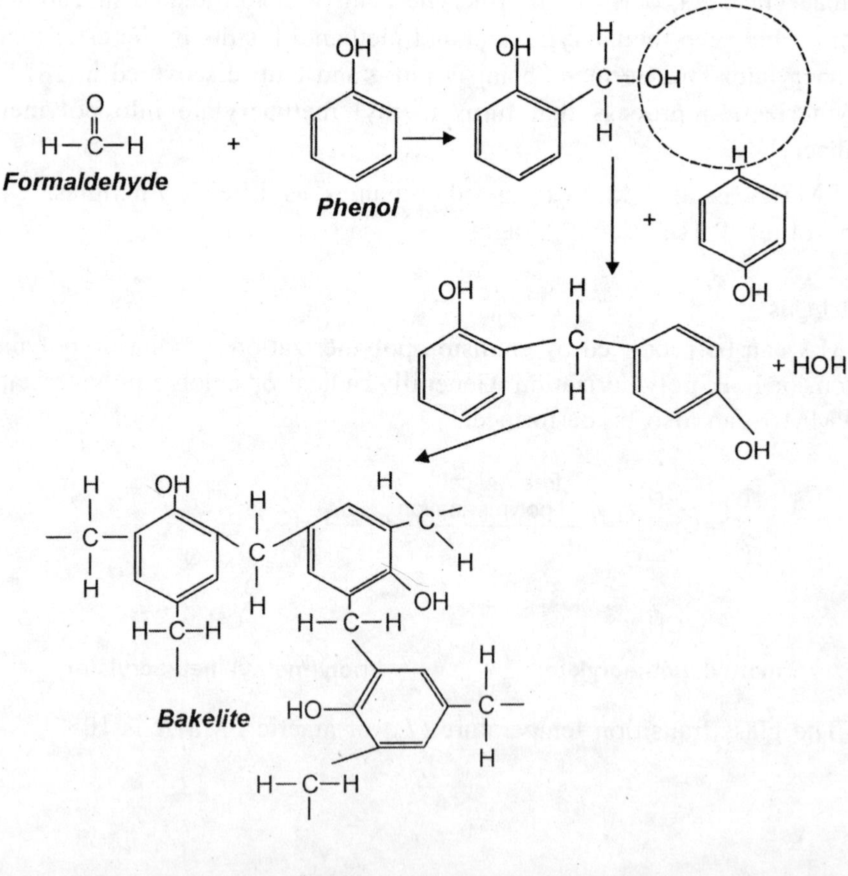

Bakelite is a three-dimensional polymer of formaldehyde and phenol. The reaction in very broad terms is illustrated in the graph. Note that the structure of Bakelite depends on ortho-para substitution and on the fact that substituting units don't lie in the identical plane as other substituting units. All of this gives Bakelite its 3-D structure.

Its industrial applications, Bakelite was particularly suitable for the emerging electrical and automobile industries because of its extraordinarily high resistance-not only to electricity, but to heat and chemical action. Now it is being used for all nonconducting parts of radios and other electrical devices, insulation of wires, boards, construction of brake pads an ' related automotive components as well as industrial electrical related applications.

POLYURETHANE

A **polyurethane (PU)** is polymer composed of a chain of organic units joined by carbamate (urethane) links. Polyurethane polymers are formed by combining two bi- or higher functional monomers. One contains two or more isocyanate functional groups (with formula –N=C=O) and the other contains two or more hydroxyl groups (with formula –OH). The alcohol and the isocyanate groups combine to form a urethane linkage:

ROH + R'NCO → ROC(O)N(H)R' (R and R' are alkyl or aryl groups)

This combining process, sometimes called condensation, typically requires the presence of a catalyst. More complicated monomers are also used.

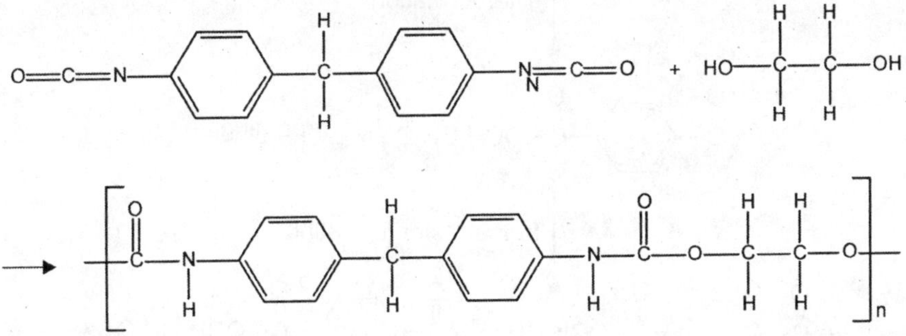

Polyurethanes are used in the manufacture of flexible, high-resilience foam seating; rigid foam insulation panels; microcellular foam seals and gaskets; durable elastomeric wheels and tires; automotive suspension bushings; electrical potting compounds; high performance adhesives; surface coatings and surface sealants; synthetic fibers (e.g., Spandex); carpet underlay; and hard-plastic parts (i.e., for electronic instruments). Polyurethane is also used for the manufacture of hoses and skateboard wheels as it combines the best properties of both rubber and plastic.

Polyester

Polyester is a category of polymers which contain the ester functional group in their main chain, which is shown below. The term "polyester" as a specific material most commonly refers to polyethylene terephthalate (PET). Depending on the chemical structure, polyester can be a thermoplastic or thermoset; however, the most common polyesters are thermoplastics.

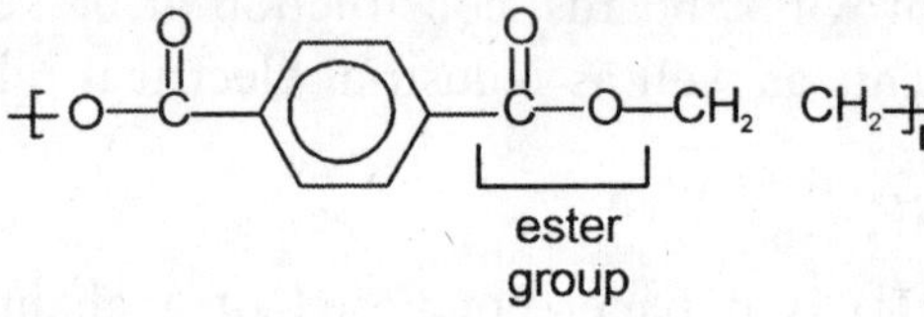

ester
group

Characteristics of polyester

Polyester fabrics and fibers are extremely strong.Polyester is very durable: resistant to most chemicals, stretching and shrinking, wrinkle resistant, mildew and abrasion resistant. Polyester is hydrophobic in nature and quick drying. Polyester retains its shape and hence is good for making outdoor clothing for harsh climates. It is easily washed and dried.

Preparation

PET is prepared by condensation of terphthalic acid and ethylene glycol in basic medium.

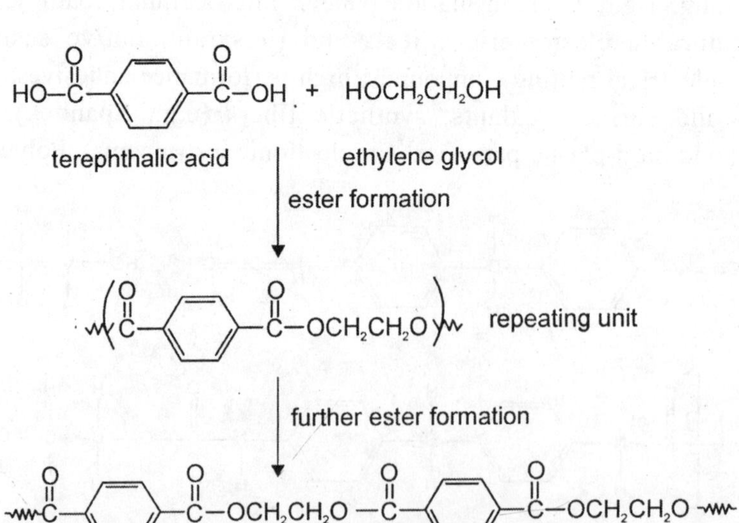

terephthalic acid   ethylene glycol

ester formation

repeating unit

further ester formation

polyethylene terephthalate (polyester)

Uses of Polyester

The most popular and one of the earliest uses of polyester was to make polyester suits and polyester clothes are made. Due to its strength and tenacity polyester is also used to make ropes in industries. PET bottles are today one of the most popular uses of polyester. Fabric balls knitted from polyester thread or yarn are used extensively in apparel and home furnishings, from shirts and pants to jackets and hats, bed sheets, blankets, upholstered furniture and computer mouse mats,etc.

Nylon (Polyamides)

Nylon is a generic designation for a family of synthetic polymers known gener as polyamides. Nylons are condensation copolymers formed by reacting equal parts of a diamine and a dicarboxylic acid, so that amides are formed at both ends of each monomer in a process analogous to polypeptide biopolymers. Chemical elements included are carbon, hydrogen, nitrogen, and oxygen. The numerical suffix specifies the numbers of carbons donated by the monomers; the diamine first and the diacid second. The most common variant is nylon 6-6 which refers to the fact that the diamine (hexamethylene diamine, IUPAC name: hexane-1,6-diamine) and the diacid (adipic acid, IUPAC name: hexanedioic acid) each donate 6 carbons to the polymer chain.

For, Nylon The general reaction is:

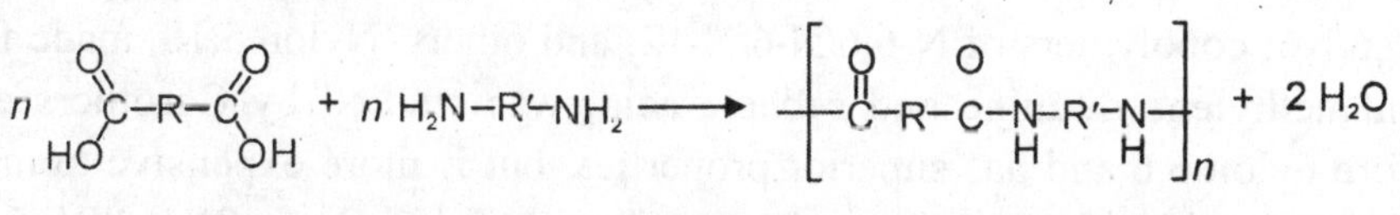

A molecule of water is given off and the nylon is formed. Its properties are determined by the R and R′ groups in the monomers. In nylon 6, 6, R = 4C and R′ = 6C alkanes, but one also has to include the two carboxyl carbons in the diacid to get the number it donates to the chain. In Kevlar, both R and R′ are benzene rings

For Nylon 66 chemical reaction is

nHOOC − $(CH_2)_4$ − COOH + n H_2N − $(CH_2)_6$ − NH_2 → [−OC − $(CH_2)_4$ − CO − NH − $(CH_2)_6$ − NH−] n + 2nH_2O and the part −CO − NH − will stick together becoming Nylon 6, 6

Nylon 6 or **polycaprolactam** is a polymer developed by Paul Schlack to reproduce the properties of nylon 6, 6. Unlike most other nylons, nylon 6 is not a condensation polymer, but instead is formed by ring-opening polymerization by using monomer, caprolacum. (alternatively made by polymerizing aminocaproic acid). The peptide bond within the caprolactam is broken with the exposed active groups on each side being incorporated into two new bonds as the monomer becomes part of the polymer backbone. In this case, all amide bonds lie in the same direction, but the properties of nylon 6 are sometimes indistinguishable from those of nylon 6, 6–except for melt temperature and some fiber properties in products like carpets and textiles. The 428°F (220°C) melting point of nylon 6 is lower than the 509°F (265°C) melting point of nylon 6,6. Its competition with nylon 6,6 and the example it set have also shaped the economics of the synthetic fiber industry. It was given the trademark Perlon in 1952. It is a semicrystalline polyamide.

Other nylons

Other nylons include copolymerized dicarboxylic acid/diamine products. For example, some aromatic nylons are polymerized with the addition of diacids like terephthalic acid (→ Kevlar, Twaron) or isophthalic acid (→ Nomex), more commonly associated with polyesters. There are copolymers of N-6,6/N6; copolymers of N-6,6/N-6/N-12; and others. Nylon 5,10, made from pentamethylene diamine and sebacic acid, was studied by Carothers even before nylon 6,6 and has superior properties, but is more expensive to make. In keeping with this naming convention, "nylon 6,12" (N-6,12) or "PA-6,12" is a copolymer of a 6C diamine and a 12C diacid. Similarly for N-5,10 N-6,11; N-10,12, etc. Because of the way polyamides are formed, nylon would seem to be limited to unbranched, straight chains. But "star" branched nylon can be produced by the condensation of dicarboxylic acids with polyamines having three or more amino groups.

Characteristics

The characteristic features of nylon 6,6 include:
- Pleats and creases can be heat-set at higher temperatures
- More compact molecular structure
- Better weathering properties; better sunlight resistance
- Softer "Hand"
- Higher melting point (256 °C/492.8 °F)
- Superior colorfastness

- Excellent abrasion resistance

On the other hand, nylon 6 is easy to dye, more readily fades; it has a higher impact resistance, a more rapid moisture absorption, greater elasticity and elastic recovery.

RUBBER OR ELASTOMER

It is a polymer which is capable of returning to its original length, shape or size after being stretched or deformed. It is the example of elastomer. Rubber are of two types.

(1) Natural rubber

(2) Synthetic rubber

(1) **Natural rubber: It is** also called **India Rubber** or **caoutchouc,** is an elastomer (an elastic hydrocarbon polymer) that was originally derived from latex, a milky colloid produced by some plants. The plants would be 'tapped', that is, an incision made into the bark of the tree and the sticky, milk colored latex sap collected and refined into a usable rubber. The purified form of natural rubber is the chemical polyisoprene, which is the polymer of isoprene (2 methyl, 1,3butadiene) unit. It is obtained as latex from rubber trees.The latex is coagulated with acetic acid or formic acid. The coagulated mass is then squeezed.The raw natural rubber is a soft gummy and sticky mass. It is insoluble in water, dil. Acids and alkalies but soluble in benzene, chloroform, ether, petrol and carbon disulphide. It absorb a large amount of water. It has low elasticity and tensile strength. Destructive distillation of natural rubber gives mainly isoprene (2-methyl butadiene). Thus isoprene is a monomer of natural rubber the no. of isoprene unit are 11,000 to 20,000 which linked together in a chain.

$$n CH_2 = \overset{\overset{\displaystyle CH_3}{|}}{C} - CH = CH_2 \xrightarrow{\text{Polymerisation}} \left[- CH_2 - \overset{\overset{\displaystyle CH_3}{|}}{C} = CH - CH_2 - \right]_n$$

Isopreme

Natural rubber

Natural rubber is used extensively in many applications and products. It is normally very stretchy and flexible and extremely waterproof.

- Natural rubber coming from latex is mostly polymerized isoprene with a small percentage of impurities in it. This limits the range of properties available to it. Also, there are limitations on the proportions of *cis* and *trans* double bonds resulting from methods of polymerizing natural latex. This also limits the range of properties available to natural rubber, although addition of sulfur and vulcanization are used to improve the properties.

(2) Synthetic rubber: The synthetic rubber is obtained by polymerising certain organic compounds which may have properties similar to rubber and some desirable properties. Most of these are derived from butadiene derivatives and contain carbon-carbon double bonds. The synthetic rubbers are either homopolymers of 1, 3 butadiene or copolymer in which one of the monomers is 1, 3 butadiene or its derivative so that the polymer has the availability of double bonds for its vulcanization. Some important examples are Neoprene, styrene, butadiene rubber (SBR) thiokol, silicones, polyurethane, rubber etc.

- Synthetic rubber can be made from the polymerization of a variety of monomers including isoprene (2-methyl-1,3-butadiene), 1,3-butadiene, chloroprene (2-chloro-1,3-butadiene), and isobutylene (methylpropene) with a small percentage of isoprene for cross-linking. These and other monomers can be mixed in various desirable proportions to be copolymerized for a wide range of physical, mechanical, and chemical properties. The monomers can be produced pure and the addition of impurities or additives can be controlled by design to give optimal properties. Polymerization of pure monomers can be better controlled to give a desired proportion of *cis* and *trans* double bonds.

Natural rubber
All cis configuration

Vulcanization of rubber

The process of heating natural rubber with sulphur to improve its properties is called vulcanization. Vulcanization was introduced by Charles Goodyear.

Although natural rubber is thermoplastic substance in which there are no cross link between the polymer chain and it on vulcanization set into a given shape which is retained.

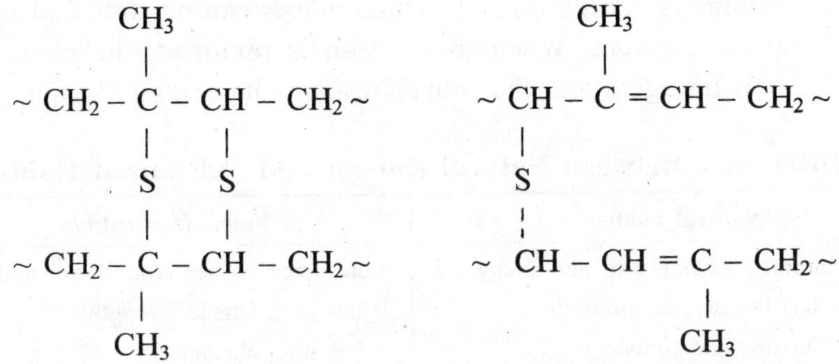

$$
\begin{array}{cc}
\quad CH_3 & \quad CH_3 \\
\quad | & \quad | \\
\sim CH_2 - C - CH - CH_2 \sim & \sim CH - C = CH - CH_2 \sim \\
\quad | \quad | & \quad | \\
\quad S \quad S & \quad S \\
\quad | \quad | & \quad \vdots \\
\sim CH_2 - C - CH - CH_2 \sim & \sim CH - CH = C - CH_2 \sim \\
\quad | & \quad | \\
\quad CH_3 & \quad CH_3
\end{array}
$$

- The vulcanization process performed originally was slow. Now a days, some additives such as zinc oxide etc. are used to accelerate the rate of vulcanization. During vulcanization, sulphur cross links are formed (shown in figure) the double bonds in the rubber molecule acts as reactive sites. The allylic $-CH_2$, alpha to double bond is also very reactive. During vulcanization, sulphur forms cross links at these reactive sites. As a result, rubber gets stiffened and intermolecular movement of rubber springs is prevented resulting in physical character of rubber. The extent of stiffness of vulcanized rubber depend upon the amount of sulphur added. For cxample about 5% sulphur is used for making tyre rubber while 30% of the sulphur is used for making battery case rubbcr.

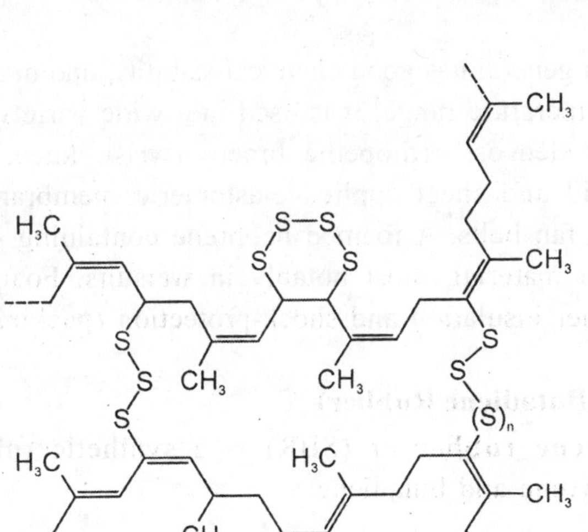

In a polymer, the chains are normally tangled up with each other. When the rubber is stretched, the chains straighten out to some extent. The chains cannot slip past each other because of the polysulphide bridges. Thus, rubber can be stretched only to a limited extent. When the tension is removed, the chains try to coil up again and the rubber resumes its original shape.

Difference Between Natural Rubber and Vulcanized Rubber

Natural rubber	Vulcanized rubber
(1) Natural rubber is soft and sticky	Vulcanized rubber is hard and non-sticky.
(2) It has low tensile strength.	It has high tensile strength.
(3) It has low elasticity.	It has high elasticity.
(4) It can be used over a narrow range of temperature (from 10° to 60°C).	It can be used over a wide range of temperature (–40° to 100°C).
(5) It has low wear and tear resistance.	It has high wear and tear resistance.
(6) It is soluble in solvents like ether, carbon, tetrachloride, petrol, etc.	It is insoluble in all the common solvents.

Neoprene

Neoprene or polychloroprene is a family of synthetic <u>rubbers</u> that are produced by polymerization of <u>chloroprene</u>.

$$n\left(\begin{matrix} H & H & Cl & H \\ | & | & | & | \\ C{=}C{-}C{=}C \\ | & & & | \\ H & & & H \end{matrix}\right) \rightarrow \left(\begin{matrix} H & H & Cl & H \\ | & | & | & | \\ {-}C{-}C{=}C{-}C{-} \\ | & & & | \\ H & & & H \end{matrix}\right)_n$$

Neoprene in general has good chemical stability, and maintains flexibility over a wide temperature range. It is used in a wide variety of applications, such as laptop sleeves, orthopedic braces (wrist, knee, etc.), electrical insulation, liquid and sheet applied elastomeric membranes or flashings, and automotive fan belts. A foamed neoprene containing gas cells is used as an insulation material, most notably in wetsuits. Foamed neoprene is also used in other insulation and shock-protection (packing) applications.

SBR-(Styrene-Butadiene Rubber)

Styrene-butadiene rubber or (SBR) is a synthetic rubber copolymer consisting of styrene and butadiene.

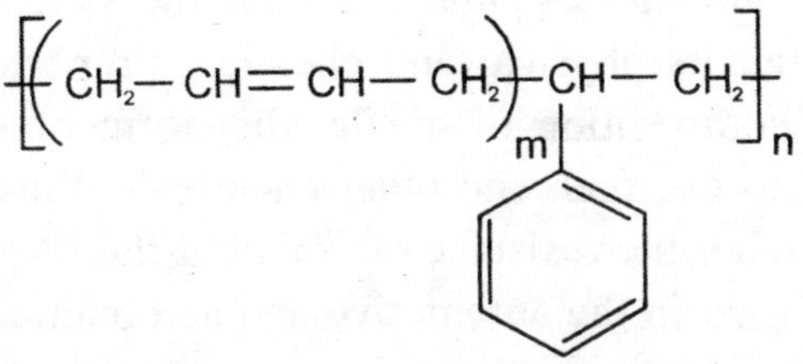

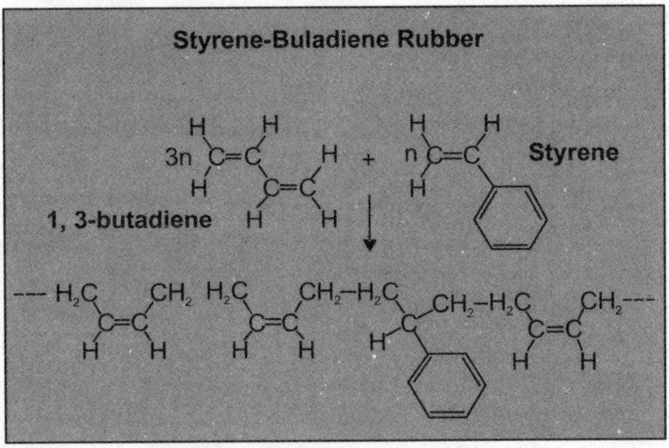

$$\left[\!\!\left(CH_2\!-\!CH\!=\!CH\!-\!CH_2\right)_{\!m}\!\!-\!CH\!-\!CH_2\!\right]_n$$

Styrene-Buladiene Rubber

It has good abrasion resistance and good aging stability when protected by additives, and is widely used in car tires, where it may be blended with natural rubber. It was originally developed prior to World War II in Germany,. Industrial manufacture began during World War 2, where it was used extensively by the USA to replace the Far-East natural rubber supplies captured by the Japanese. The elastomer is used widely in pneumatic tires, shoe heels and soles, gaskets and even chewing gum. It is a commodity material which competes with natural rubber. Latex (emulsion) SBR is extensively used in coated papers, being one of the most cost-effective resins to bind pigmented coatings. It is also used in building applications, as a sealing and binding agent behind renders as an alternative to PVA, but is more expensive.

Buna N-Rubber

It is also known as Buna-N, Perbunan, or NBR, is a synthetic rubber copolymer of acrylonitrile (ACN) and butadiene. Trade names include Nipol, Krynac and Europrene.

Nitrile butadiene rubber (NBR) is a family of unsaturated copolymers of 2-propenenitrile and various butadiene monomers (1,2-butadiene and 1,3-butadiene). Although its physical and chemical properties vary depending on the polymer's composition of nitrile, this form of synthetic rubber is generally resistant to oil, fuel, and other chemicals (the more nitrile within the polymer, the higher the resistance to oils but the lower the flexibility of the material). It is used in the automotive and aeronautical industry to make fuel and oil handling hoses, seals, and grommets. It is used in the nuclear industry to make protective gloves. NBR's ability to withstand a range of temperatures from −40°C to +108°C makes it an ideal material for aeronautical applications. Nitrile butadiene is also used to create moulded goods, footwear, adhesives, sealants, sponges, expanded foams, and floor mats. Its resilience makes NBR a useful material for disposable lab, cleaning, and examination gloves. Nitrile rubber is more resistant than <u>natural rubber</u> to <u>oils</u> and <u>acids,</u> but has inferior strength and flexibility. Nitrile gloves are nonetheless three times more <u>puncture-resistant</u> than natural rubber gloves.

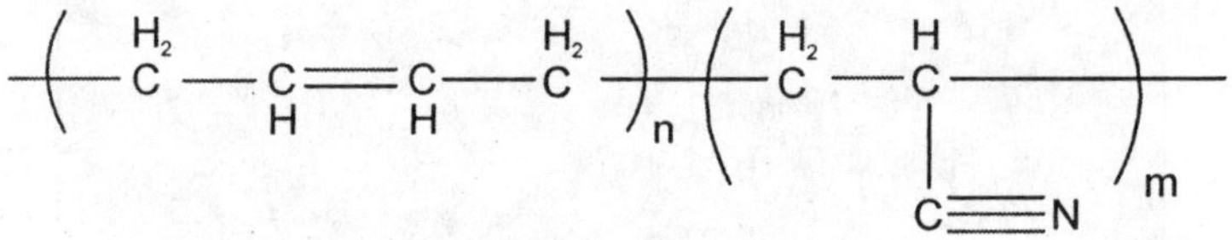

Fig. 8.4: Nitrile rubber

Biodegradable Polymers

These are the polymers which gets decomposed by the process of biodegradation. Biodegradation is defined as a process carried out by biological systems usually fungi or bacteria wherein a poly chain is cleaved via enzymatic activity. Different polymers are degraded at different rate depending upon its structure. Degradation consists of

- Enzymatic degradation
- Hydrolysis
  (depend on main chain structure: anhydride > ester > carbonate)

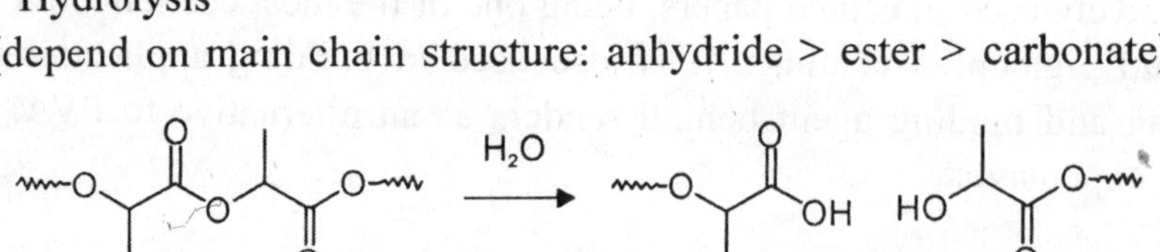

Requirement for biodegradation

— **Micro-organisms:** These micro-organisms must exist with the appropriate biochemical machinery to synthesize enzymes specific for the target polymer to initiate the depolymerization process.

— **Environment:** Temperature, Pressure, Moisture, Oxygen, Type and concentration of salts, Light etc.

— **Substrate:**

  (i) Suitable functional groups

  (ii) Hydrophilicity

  (iii) Low molecular weights

  (iv) Less crystallinity

Natural rubber, collagen, lignin, poly (gamma-glutamic acid), starch, cellulose, gelatin, silk, wool are natural biodegradable polymers while synthetic biodegradable polymers are Polyvinyl alcohol, polyanhydrides, PHBV or poly-(3-Hydroxybutyrate–CO–3–Hydroxyvalerate), Polycaprolactum, Polylactic acid, Polyglycolide.

Applications of biodegradable problems

— The use of packaging materials produced from biopolymers (bio based polyesters) offers ecological advantages over synthetic plastic packaging because they can be produced from renewable

— PHB or poly (β-hydroxy butyrate) is used in the manufacture of shampoo bottles.

— **PLA or poly lactic acid:** It breaks down in the environment back to lactic acid which can be metabolized which has application in medical science such as sutures, drug delivery systems and wound clips. It has also agricultural applications such as time release coatings for fertilizers and pesticides.

Limitations

— Biodegradable polymers are very expensive.

— They are not easily available.

— In order to store potentially hazardous materials, landfills are built to be free of moisture and air tight. These anaerobic conditions which serve to guard against the release of hazardous chemicals from landfills also retard biodegradation.

— Biodegradable polymers are not suitable candidates in the recycling of commingled plastics.

Examples of biodegradable polymers

  (i) **Polyhydroxy butyrate (PHB):** Polyhydroxy butyrate (PHB) is obtained from hydroxy butyric acid (3-hydroxy butanoic acid)

$$nHO \ CHCH_2C \ OH \xrightarrow{\text{Condensation}} \left\{ -O-CHCH_2C- \right\}_n$$

3-Hydroxy butanoic acid   Polyhydroxybutyrate (PHB)

(ii) **Poly-Hydroxybutyrate-co-b-Hydroxy valerate (PHBV)** : It is copolymer of 3-hydroxy butanoic acid and 3-hydroxy pentanoic acid, in which the monomer units are joined by ester linkages.

$$nCH_3-CH-CH_2COOH + nCH_3-CH_2-CH-CH_2-COOH \rightarrow \left(-O-CH-CH_2-CO- \right)_n, R = CH_3, C_2H_5$$

3-Hydroxy butanoic acid   3-Hydroxy pentanoic acid   PHBV

The properties of PHBV vary according to the ratio of both the acids. 3-Hydroxy butanoic acid provides stiffness while 3-Hydroxypentanoic acid gives flexibility to the copolymer.

(iii) **Polyglycolic acid (PGA)** : Polyglycolic acid (PGA) is obtained by the chain polymerisation of cyclic dimer of glycolic acid, .

$$nHO-CH_2COOH \xrightarrow{\text{Heat}} \left(-OCH_2 \ C- \right)_n$$

Glycolic acid   Polyglycolic acid (PGA)

(iv) **Polylactic acid (PLA):** Polylactic acid (PLA) is obtained by polymerisation of the cyclic dimer of lactic acid or by microbiological synthesis of lactic acid followed by the polycondensation and removal of water by evaporation.

$$nHOCHC-OH \xrightarrow{\text{Condensation}} \left(-OCH-C- \right)_n$$

Lactic acid   Polylactic acid (PLA)

Conducting polymer

Generally, the polymers are not assumed to be conductor of current but there are many polymers which can conduct electricity are known as conducting polymers e.g. polyaniline, polyacetylene, polypyrrole. Normal polymers do not have so much conductance as metals, however by doing some modifications like blending with metals or by oxidation or reduction method, conductance of some polymers can be increased up to great extent, on this basis polymer can be classified as follows-

1. Intrinsic conducting polymers
2. Doped conducting polymers
3. Extrinsic conducting polymers

1. **Intrinsic Conductive polymers** (ICPs) are organic polymers that conduct electricity mainly due to conjugation (π electrons) present in the backbone of the molecule like polyacetylene. Such compounds may have metallic conductivity or can be semiconductors. The biggest advantage of conductive polymers is their processability, mainly by dispersion. Conductive polymers are generally not thermoplastics, i.e., they are not thermoformable. But, like insulating polymers, they are organic materials. They can offer high electrical conductivity but do not show similar mechanical properties to other commercially available polymers. The electrical properties can be fine-tuned using the methods of organic synthesis and by advanced dispersion techniques.

(X = NH/N, S)   (X = NH, S)

Chemical structures of some conductive polymers

From top left clockwise: polyacetylene; polyphenylene vinylene; polypyrrole (X = NH) and polythiophene (X = S); and polyaniline (X = NH/N) and polyphenylene sulfide (X = S).

The linear-backbone "polymer blacks" (polyacetylene, polypyrrole, and polyaniline) and their copolymers are the main class of conductive polymers. Historically, these are known as melanins. Poly(p-phenylene vinylene) (PPV) and its soluble derivatives have emerged as the prototypical electro-luminescent semiconducting polymers. Today, poly(3-alkylthiophenes) are the archetypical materials for solar cells and transistors.

2. **Doped conducting polymers-** These polymers are obtained by doing some modifications like oxidation or reduction .On this basis further it may be of two types-

(i) **p doped polymer-** These polmers are obtained by oxidation process. Conducting polymer like polyacetylene is treated with lewis acid or with iodine vapours, which creates positive charge on polymer back bone. This positive charge is mainly responsible for conduction.

$$(C_2H_2)_n + A(\text{Lewis acid}) = (C_2H_2)^+_n A^- (\text{Oxidation Process})$$

(ii) **n doped polymer:** This type of polymer is obtained by reduction process, i.e polymers are treated with lewis base (Li or Na reductant)

$$(C_2H_2)_n + B(\text{Lewis base}) = (C_2H_2)^-_n B^+ (\text{Reduction Process})$$

By doing such type of doping, conductivity of polymers can be increased in the order of 10^5 to ^{15} times, conductivity of polyaniline is increased from 10^{-11} SCm^{-1} to 10^{-5} SCm^{-1}.

3. **Extrinsic conducting polymer:** These conducing polymers have conductivity due to the externally added materials into the polymer, on the basis of externally added material these can be divided into two types:

(i) **Conducting element filled polymers:** The polymers are filled with conducting materials like carbon black, metallic oxides, metallic fibres etc. The polymers have conductivity mainly due to externally added material. Minimum concentration of conductive element (material) required to added so that polymer starts conducting is known as percolation threshold. Such type of polymer have low cost and high weight with good conductivity.

(ii) **Blended conducting polymers:** This type of polymer is obtained by blending a metal with the conventional polymer. This blending is done by mechanical and chemical action. In this way they have better physical, chemical and mechanical properties.

Molecular basis of electrical conductivity

The conductivity of such polymers is the result of several processes. E.g., in traditional polymers such as polyethylenes, the valence electrons are bound in sp^3 hybridized covalent bonds. Such "sigma-bonding electrons" have low mobility and do not contribute to the electrical conductivity of the material. However, in conjugated materials, the situation is completely different. Conducting polymers have backbones of contiguous sp^2 hybridized carbon centers. One valence electron on each center resides in a p_z orbital, which is orthogonal to the other three sigma-bonds. The electrons in these delocalized orbitals have high mobility when the material is "doped" by oxidation, which removes some of these delocalized electrons. Thus, the conjugated p-orbitals form a one-dimensional electronic band, and the electrons within this band become mobile when it is partially emptied. The band structures of conductive polymers can easily be calculated with a tight binding model. In principle, these same materials can be doped by reduction, which adds electrons to an otherwise unfilled band. In practice, most organic conductors are doped oxidatively to give p-type materials. The redox doping of organic conductors is analogous to the doping of silicon semiconductors, whereby a small fraction silicon atoms are replaced by electron-rich (e.g., phosphorus) or electron-poor (e.g. boron) atoms to create n-type and p-type semiconductors, respectively. Although typically "doping" conductive polymers involves oxidizing or reducing the material, conductive organic polymers associated with a protic solvent may also be "self-doped."

The most notable difference between conductive polymers and inorganic semiconductors is the electron mobility, which historically was dramatically lower in conductive polymers than their inorganic counterparts. This difference is diminishing with the invention of new polymers and the development of new processing techniques. Low charge carrier mobility is related to structural disorder. In fact, as with inorganic amorphous semiconductors, conduction in such relatively disordered materials is mostly a function of "mobility gaps"with phonon-assisted hopping, polaron-assisted tunneling, etc., between localized states. Undoped conjugated polymers state are semiconductors or insulators. In such compounds, the energy gap can be > 2 eV, which is too great for thermally activated conduction. Therefore, undoped conjugated polymers, such as polythiophenes, polyacetylenes only have a low electrical conductivity of around $10^{"10}$ to $10^{"8}$ S/cm. Even at a very low level of doping (< 1%), electrical conductivity increases several orders of magnitude up to values of around 0.1 S/cm. Subsequent doping of the conducting polymers will result in a saturation of the conductivity at values around 0.1–10 kS/cm for different polymers. Highest values reported up to now are for the conductivity of stretch oriented polyacetylene with confirmed values of about 80 kS/cm. Although the pi-electrons in polyactetylene are delocalized along the chain, pristine polyacetylene is not a metal. Polyacetylene has alternating single and double bonds which have lengths of 1.44 and 1.36 Å, respectively. Upon doping, the bond alteration is diminished in conductivity increases. Non-doping increases in conductivity can also be accomplished in a field effect transistor and by irradiation. Some materials also exhibit negative differential resistance and voltage-controlled "switching" analogous to that seen in inorganic amorphous semiconductors.

Properties and applications

Due to their poor processability, conductive polymers have few large-scale applications. They have promise in antistatic materials and they have been incorporated into commercial displays and batteries, but there have had limitations due to the manufacturing costs, material inconsistencies, toxicity, poor solubility in solvents, and inability to directly melt process. Literature suggests they are also promising in organic solar cells, printing electronic circuits, organic light-emitting diodes, actuators, electrochromism, super-capacitors, chemical sensors and biosensors[14], flexible transparent displays, electromagnetic shielding and possibly replacement for the popular transparent conductor indium tin oxide. Conducting polymers are rapidly gaining attraction in new applications with increasingly processable materials with better electrical and physical properties and lower costs. The new nanostructured forms of conducting polymers particularly, provide fresh air to this field with their higher surface area and better dispersability.

With the availability of stable and reproducible dispersions, polyaniline have gained some large scale applications. While PEDOT (poly(3,4-ethylene-dioxythiophene)) is mainly used in antistatic applications and as a transparent conductive layer in form of PEDOT:PSS dispersions (PSS=polystyrene sulfonic acid), polyaniline is widely used for printed circuit board manu-facturing – in the final finish, for protecting copper from corrosion and preventing its solderability.

Chapter 9
ENGINEERING MATERIALS

- ➤ **Alloys**
- ➤ **Ceramics-glass**
- ➤ **Refractory**
- ➤ **Nano Compsites and Organomettalics**

ALLOY

An alloy is a partial or complete solid solution of one or more elements in a metallic matrix. Complete solid solution alloys give single solid phase microstructure, while partial solutions give two or more phases that may be homogeneous in distribution depending on thermal properties. Alloys usually have different properties from those of the component elements. For examples, steel is a metal alloy whose major component is iron, with carbon content between 0.02 and 2.14% by mass, brass is an alloy made from copper and zinc. Bronze, used for bearings, statues, ornaments and church bells, is an alloy of copper and tin.

Important Alloys

1. Brass

Brass is an alloy of copper and zinc. The proportions of zinc and copper can be varied to create a range of brasses with varying properties. Brass has a muted yellow colour, somewhat similar to gold. It is relatively resistant to tarnishing, and is often used as decoration and for coins. In antiquity, polished brass was often used as a mirror.

Type of Brasses

Types of Brasses	Composites	Properties
Admiralty brass	30% zinc, and 1% tin,	Dezincification in most
Arch alloy	60.66% copper, 36.58% zinc, 1.02% tin, and 1074% iron	Corrosion resistance, hardness and toughness

Alpha brasses	75% copper and 25% zinc	Imitation of gold
Alpha-beta brass	35-45 zinc	Harder and stronger
Beta brasses	45-50% zinc brass	Harder, stronger and suitable for casting.
Cartridge brass	30% zinc brass properties	Good cold working
Common brass, or river brass	37% zinc brass	Standard for cold working
Gilding metal	95% copper and 5% zinc components	Used for ammunition
High brass	65% copper and 35% zinc used for springs, screws	High tensile strength and is rivent

Characteristics

- Brass has higher malleability than copper or zinc.
- The relatively low melting point of brass (900 to 940^{0}C, depending on composition) and its flow characteristics make it a relatively easy material to cast.
- By varying the proportions of copper and zinc, the properties of the brass can be changed, allowing hard and soft brasses.
- The density of brass is approximately 8400 to 8730 kilograms per cubic meter (equivalent to 8.4to 8.73 grams per cubic centimeter).
- Brass alloy are recycled. Because brass is not ferromagnetic, it can be separated from ferrous scraps by passing the scraps near a powerful magnet. Brass scrap is collected and transported to the foundry where it is melted and recast into billets. Billets are heated and extruded into the desired form and size.
- Aluminium makes brass stronger and more corrosion resistant. Aluminium also causes a highly beneficial hard layer of aluminium oxide (Al_2O_3) to be formed on the surface that is thin, transparent and self healing.
- Tin has similar effects & finds its use especially in sea water applications (naval brasses).
- Combinations of iron, aluminium, silicon and manganese make brass wear and tear resistant.

Uses

Brass is a substitution Alloy. It is used for:

- Decoration for its bright gold-like appearance.
- For applications where low friction is required such as locks, gears, bearings, doorknobs, ammunition and valves.
- For plumbing and electrical applications; and extensively in musical instruments such as horns and bells for its acoustic properties.

- Used in zippers. Because it is softer than most other metals in general use.
- Used in situations where it is important that sparks not be struck, as in fitting and tools around explosive gases.
- Used for fixings for use in cryogenic systems.

2. Bronze

Bronze is a metal alloy consisting of copper, with tin as the main additive, but sometimes with other elements such as phosphorous, manganese, aluminium or silicon. Bronze is typically contains 88% copper and 12% tin. It is one of the most innovative alloys of humankind. Tools, weapons, armor and various building materials like decorative tiles made of bronze were harder and more durable.

Type of Bronze

(a) Alpha bronze consist of the alpha solid solution of tin in copper. Alpha bronze alloy of 4-5% tin are used to make coins, springs, turbines and blades.

(b) Commercial bronze (90% copper and 10% zinc) and Architectural bronze (57% copper, 3% lead, 40% zinc) are actually brass alloy because they contain zinc as the main alloying ingredient. They are commonly used in architectural applications.

Characteristics

- Bronze can be superior to iron in many applications. It is considerer ably less brittle than iron.
- Bronze only oxidized superficially; once a copper oxide (eventually becoming copper carbonate) layer is formed, the underlying metal is protected from further corrosion.
- Copper–based alloys have lower melting points than steel or iron, and are more readily produced from their constituent metals.
- Bronzes are softer and weaker than steel.

Uses

- Bronze is especially suitable for use in boat and ship fitting.
- It is also widely used for cast bronze sculpture.
- Bronze parts are tough and typically used for bearings, clips, electrical connectors and spring.
- It is used in building restoration and custom construction.

- Bronze also has very little metal –on –metal friction, which made it invaluable for the building of cannon.

3. Duralumin

Duralumin (also called duraluminum and duraluminium or dural) is the trade name of the aluminium alloys. The main alloying constituents are copper, manganese and magnesium. Duralumin alloy which contain 44% copper, 1.5% magnesium, 0.6% manganese and 93.5% aluminium by weight.

Properties

- Good conductor of heat and electricity.
- High tensile strength. Strength comparable to steel but density is one-third of steel.
- Tough, ductile, easily cast able and possess high machinability.

Application

- Wire, rod and bar for screw machine products.
- Heavy-duty forgings, plate, and extrusions for aircraft fittings, wheels and major structural components, apace booster tankage and structure, truck frame.
- Welded space booster oxidizer and fuel tanks.

4. Steel

Iron containing 0.15 to 1.5% carbon is called steel. Steels can be broadly subdivided into two categories:

    (a) Plain- carbon steels and

    (b) Alloy or special steels.

These are briefly described below:

Plain-Carbon Steels

These steels owe their distinctive properties to their carbon contents. In addition to carbon, these steels may contain Si (upto 0.03%), S (upto 0.5%) and Mn (upto 1%).

The increase in carbon content changes the following properties in steels:

    (a) The susceptibility to heat treatment increases.

    (b) The hardness increases.

    (c) Strength of steel increases, till 0.83% carbon after which the strength decreases.

    (d) The ductility decreases.

There are three classes of steel depending on the carbon content.

Classification of steels based on carbon content

Steel	Low- Carbon or Mild or Soft Steel	Medium- Carbon Steel	High-Carbon Steel
% of C- content	0.15 to 0.3	0.3 to 0.8	0.8 to 1.5
Properties			
i. Strength	-40 kg/mm^2	-50kg/mm^2	-65kg/mm^2
ii Weldability by forging	Possible	Difficult	Difficult
iii. Ability to with stand shock	Good	Better	Best
iv. possibility of hardening and tempering	Yes, but with difficulty	Yes, to some extent	Yes, easily
v. Structure	Fibrous	—	Granular
vi. Toughness	Quite tough	Tougher than mild steel	

Steel	Low- Carbon or Mild or soft Steel	Medium- Carbon Steel	High- Carbon Steel
% of C- content	0.15 to 0.3	0.3 to 0.8	0.8 to 1.5
Applications	Mild steel (M-S) round bars are used for reinforcement in reinforced cement concrete (RCC). M.S. sheets are used for roof covering. M.S. is also also used for the manufacture of bolts, nuts, rivets, screws etc. M.S. (in the form of I- or T-sections, angle irons, plates, channel sections) is used in the manufacture of rail tracks. Industrial building structures etc.	Medium carbon steels are used for Hydraulic fittings (like cylinder, rams, shafts, turbine rotors etc.) Agricultural tools and implements.Heavily stressed Parts in general engineering casting for automobile engine components. Riffle barrels, gun parts wheels, gears, clutch plates etc.	High carbon steels are used for metal cutting tools (for lathes planers and slotters). Smith's cutlery, knives wear resistant forgings, Boring and engraving tools. Wood working tools like saws, drills, files, chisels, hammers etc.

Alloy Steels or Special Steels

The properties of steel can be greatly improved by the presence of some alloying elements like Ni, Cr, Co etc. Such are called alloy steels or special steels.

Specific Effects of Alloying Elements

(a) **Chromium (Cr):** It improves hardness and toughness simultaneously. When added upto12%; it imparts high corrosion resistance.

When added upto15%; Cr enhances tensile strength.

(b) **Manganese (Mn):** When Mn is added upto 1-1.5%, it increases toughness, strength and brittleness. But when added 11 to 14% Mn imparts high degree of hardness.

(c) **Nickle (Ni):** Ni improves corrosion and heat resistance, elasticity, toughness, ductility and tensile strength.

(d) **Molybdenum (Mo):** Mo improves corrosion and abrasion resistance and strength at elevated temperature. By incorporating Mo, temper-brittleness can be eliminated.

(e) **Tungsten (W):** It improves toughness, abrasion and shock resistance and hardness at higher temperatures.

(f) **Vanadium (V):** It improves tensile strength, ductivity and shock-resistance.

5. Magnalumin

Composition

Magnalumin contains about 30-10% magnesium and 70- 90% aluminium.

Properties

Mangnalumin possesses similar mechanical properties like brass. It is strong, tough and higher than Al.

Applications

Mangnalumin is used for making scientific instruments, airplane parts and low cost balances.

6. Alloys of Lead and Tin

Solders (have low melting point), Type metal (on solidification it expands and gives good castings), Wood's metal (easily fusible) and Rose metal (easily fusible) are some of the commercially available alloys of Lead and Tin.

Their composition and uses are briefly summarized below:

Pb-Sn Alloy	Composition	Uses
(A) Solders		
(a) Soft solders	Pb (37- 67%) Sn (31- 60%) Sb (0.12- 2%)	Used for joining lead pipes, sealing tin cans and soldering electrical connections.
(b) Brazing alloys	Pb (505%) Sn (92%) Cu (2.5%)	Used for soldering steel joints by fusion process.
(c) Tinman's solders	Pb (34%) Sn (66%)	Used for soldering and tinning.
(B) Type Metal Alloys	Pb (75%) Sn (5%) Sb(20%)	Used for the manufacture of priter's type (on solidification it expands and gives good casting)
(C) Low Melting Alloys	Pb (25%) Sn (12.5%)	Used for soldering and tinning. Used for making fire- alarms, safety
(a) Wood's Metal (m.p. = 70⁰C)	Bi (50%) Cd (12.5%)	plugs for cookers, as a soft solder for joining two metallic parts/ pieces, for boiler and electric fuses, as castings for dental works.
(b) Rose metal (m.p. = 89⁰C	Pb (28%) Sn (22%) Bi (50%)	Used for making fire- alarms, fuse-wires, castings for dental works and in automatic sprinkler systems.

NANO COMPOSITES

Nenocomposite materials is a multiphase solid material in which nano-dimensional additive is reinforced in bulk matrix phase.

i.e. Minimum two solid phases will be mixed the materials which is added in nanosize (less than 100 nm) with pressure is known as reinforcement material or nanoaddetive, while other material which is taken as major phase is known as Bulk Matrix phase.

Small quantity of reinforcement material is required by doing this. Nanocomposite material is observed to none significant variation in the mechanical, electrical, thermal, optical, electrochemical, catalytic properties from that of the component materials.

Variation in the nanosize after the preparation of composite in general size limits are:

5 nm for catalytic activity

20 nm for magnetic material

50 nm for refractive index

100 nm for supermagnetisim

Classification

On the basis of bulk matrix phase, Nano Composites can be classified three types:

(a) **Ceramic – matrix Nanocomposites:** In this type of nano composite major part of the volume is occupied by a ceramic material and reinforcement material is generally metal phase. Metal particles in nanosize are dispersed to get particular / specific property. Generally in this optical, electrical, corrosion resistance, magnetic etc properties are gained.

(b) **Metal – Matrix Nanocomposites:** When metal material is taken as major part in the composition and some other material like ceramic is added as reinforcement material in nano size than composite is metal matrix. Hybrid sole get with a silica base is dispersed in metal like Aluminum powder to form superthermic materials.

(c) **Polymer – Matrix Nanocomposite :** In this composite, Polymer phase is major phase and some other material like metals are added in nanosize than composite is polymer – matrix. Flame retardency can be introduced in polymer matrix by reinforcing some ceramic material in nano size. Similarly biodegradability can be enhanced in the polymer.

REFRACTORIES

Refractories are ceramic materials which can withstand high temperatures without suffering a deformation in shape. The main objective of refractory is to confine heat.

Classification of Refractories

On the basis of the chemical properties of their constituent substance, refractories are classified into three categories :

(a) **Neutral Refractories :** The ceramic material which has almost neutral pH are neutral refractory, like graphite, zirconia and SIC (carborandum). These refractories are made from weakly basic/acidic materials like carbon, zirconia (ZrO_2) and chromite ($FeO.CrO_2$). Neutral Refractory (Graphite) has highest fusion temperature (3500^0C).

(b) **Acid refractories**: The ceramic material which has acidic nature, like alumina, silica and fire clay refractories. These refreactories consist of acidic materials like alumina (Al_2O_3) and silica (SiO_2). These refractory materials are resistant to acid slags (like silica) and are often used as containment vessel for them. On the other hand, they are readily attacked by basic slags (like CaO, MgO etc.) and contact with these oxide materials should be avoided.

(c) **Basic refractories:** Alumina (fusion temperature 2050^0C) like magnestic and dolomite refractories. These refractories consist of basic materials like CaO, MgO etc. and are especially resistant to basic slags. That's why they find extensive use in some steel making open hearth furnaces. The presence of acidic materials like silica is deleterious to their high-temperature performance.

Characteristics of refractory materials

(i) A good refractory material should have excellent heat, corrosion and abrasion resistance;

(ii) It should possess low thermal coefficient of expansion and should expand and contract uniformly, with increase and decrease of temperature respectively;

(iii) It should possess high fusion temperature. It should be infusible at the temperature to which it is liable to be exposed;

(iv) It should be able to withstand the overlying load of structure, at operating temperatures;

(v) They should be chemically inert towards corrosive action of molten metal, gases and slags, produced in its immediate contact in furnaces.

(vi) They should not crack at the operating temperatures.

If given refractory material does not have the above mentioned characteristics, it will fail in service.

Conditions which lead to failure of a refractory material

(i) Using a refractory material which do not have required heat, corrosion and abrasion resistance;

(ii) Using refractory material of higher thermal expansion;

(iii) Using a refractory of refractoriness less than that of the operating temperature;

(iv) Using lower-duty refractory bricks in a furnace than the actual load of raw materials in products;

(v) Using basic refractory in a furnace in which acidic reactants and/ or products are being processed and vice-versa;

(vi) Using refractories which undergo considerable volume changes during their use at high termperature.

Properties of Refractories

The important properties are summarized and discussed as under.

Refractoriness

It is the ability of a refractory material to withstand the heat without appreciable softening or deformation under given service conditions.

S.No.	Refractory Type	Refractory Material	Fusion Temperature (^{0}C)
1.	Neutral	Graphite (C)	3500
2.	Neutral	Zirconia (ZrO_2)	2710
3.	Neutral	Silicon carbide (SiC)	2700
4.	Acidic	Alumina (Al_2O_3)	2050
5.	Acidic	Silica brick (SiO_2)	1700
6.	Acidic	Fire clay brick	1600-1750
7.	Basic	Magnesia brick	2200

Dimensional Stability

Dimensional stability is the resistance of a material to any change in volume when it is exposed to high temperatures, over a prolonged time.

Chemical inertness

The refractory material which is used as liner for furnace walls should be chemically inert to the chemicals charged into a furnace. It should not react with the reactants, slags, furnace gases, fuel ashes and the products involved inside the furnace. Such reactions can contaminate the product and/or gradually corrode the furnace. Hence, it is inadvisable to employ an acid refractory in contact with an alkaline product or vice-versa.

Thermal expansion and contraction

A good refractory material should have least possible coefficient of thermal expansion. Since like other materials, refractory also expands when heated and contract when cooled. Repeated expansion and contraction contribute much towards rapid wear and tear of the refractory structure and its rapid breakdown. Sustained strong binding between the refractory lining and base structure and within the refractory matter is possible only when the thermal effect or volume (coefficient of expansion) is negligible. Due to thermal shock, a substandard refractory develops cracks and then detaches itself from the furnace wall. It is essential therefore, allowance has to be made for thermal expansion.

Thermal conductivity

It is amongst one of the important properties of refractory material since it determines the amount of heat transmission or heat loss due to radiation through it.

Refractories with low thermal conductivities are used for lining the walls of blast furnace, copper hearth furnace etc., because they minimize the heat losses to outside by radiation and help in the maintenance of high temperatures inside the furnace. On the other hand, refractories with high thermal conductivities are used for lining the walls of muffle furnace, coke-oven retorts etc., because in these cases efficient heat transfer from the outer surface to charge is needed.

Hence, depending upon the type of furnace, refractory materials of high or low thermal conductivities are required by industrial operations.

Resistance to Corrosion and Erosion

The higher temperatures at which the furnace is operated, viscosity of slag decreases which accelerate the chemical reaction between the slag and refractory lining. This might lead to corrosion of refractory lining. Greater wetting of the refractory by the slag also increases corrosion. Erosion is gradual wearing away of a material from its surface due to the mechanical action of flue gases escaping at high velocities, carbon-particles and descending hard charge inside the furnace. Erosion produces cavities on the surface of refractories which in turn increase the probability of corrosion.

For a refractory to last longer, it is desirable that it should have excellent corrosion and erosion resistance. This property is very important for the selection of refractory material for by product coke-oven wall and lining of discharge ends of rotary cement kilns etc.

Electrical conductivity

A refractory material of low electrical conductivity is desired for lining the walls of electrical furnace. For proper selection of refractory material it should be always remembered that electrical conductivities of these material increases with rise in temperature. In general, all refractory materials (except graphite), are poor conductors of electricity.

Porosity

Porosity of a refractory material is the ration of its pore's volume to the bulk volume. Pores are present in all refractory material and these can be open or closed. Porosity affects many characteristics of a refractory material. For instance, flue gases, slag and/or molten charge can penetrate to greater depth and may react and reduce the life of refractory material of porous refractory. Porosity can also increase the thermal shock resistance. In addition, air is entrapped in the pores and increase the insulation characteristics of porous bricks. In contrast, the densest and least porous bricks have the highest thermal conductivity, strength, resistance to abrasion and corrosion.

Thermal spalling

Rapid changes in temperature, cause uneven expansion and contraction of refractory material, thereby leading to development of internal stresses and strains. This in turn are responsible for cracking, breaking or fracturing of a refractory brick or block under high temperature, collectively known as thermal spalling. Thermal spalling can also be caused by the variation in the coefficient of expansion due to slag penetration in the refractory brick. A good refractory must show a good resistance to thermal spalling. Thermal spalling can be decreased by minimizing the development of internal stresses by:

    (i) Using a refractory with high porosity, good thermal conductivity and low coefficient of expansion,

    (ii) Avoiding sudden temperature changes, and Proper furnace design.

Permeability

It is measure of rate of diffusion of molten solids, liquids and gases through the connected pores of refractory. The higher the porosity of a refractory bricks, the more easily it is penetrated by gases and molten fluxes. Permeability depends on the size and number of connected pores. A good refractory material should show low permeability.

Texture

Texture can be coarse or fine. Porosity of coarse or light textured bricks are higher than fine or dense-textured bricks. That's why coarse textured refractory bricks have

(i) good resistance to thermal spalling,

(ii) low crushing strength, and

(iii) low abrasion and corrosion resistance.

Heat capacity

The dense and heavy fire-clay bricks have higher heat capacity and as such are best suited for regenerators, checker-works as in stoves for blast furnaces, coke ovens, glass furnaces etc. In contrast, intermittently operated furnaces require refractory material of low heat capacity (i.e. light weight refractory brick). Because in them working temperature of the furnace is achieved with lesser consumption of fuel and in lesser time.

NEUTRAL REFRACTORIES

Silicon carbide (carborundum) Refractories

Preparation

Carborundum is made by heating a mixture of coke (40%) and sand (60%) together with some saw dust (it helps in increasing the porosity) and salt (it helps in the removal of iron etc., in the form of volatile chlorides) in an electric furnace at 1500^0C. The SiC in the form of interlocked crystals are formed by this method. These interlocked crystals are crushed; sized and suitably graded for getting dense packing. These are then mixed with bonding agents (10%) like plastic, fire clay, graphite or silicon nitride for imparting superior oxidation resistance. After mixing with bonding agent, final firing is done in reducing atmosphere at about 1500^0C. It is interesting to note here that if SiC particles are mixed with glue (temporary binding agent) and fired at 2000^0C, self-bonding type of SiC refractory bricks (having intercrystalline bonds) results.

Properties

(a) SiC refractories have high thermal conductivity, low thermal coefficient of expansion and thus have ability to withstand sudden temperature fluctuations.

(b) The SiC bricks are extremely refractory and possess high mechanical strength. They can withstand loads in furnaces even at higher temperatures (e"1650^0C). They possess excellent resistance to spalling and abrasion.

(c) Chemical resistance of SiC refractories are also good. They have high resistance to reducing atmosphere and acid slag, medium resistance to oxidizing atmosphere and low resistance to basic slag.

In oxidizing atmosphere, at temperature of about 950^0C, SiC bricks have a tendency to oxidize to Si. This tendency can be minimized by thin layer of zirconium coating.

Chromite Bricks

Preparation: Chromite ($Cr_2O_3.FeO$) is blended with clary and then firing is done at a temperature of 1500 to 1700^0C for the manufacture of chromite bricks.

Properties

(a) Chromite bricks are neutral refractories having good slag resistance.

(b) Their spalling resistance is moderate.

(c) They possess moderate thermal conductivity and high density.

(d) Their use temperature is limited to 1800^0C.

(e) They have good crushing strength and refractoriness under load.

Applications

Chromite bricks are used in—

(a) Furnace linings,

(b) Sodium carbonate recovery furnaces

(c) Bottom of soaking pits.

ACID REFRACTORIES

Fire clay refractories

Preparation

Fire clay refractories are made from raw and calcined alumino silicate which are known as fire clays because they can withstand high temperatures. Calcined fire clay, known as the "Grog", accounts for 50% or more of the batch mix. The exact properties of the constituents depend on the type of bricks to be made. For example, feebly acidic fireclay bricks contain 55% SiO_2 and 35% Al_2O_3 while nearly neutral fire clay bricks contain 40% SiO_2 and 55% Al_2O_3. The balance in both of them consists of K_2O, FeO, CaO, MgO etc. (Accessory oxides in the clay).

Properties

(a) Depending on the content of iron oxides, fireclay bricks are light yellow to reddish-brown in colour.

(b) Depending on the SiO_2 content, the fireclay bricks show acidic character.

(c) Depending on the percentage of grog, these materials show resistance to thermal spalling. Greater is the % of grog, greater will be the resistance to thermal spalling.

(d) They also have high crushing strength (about 200 kg/cm^2) which goes down with increasing temperatures.

(e) Properly fired bricks are as hard as steel.

Applications

(a) Fire clay refractories are mostly consumed by steel industries as they are used for the lining of blast furnaces, open hearths, stoves, ovens, crucible furnaces etc.

(b) These are also widely used in foundries; lime, continuous ceramic, pottery and metallurgical kilns; glass, brass and copper furnaces; cupolas etc.

Basic Refractories

Magnestic Refractories

It is made from dead-burnt magnesite grain which are property crushed into powder form of proper size. Molasses or sulphite lye is used as a binder. Thermal shock resistance is imparted to the magnesite refractory by adding 2 to 6% of alumina. The ingredients are blended after adding requisite quantity of water and the mix is aged for 1 to 10 days to ensure complete hydration of any free lime present. The mix is then moulded into bricks and temperature is slowly increased to 1500^0C. The bricks are kept at this temperature for about 8 hrs and then slowly cooled.

Properties

(a) Magnesite refractories have high resistance to basic slag and low resistance to acid slag.

(b) They possess good crushing strength.

(c) It can be used up to 2000^0C without load and under a load of 3.5 kg/cm^2, it can be used upto 1500^0C.

(d) It has poor resistance to abrasioin and spalling.

Applications

(a) Mainly used in steel industry for the lining of basic converters and open-hearth furnaces.

(b) These refractories are also used in the roofs of non-ferrous reverberating furnaces e.g., those used for Pb, Cu and Sn.

(c) Also used for the lining of refining furnaces for gold, silver and platinum etc.

Ceramics: Glass

Glass is a super cooled liquid consisting of a mixture of silicates. The basic building block of ordinary glass is a tetrahedron built from a silicon atom at the centre and four oxygen atoms directed along the four corners of tetrahedron. The tetrahedral join together to give a three-dimensional interlocking structure that gives glass its high viscosity. However, glass is entirely lacking in the ordered internal structure of characteristic crystals. When heated, glass does not melt sharply but it gradually softens until it becomes liquid. Thus, glass can be moulded into any desired shape. It is this property of glass which makes it a highly useful material since a number of objects of different shapes and forms can be made out of it.

Silica glass as described above, has excellent properties but for its production very high temperatures are needed. This makes it too expensive for general use. However, it is used in scientific instruments of chemical laboratories, and electrical insulating materials in electrical heaters, furnaces etc.

We can incorporate various oxides in the melt of reducing the temperature required for melting. Most commonly used oxides are Na_2O, K_2O, MgO, CaO, BaO, B_2O_3, Al_2O_3, PbO and ZnO and the corresponding glasses are commonly known as silicate glasses. It is to be noted that above mentioned oxides are added in very small amount and thus SiO_4 tetrahedra have a significant role in the structure.

Since glass is a solid solution, its composition may vary.

In general it may be represented as

$$xR_2.yMO. 6SiO_2$$

where x and y are whole numbers,

R is an atom like Na, K etc., i.e. a monovalent alkali metal atom,

M is an atom like Pb, Ca, Zn etc. i.e. a bivalent metal atom.

Manufacture of Glass

Raw Materials

Broadly speaking, two types of raw materials are used for the manufacture of glass viz. (i) Glass forming oxides like acid, alkaline and alkanile-earth metal oxides and (ii) Oxides which form the glass body.

The raw materials for incorporating:

(a) Sodium is a soda ash (Na_2CO_3). Soda ash is used as a source of Na_2O to prepare soft glass.

(b) Potassium is potash (K_2CO_3) or feldspar (K_2O, Al_2O_3, GH_2O). These are used to give K_2O required for hard and superior glass.

(c) Calcium are limestone ($CaCO_3$) or chalk or lime $Ca(OH)_2$. Sometimes burnt dolomite containing CaO and MgO is used as a substitute of lime.

(d) Lead are litharge and red lead. They are used as source of PbO for making flint glass.

(e) Silica and quartz, white sand, and ignited flint. Sand is washed before use in order to make it free from impurities. Especially, sand should be free from iron because it can impart colour to glass.

(f) Zinc is zinc oxide. It is used for making heat and shock proof glass.

(g) Borate are borax and boric acid, these are incorporated to make glass heat and shock proof.

(h) Phosphorus is P_2O_5, it provides brightness to table ware.

Some other raw materials are incorporated. There roles are summarized below :

(i) Modifiers like alkalies, the alkali earths, PbO, ZnO etc. are incoroporated to reduce the melting and working temperature otherwise pure silic glass requires an extremely high temperature to melt and work.

(j) Melting and refining agents like sodium sulphate, sodium nitrate, sodium chloride, C, CaF, As_2O_3 etc. are added in small quantities to the glass batch in order to promote refining, i.e. the removal of small gas bubble from the glass.

(k) Colouring and decolouring agents :

Colouring agents impart a definite colour to glass. Important colouring agents are: Cr_2O_3 (green), CrO_3 (Yellow-green), CoO

(blue), CuO (red), Fe_2O_3 (brown), CdS (lemon-yellow), Na_3AlF_6 (opaque milky white), MnO_2 (purple) etc.

Decolouring agents neutralize an undesired colour which would otherwise be obtained when sand of less purity is used. Important decolouring agents are : Se, CeO etc.

(l) **Cullet.** Cullet is a crushed glass from defective or broken glass articles. It makes the melting easy and utilizes waste glass.

Manufacturing steps

The manufacture of glass can be divided into four steps viz.

1. Melting
2. Shaping and Forming
3. Annealing
4. Finishing

These steps are briefly discussed below :

Step 1:Melting: Raw materials in proper proportions mixed with cullets and finely powdered to get an intimate mixture (called 'batch'). Melting of glass batches is carried out either in Pot furnace or in Tank furnace.

Selection Criteria of Furnace

Pot Furnace: As pots in pot furnace can be stirred so a great uniformity (as is required in optical glass) is achieved. Moreover, pots are closed so glass melt is completely protected from combustion products impurities are required for special glasses. Thus, pot furnace is used for special glasses, optical glasses, art glasses etc.

Tank Furnace: Tank Furnace is used for large scale production of sheet glass, bottle glass and other common glasses. There are two limitations of the tank furnace viz. stirring is not possible and glass melt is not completely protected from combustion, impurities. Because of these impurities, special glasses can not be made by using tank furnace.

It is to be noted that both pot furnace as well as tank furnaces can be Regenerative or Recuperative type.

Regeneration: It means the utilization of the heat of flue (waste) gases for heating the incoming gaseous fuel and air mixture. By regeneration, flame of greater intensity and flame is produced.

Recuperation: In recuperation, although the purpose is same as that of regeneration viz., utilization of sensible heat of the waste gases and production of higher temperatures in the furnace. However, it is different in the sense that incoming gases flow continuously in one direction only. The hot flue gases and air are simultaneously and continuously made to pass in opposite directions in adjacent passages.

Step-1: Melting of glass is a high temperature process. It takes place through number of intermediate steps. The nature of the steps vary with the composition of the raw materials and temperature of the mixture at a particular stage of glass formation. This is illustrated below for the melting of soda glass and flint glass respectively.

Step 2: Shaping and Forming: Desired shaped articles are made from molten glass by blowing or by pressing between rollers or by moulding.

Step 3: Annealing: Annealing is the very slow cooling of manufactured glass articles, in order to reduce strain, either in annealing lehrs or annealing chambers.

If glass articles are allowed to cool rapidly, their outer surfaces cool more quickly than the internal portions because glass is a poor conductor of heat. This creates strain in the interior portion of glass articles so they are likely to crack to pieces if subjected to shock or change of temperature.

It is to be noted that quality of glass is better if it is annealed at its annealing temperature and for longer period.

Step 4: Finishing: After annealing, all glass articles are subjected to finishing processes such as cleaning, polishing, cutting, grinding, sand-blasting etc.

Note: For the manufacture of glass, when its ingredients are heated, a transparent and viscous liquid is formed. This on careful and slow cooling assume the form of a transparent amorphous solid. The whole process of not forming the crystalline solid is known as devitrification of glass.

Types of Glasses

Some commercial glasses are discussed below:

Soda-lime glass or soft glass

It is the simplest silicate glass in which Na_2O is added to the melt for lowering down the temperature for melting of silica glass.

Preparation: It is made by fusing the sodium carbonate, calcium carbonate and SiO_2. It's approximate composition is

$$Na_2O, Cao, 6SiO_2$$

As the carbonates decompose to oxides on heating.

Properties

(a) Low melting point and thus can be hot-worked easily.

(b) Resistant to water and devitrification.

(c) Low cost.

(d) Attacked by common reagents like acids and hence limited chemical stability and

(e) Poor high temperature resistance.

Applications: Soda-lime glass is widely used for

(a) Window glasses,

(b) Cheapter tablewares like bottles, jars etc.

(c) Cheap laboratory glassware.

Potash glass or Hard glass

Preparation: It is made by fusing K_2CO_3, $CaCO_3$ and SiO_2. Its average composition is K_2O, CaO, $6SiO_2$.

Compared to soda glass, potash glass :

(a) Possesses high melting point and can withstand high temperature.

(b) Is more harder

(c) Fuse with difficulty

(d) More resistant to acids, alkalis and other solvents.

(e) More costly.

Applications: It is used for heating operations like Chemical apparatus and combustion tubes

Lead glass or flint glass

Preparation: It is made by fusing K_2CO_3, red lead and SiO_2. The approximate composition is K_2O, PbO, $6Si_2$. As much as 80% PbO is incorporated for dense optical glasses.

Properties

(a) Lead glass is bright and lustrous due to its higher refractive index.

(b) Its softening temperature is lower than soda-glass and thus it is much easjer to shape and work with it.

(c) Its specific gravity is high (3 to 33).

Applications

Lead glass is widely used for

(a) Making prisms, lenses and other optical devices.

(b) Making high-quality table wares and art-objects, because of high lusture.

Borosilicate glass or Pyrex glass or jena glass

Borosilicate glass contains born trioxide (B_2O_3) and is very rich in silica and little amounts of alumina and alkali metal oxide.

Al_2O_3 and B_2O_3 provide Al^{3+} and B^{3+} ions for pyrex glass. Al^{3+} may be present in structure as a free metal ion, or it may replace Si^{4+} in SiO_4 tetrahedra. Similarly, B^{3+} replaces some Si^{4+} in the tetrahedral skeleton.

The percentage composition of different components would be

Component	SiO_2	B_2O_3	Al_2O_3	K_2O	Na_2O
%	80.5	13	3	3	0.5

Properties

Borosilicate glass has

(a) Low thermal coefficient of expansion;

(b) High softening point;

(c) High chemical resistance;

(d) Excellent shock-resistance (shock-proof).

Applications

Borosilicate glass is widely used in

(a) Industry for pipelines for corrosive liquids,

(b) Superior laboratory apparatus like flasks, beakers, etc.

(c) Kitchenware,

(d) Television tubes, electrical insulators etc.

Optical or Crooks Glass

As the name indicate, optical glasses are used in optical instruments.

Optical glasses contain phosphorus and lead silicate in which calcium oxide is replaced by oxides of Pb, phosphorus etc. They have high refractive indicates and used for the manufacture of lenses.

Crooke's glass is a special type of optical glass which contains little cerium oxide which is capable of absorbing ultraviolet light (which is injurious to eyes).

Safety glass or laminated glass

Preparation

Safety glass is made by placing a thin layer of plastic (either acetal resin or cellulose acetate) between two sheets of ordinary glass. This sandwiched structure is then heated under slight pressure till the glass layers and plastic layers merge into one another.

Properties

Safety of glass is quite touch and It is shatter-proof.

When it breaks, it does not allow its broken pieces to fly apart, since the inner plastic layer tends to hold back the broken pieces of glass. That's why broken pieces does not cause any harm to the people around. Three-layer laminated (safety) glass is used as wind-shields in automobile and aero plane industries. Five layer laminated glass is used in building construction. Several layered laminated glass is bullet-proof and is used for making automobile wind screens, looking windows etc.

Toughened Glass

Preparation

After conversion of glass into desired shape articles, the hot articles are dipped in oil-bath so that some chilling takes place. By doing so the outer layers of the articles acquire a state of compression because of shrinkage; while the inner layers are in a state of tension.

Properties

   (a) Toughened glass is more elastic;

   (b) It is capable of withstanding thermal and mechanical shocks;

   (c) When toughened glass breaks it is reduced to fine powder and the pieces do not fly away.

Applications

Toughness glass is used for making

   (a) Window shields of trucks, cars, aero planes, and other fast moving vehicles;

   (b) Window shields of furnaces;

   (c) Automatic opening doors and

   (d) Large show-cases.

Glass Wool

It is intermingled fine threads or flaments of glass.

Preparation

It is obtained by forcing molten mass of completely alkali-free glass through small holes (Average diameter of 0.0005 to 0.007 mm) continuously. The filaments of glass are then thrown over a rapidly revolving drum to get the material in the form of intermingled fine threads or filaments of glass.

Properties

Glass wool is

(a) Resistant to heat, fire and chemicals.

(b) It is having low thermal and electrical conductivity.

(c) Its density is quite low (about 65 kg/m^3) but tensile strength is about eight times that of steel.

Applications

(a) It is used in domestic and industrial appliances like oven, insulation of metal pipe-lines, motors, vacuum-cleaners, etc. where heat insulation is required.

Photochromic Glass

Photochromic glasses change colour in the presence of high-energy radiation (usually ultra-violet radiation) but reverts back to their original appearance in the absence of this radiation.

Preparation

With the base composition of borosilicate glass, silver, copper nitrate and a metal halide is mixed and heated until the solid melt, at approximately 1200^0C. As the glass cools, small crystals of silver halide form, along with a small portion of copper halide. The crystallites (approximate 10 nm in diameter and 100 nm apart) are too small to scatter or absorb visible light and thus the glass appears transparent.

How photochromic glasses change colour?

When the glass is exposed to ultraviolet radiation (UV), an electron is removed from the Cu^+, ion and accepted by the Ag^+ ion:

$$Cu^+ + Ag^+ \rightarrow Cu^{2+} + Ag$$

Tiny clusters of various dimensions containing the Ag atoms absorb most wavelengths from the near UV through the visible region and i9nto the near infrared, depending on the halide. When the halide is the chloride, the absorption is especially effective in the 300 – 400 nm region. With the bromide, this range extends up to 550 nm and results in a gray appearance. Maximum absorption occurs within about 1 min. In the absence of uv radiation, the silver atoms quickly revert to silver ions, thereby causing the reduction of the Cu^{2+} ions and restoring the transparency of the original glass.

$$Cu^{2+} + Ag \rightarrow Cu^+ + Ag^+$$

This apparent reversibility means that there is no loss or migration of the reaction products away from the reaction zone.

Applications

(a) Photochromic glass is used in the manufacture of lenses of spectacles.

(b) It may also be used for automobile safety glass, automobile sunroofs, light control devices, and window glass in homes for better climate control.

ORGANOMETALLIC CHEMISTRY: ORGANOMETALLICS

Organometallic chemistry is the study of chemical compounds containing bonds between carbon and a metal.

Organometallic compounds

The compound in which at least one metal atom is directly attached to Carbon is known as Organometallic compound. Compounds like organolithium, organopalladium compound and Ferrocene are examples of organometallic compounds containing transition metals. Other examples include organomagnesium compounds like iodo(methyl)magnesium MeMgI, diethylmagnesium (Et_2Mg), and all Grignard reagents; organolithium compounds such as n-butyllithium (n-BuLi), organozinc compounds such as diethylzinc (Et_2Zn) and chloro(ethoxycarbonylmethyl)zinc ($ClZnCH_2C(=O)$ OEt); and organocopper compounds such as lithium dimethylcuprate ($Li^+[CuMe_2]^-$).

The term "metalorganics" usually refers to metal-containing compounds lacking direct metal-carbon bonds but which contain organic ligands. Metal beta-diketonates, Na-alkoxides (RoNa) and dialkylamides are representative members of this class.

In addition to the traditional metals, lanthanides, actinides, and semimetals, elements such as boron, silicon, arsenic, and selenium are considered to form organometallic compounds, e.g. organoborane compounds such as triethylborane (Et_3B).

Many complexes feature coordination bonds between a metal and organic ligands. The organic ligands often bind the metal through a heteroatom such as oxygen or nitrogen, in which case such compounds are considered coordination compounds. However, if any of the ligands form a direct M-C bond, then complex is usually considered to be organometallic, e.g., $[(C_6H_6)Ru(H_2O)_3]^{2+}$. Furthermore, many lipophilic compounds such as metal acetylacetonates and metal alkoxides are called "metalorganics."

Many organic coordination compounds occur naturally. For example, hemoglobin and myoglobin contain an iron center coordinated to the nitrogen atoms of a porphyrin ring; magnesium is the center of a chlorin ring in chlorophyll. The field of such inorganic compounds is known as bioinorganic chemistry. In contrast to these coordination compounds, methylcobalamin (a form of Vitamin B_{12}), with a cobalt-methyl bond, is a true organometallic complex, one of the few known in biology.

The status of compounds in which the canonical anion has a delocalized structure in which the negative charge is shared with an atom more electronegative than carbon, as in enolates, may vary with the nature of the anionic moiety, the metal ion, and possibly the medium; in the absence of direct structural evidence for a carbon–metal bond, such compounds are not considered to be organometallic.

Structure and properties

The metal-carbon bond in organometallic compounds is generally of character intermediate between ionic and covalent. Primarily ionic metal-carbon bonds are encountered either when the metal is very electropositive (as in the case of Group 1 or Group 2 metals) or when the carbon-containing ligand exists as a stable carbanion. Carbanions can be stabilized by resonance (as in the case of the aromatic cyclopentadienyl anion) or by the presence of electron-withdrawing substituents (as in the case of the triphenylmethyl anion). Hence, the bonding in compounds like sodium acetylide and triphenylmethylpotassium is primarily ionic. On the other hand, the ionic character of metal-carbon bonds in the organometallic compounds of transition metals, poor metals, and metalloids tends to be intermediate, owing to the middle-of-the-road electronegativity of such metals.

Organometallic compounds with bonds that have characters in between ionic and covalent are very important in industry, as they are both relatively stable in solutions and relatively ionic to undergo reactions. Two important classes are organolithium and Grignard reagents. In certain organometallic compounds such as ferrocene or dibenzenechromium, the pi orbitals of the organic moiety ligate the metal.

Applications

Organometallics find practical uses in stoichiometric and catalytic processes, especially processes involving carbon monoxide and alkene-derived polymers. All the world's polyethylene and polypropylene are produced via organometallic catalysts, usually heterogeneously via Ziegler-Natta catalysis. Acetic acid is produced via metal carbonyl catalysts in the Monsanto process and Cativa process. Most synthetic aldehydes are produced via hydroformylation. The bulk of the synthetic alcohols, at least those larger than ethanol, are produced by hydrogenation of hydroformylation derived aldehydes. Similarly, the Wacker process is used in the oxidation of ethylene to acetaldehyde.

Organolithium, organomagnesium, and organoaluminium compounds are highly basic and highly reducing. They catalyze many polymerization reactions, but are also useful stoichiometrically.Semiconductors are produced from trimethylgallium, trimethylindium, trimethylaluminum and related nitrogen / phosphorus / arsenic / antimony compounds. These volatile compounds are decomposed along with ammonia, arsine, phosphine and related hydrides on a heated substrate via metalorganic vapor phase epitaxy (MOVPE) process for applications such as light emitting diodes (LEDs) fabrication. Organometallic compounds may be found in the environment and some, such as organo-lead and organo mercury compounds are a toxic hazard

Physical Properties

- Organometallic are usually kept in solution in organic solvents due to their very high reactivity (especially with H_2O, O_2 etc.)

Structure

- Organosodium and organopotassium compounds are essentially ionic compounds.
- Organolithiums and organomagnesiums have a s bond between a C atom and the metal.
- These are very polar, covalent bonds due to the electropositive character of the metals.

Therefore, organometallic compounds react as electron rich or anionic carbon atoms *i.e.* as carbanions, which means they will function as either **bases** or **nucleophiles**.

It is reasonable to think of these organometallic compounds as $R^- M^+$

Basicity

The following equation represents the loss of a proton from a generic hydrocarbon forming a carbanion:

$$R-H \underset{}{\overset{pKa}{\rightleftharpoons}} R^- : \qquad H^+$$
$$\text{carbanion}$$

- Organolithium and organomagnesium compounds are strong bases since the negative charge is on carbon.
- Simple carbanions are strong bases, (see pKa's below) since the C is not very electronegative (compared to N or O)
- In the presence of weak acids, **RLi** and **RMgX** protonate giving the hydrocarbon.

$$RLi + HOR \rightarrow R + Li^{+-}OR$$

- In the presence of weak acids, **RLi** and **RMgX** protonate giving the hydrocarbon.

$$RLi + HOR \rightarrow R + Li^{+-}OR$$

$$RMgX + HOR \rightarrow RH + Mg^{2+-}OR \; X^-$$

Classification of organometallic compounds

On the basis of bonding Organometallics have been classified as :

(1) **σ–(sigma)bonded organometallic compounds:** Compounds such as $RMgX$, R_2Zn, R_3Pb, R_3Al, R_4Sn etc, contains $M - C$ σ–bond and are called **σ-bonded** organometallic compound.

(2) **π-(pi) bonded organometallic compounds:** The transition metals binds to unsaturated hydrocarbons and their derivatives using their d-orbitals. Here metal atom is bonded to ligands in such a way that donations of electrons and back acceptance by the ligand is feassible. These are called **π–orbitals** of the ligand. These are called **π–complexes**.

Examples

(i) **π – cyclopentadienyl – iron complex**

Ferrocene [$Fe(\eta^5 - CH_5)_2$], Bis (cyclopentadienyl) iron (II)

It is a π bonded sandwitch compound. The number of carbon

atoms bonded to the metal ion is indicated by superscript on eta (η^x) i.e. η^5 in this complex.

(ii) Dibenzene chromium (π–complex)

It is also a bonded sandwitch compound. Its formula is [Cr(η^6 – $C_6H_6)_2$]

(iii) Alkene complex (π–complex): Zeise's salt K PtCl$_3(\eta^2 - C_2H_4)$; Potassium trichloroethylene platinate (IV).

It is a bonded complex. μ^2 indicates that two carbons of ethylene are bonded to metals.

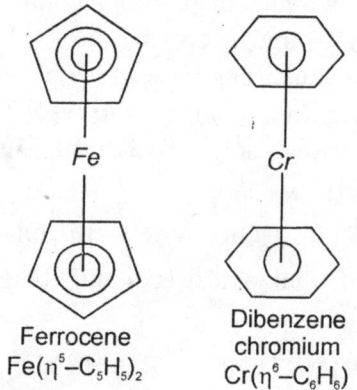

Ferrocene
Fe(η^5–C$_5$H$_5$)$_2$

Dibenzene
chromium
Cr(η^6–C$_6$H$_6$)

(3) **Complexes containing both σ– and π–bonding characteristics:** Metal carbonyls, compounds formed between metal and carbon monoxide belong to this class. Metal carbonyls have been included in organometallics.

(i) Mononuclear carbonyls : Contain one metallic atom per molecule. e.g Ni (CO)$_4$.Fe(CO)$_5$, Cr(CO)$_6$

(ii) Polynuclear carbonyls : Contain two or more metallic atoms per molecule. e.g., Mn$_2$(CO)$_{10}$, Fe(CO)$_9$, Fe(CO)$_{12}$

Applications of organometallics

(1) Grignard reagent (RMgX) has been extensively used for synthesis of various organic compounds.

(2) Wilkinson's catalyst [(PH$_3$P)$_3$RhCl] i.e. tris (triphenylphosphine) chlororhodium (I) is used as a homogeneous catalyst for the hydrogenation of alkenes.

(3) Zeigler Natta catalyst (composed of a transition metal salt, generally TiCl$_4$ and trialkyl aluminium) are used as heterogeneous catalysts in the polymerisation of alkenes.

Chapter 10
LUBRICANTS

> ➤ **General Definition**
> ➤ **Types**
> ➤ **Mechanism**
> ➤ **Properties**

GENERAL DEFINITION

A **lubricant** is a substance introduced between two moving surfaces to reduce the friction between them, improving efficiency and reducing wear. It may also have the function of dissolving or transporting foreign particles and of distributing heat. A lubricant's ability to lubricate moving parts and reduce friction is the property known as lubricity. One of the single largest applications for lubricants is protecting the internal combustion engines in motor vehicles and powered equipment.

Typically lubricants contain 90% base oil (most often petroleum fractions, called mineral oils) and less than 10% additives. Vegetable oils or synthetic liquids such as hydrogenated polyolefins, glycolic esters, silicones, fluorocarbons and many others are sometimes used as base oils. Additives deliver reduced friction and wear, increased viscosity, improved viscosity index, resistance to corrosion and oxidation, aging or contamination, etc. Lubricants such as 2-cycle oil are added to fuels like gasoline which has low lubricity. Sulfur impurities in fuels also provide some lubrication properties, which has to be taken in account when switching to a low-sulfur diesel; biodiesel is a popular diesel fuel additive providing additional lubricity.

Non-liquid lubricants include grease, powders (dry graphite, PTFE, Molybdenum disulfide, tungsten disulfide, etc.), teflon tape used in plumbing, air cushion and others. Dry lubricants such as graphite, molybdenum disulfide and tungsten disulfide also offer lubrication at temperatures (up to 350 °C) higher than liquid and oil-based lubricants are able to operate.

Limited interest has been shown in low friction properties of compacted oxide glaze layers formed at several hundred degrees Celsius in metallic sliding systems, however, practical use is still many years away due to their physically unstable nature.

Need for lubricant

Any metallic smooth surface even polished surface has irregularities in the form of asperities and valleys. When two metal surfaces are in contact with each other in moving condition ,then real contact occurs only at the asperities, the height and depth of asperities & valleys(Given below in the figure) differ from one place to another, in this way metal surface wears high pressure on asperities which cause cold welding. The wear of metal actually depends on the nature of two metals opposing each other.

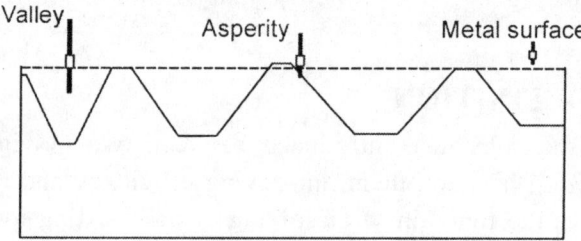

Fig. 10.1

Purpose OR Functions of Lubricant

Lubricants perform the following key functions.

- Reduce friction
- As a coolant
- Keep moving parts apart
- Transfer heat
- Carry away contaminants and debris
- Transmit power
- Protect against tear and wear
- Prevent corrosion
- Seal for gases
- Stop the risk of smoke and fire of objects

Another approach to reducing friction and wear is to use bearings such as ball bearings, roller bearings or air bearings, which in turn require internal lubrication themselves, or to use sound, in the case of acoustic lubrication.

In addition to industrial applications, lubricants are used for many other purposes. Other uses include cooking (oils and fats in use in frying pans, in baking to prevent food sticking), bio-medical applications on humans (e.g. lubricants for artificial joints), ultrasound examination, internal examinations for males and females, and the use of personal lubricant for sexual purposes.

Reduce Friction

Typically the lubricant-to-surface friction is much less than surface-to-surface friction in a system without any lubrication. Thus use of a lubricant reduces the overall system friction. Reduced friction has the benefit of reducing heat generation and reduced formation of wear particles as well as improved efficiency. Lubricants may contain additives known as friction modifiers that chemically bind to metal surfaces to reduce surface friction even when there is insufficient bulk lubricant present for hydrodynamic lubrication, e.g. protecting the valve train in a car engine at startup.

As a Coolant

Lubricant acts as a coolant in the machine, where heat is produced due to friction at the point of contact between the rubbing parts.Lubricant molecule absorbs the heat and provide the coolness to the surface.

Keep Moving Parts Apart

Lubricants are typically used to separate moving parts in a system. This has the benefit of reducing friction and surface fatigue together with reduced heat generation, operating noise and vibrations. Lubricants achieve this by several ways. The most common is by forming a physical barrier i.e. a thin layer of lubricant separates the moving parts. This is termed hydrodynamic lubrication. In cases of high surface pressures or temperatures the fluid film is much thinner and some of the forces are transmitted between the surfaces through

Transfer Heat

Both gas and liquid lubricants can transfer heat. However, liquid lubricants are much more effective on account of their high specific heat capacity. Typically the liquid lubricant is constantly circulated to and from a cooler part of the system, although lubricants may be used to warm as well as to cool when a regulated temperature is required. This circulating flow also determines the amount of heat that is carried away in any given unit of time. High flow systems can carry away a lot of heat and have the additional benefit of reducing the thermal stress on the lubricant. Thus lower cost liquid lubricants may be used. The primary drawback is that high flows typically require larger sumps and bigger cooling units. A secondary drawback is that a high flow system that relies on the flow rate to protect the lubricant from thermal stress is susceptible to catastrophic failure during sudden system shut downs. An automotive oil-cooled turbocharger is a typical example. Turbochargers get red hot during operation and the oil that is cooling them only survives as its residence time in the system is very short i.e. high flow rate. If the system is shut down suddenly (pulling into a service area after a high speed drive and stopping the engine) the oil that is in the turbo charger immediately oxidizes and will clog the oil ways with deposits. Over time these deposits can completely block the oil ways, reducing the cooling with the result that the turbo charger experiences total failure typically with seized bearings. Non-flowing lubricants such as greases and pastes are not effective at heat transfer although they do contribute by reducing the generation of heat in the first place.

Carry away contaminants and debris

Lubricant circulation systems have the benefit of carrying away internally generated debris and external contaminants that get introduced into the system to a filter where they can be removed. Lubricants for machines that regularly generate debris or contaminants such as automotive engines typically contain detergent and dispersant additives to assist in debris and contaminant transport to the filter and removal. Over time the filter will get clogged and require cleaning or replacement, hence the recommendation to change a car's oil filter at the same time as changing the oil. In closed systems such as gear boxes the filter may be supplemented by a magnet to attract any iron fines that get created.

It is apparent that in a circulatory system the oil will only be as clean as the filter can make it, thus it is unfortunate that there are no industry standards by which consumers can readily assess the filtering ability of various automotive filters. Poor filtration significantly reduces the life of the machine (engine) as well as making the system inefficient.

Transmit power

Lubricants known as hydraulic fluid are used as the working fluid in hydrostatic power transmission. Hydraulic fluids comprise a large portion of all lubricants produced in the world. The automatic transmission's torque converter is another important application for power transmission with lubricants.

Protect against tear and wear

Lubricants prevent wear by keeping the moving parts apart. Lubricants may also contain anti-wear or extreme pressure additives to boost their performance against wear and fatigue.

Prevent corrosion

Good quality lubricants are typically formulated with additives that form chemical bonds with surfaces to prevent corrosion and rust.

Seal for gases

Lubricants will occupy the clearance between moving parts through the capillary force, thus sealing the clearance. This effect can be used to seal pistons and shafts.

General composition

Lubricants are generally composed of a majority of base oil and a minority of additives to impart desirable characteristics.

TYPES OF LUBRICANTS: CLASSIFICATION

General classification is based on the type physical state viz solid, liquid etc.While two Other types of lubricants are synthetic and biodegradable. So over all lubricants can be classified into following types:

- (a) Solid Lubricants
- (b) Liquid Lubricants
- (c) Semi Solid lubricants or Greases
- (d) Emulsion Lubricants
- (e) Gaseous Lubricants

Other Types

- (f) Synthetic Lubricants
- (g) Biodegradable lubricants

Solid lubricants

Dry lubricants or **solid lubricants** are materials which despite being in the solid phase, are able to reduce friction between two surfaces sliding against each other without the need for a liquid media such as graphite, hexagonal boron nitride, molybdenum disulfide and tungsten disulfide.

Such lubricants offer lubrication at temperatures higher than that of liquid and oil-based lubricants . These lubricants are often to be found in applications such as space air crafts machines, fire fighting machines etc. Such materials can operate up to 350°C (662°F) in oxidizing environments and even higher in reducing / non-oxidizing environments (molybdenum disulfide up to 1100°C, 2012°F). The low-friction characteristics of most dry lubricants are attributed to a layered structure on the molecular level with weak bonding between layers. Such layers are able to slide relative to each other with minimal applied force, thus giving them their low friction properties. However, a layered crystal structure alone is not necessarily sufficient for lubrication. In fact, there are also some solids with non-lamellar structures that function well as dry lubricants in some applications. These include some soft metals(like Silver, Lead, Indium), PTFE, fullerene,some solid oxides, rare-earth fluorides, and even diamond.

The most commonly used solid lubricants are:

Graphite

It is structurally composed of planes of polycyclic carbon atoms that are hexagonal in orientation. The distance of carbon atoms between planes is longer and therefore the bonding is weaker.

Graphite is best suited for lubrication in a regular atmosphere. Water vapor is a necessary component for graphite lubrication. The adsorption of water reduces the bonding energy between the hexagonal planes of the graphite to a lower level than the adhesion energy between a substrate and the graphite. Because water vapor is a requirement for lubrication, graphite is not effective in vacuum. In an oxidative atmosphere graphite is effective at high temperatures up to 450°C continuously and can withstand much higher temperature peaks. The thermal conductivity of graphite is generally low: approximately 1.3 W/mK at 40°C.

Graphite is characterized by two main groups: natural and synthetic. Synthetic graphite is a high temperature sintered product and is characterized by its high purity of carbon (99.5 – 99.9%). The primary grade synthetic graphite can approach the good lubricity of quality natural graphite.

Natural graphite is derived from mining. The quality of natural graphite varies as a result of the ore quality and post mining processing of the ore.

The end product is graphite with a content of carbon (high grade graphite 96–98% carbon), sulfur, SiO_2 and ash. The higher the carbon content and the degree of graphitization (high crystalline) the better the lubricity and resistance to oxidation.

For applications where only a minor lubricity is needed and a more thermally insulating coating is required, then amorphous graphite would be chosen (80% carbon). It is used in air compressors, foodstuff industry, railway track joints, open gear, ball bearings, machine-shop works etc. It is also very common for lubricating locks, since a liquid lubricant allows particles to get stuck in the lock worsening the problem.

Molybdenum Disulfide

MoS_2 is a mined material found in the thin within granite and highly refined in order to achieve a purity suitable for lubricants. Like graphite, MoS_2 has a hexagonal crystal structure with the intrinsic property of easy shear. MoS_2 lubrication performance often exceeds that of graphite and is effective in vacuum as well whereas graphite does not. The temperature limitation of MoS_2 at 400°C is restricted by oxidation. The particle size and film thickness are important parameters that should be matched to the surface roughness of the substrate. Large particles may result in excessive wear by abrasion caused by impurities in the MoS_2, small particles may result in accelerated oxidation. It is used in CV joints and space vehicles. Does also lubricate in vacuum.

Hexagonal Boron Nitride

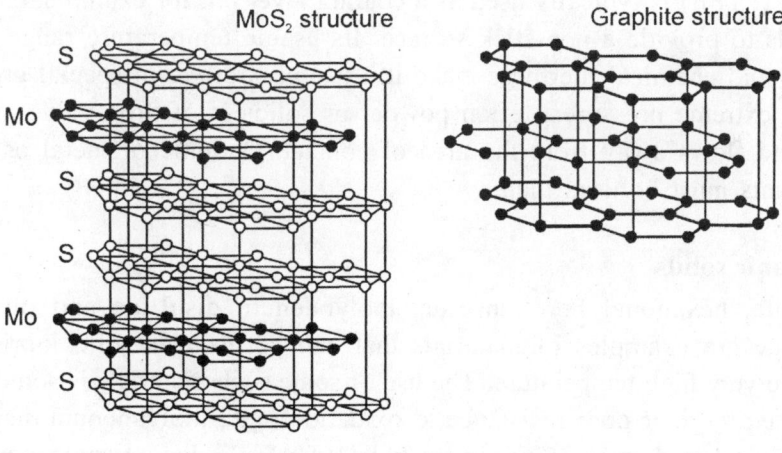

MoS$_2$ structure   Graphite structure

Fig. 10.2

Boron Nitride is a ceramic powder lubricant. The most interesting lubricant feature is its high temperature resistance of 1200°C service temperature in an oxidizing atmosphere. Furthermore, boron has a high thermal conductivity. Boron is available in two chemical structures, i.e. cubic and hexagonal where the last is the lubricating version. The cubic structure is very hard and used as an abrasive and cutting tool component. It is used in space vehicles. Also called "white graphite".

Tungsten disulfide

Similar usage as molybdenum disulfide, but due to the high cost only found in some dry lubricated bearings.

Graphite and molybdenum disulfide (MoS_2) are the predominant materials used as solid lubricant. In the form of dry powder these materials are effective lubricant additives due to their lamellar structure. The lamellas orient parallel to the surface in the direction of motion.

Even between highly loaded stationary surfaces the lamellar structure is able to prevent contact. In the direction of motion the lamellas easily shear over each other resulting in a low friction. Large particles best perform on relative rough surfaces at low speed, finer particle on relative smooth surface and higher speeds.

Other components that are useful solid lubricants include boron nitride, polytetrafluorethylene (PTFE), talc, calcium fluoride, cerium fluoride and tungsten disulfide.

Teflon or PTFE

Teflon (PTFE) is typically used as a coating layer on, for example, cooking utensils to provide a non-stick surface. Its usable temperature range up to 350°C and chemical inertness make it a useful additive in special greases. Under extreme pressures, teflon powder or solids is of little value as it is soft and flows away from the area of contact. Ceramic or metal or alloy lubricants must be used then.

Inorganic solids

Graphite, hexagonal boron nitride, molybdenum disulfide and tungsten disulfide are examples of materials that can be used as solid lubricants, often to very high temperature. The use of some such materials is sometimes restricted by their poor resistance to oxidation (e.g., molybdenum disulfide can only be used up to 350°C in air, but 1100°C in reducing environments).

Liquid Lubricants

The Primary Function of liquid lubricants is to control friction, wear, and surface damage over the intended life of a system that contains machine elements, such as gears and bearings. Wear and surface damage occur under boundary or partial boundary lubrication conditions, but not under full hydrodynamic conditions. Secondary functions are to prevent corrosion and to scavenge heat, dirt, and wear etc.

Fluid or oil lubricants are further categorised in three types as Mineral oils, Vegetable and animal oils and blended oils.

Mineral fluid lubricants are based on mineral oils. Mineral oils (petroleum oils) are products of refining crude oil. There are three types of mineral oil: paraffinic, naphtenic and aromatic.

Paraffinic oils are produced either by hydrocracking or extraction process. Most hydrocarbon molecules of paraffinic oils have non-ring long-chained structure. Paraffinic oils are relatively viscous and resistant to oxidation. They possess high flash point and high pour point. Paraffinic oils are used for manufacturing engine oils, industrial lubricants and as processing oils in rubber, textile, and paper industries.

Naphtenic oils are produced from crude oil distillates.

Most hydrocarbon molecules of naphtenicnic oils have saturated ring structure. Naphtenic oils possess low viscousity, low flash point, low pour point and low resistance to oxidation.

Naphtenic oils are used in moderate temperature applications, mainly for manufacturing transformer oils and metal working fluids.

Aromatic oils are products of refining process in manufacture of paraffinic oils.

Most hydrocarbon molecules of aromatic oils have non-saturated ring structure.

Aromatic oils are dark and have high flash point.

Aromatic oils are used for manufacturing seal compounds, adhesives and as plasiticezers in rubber and asphalt production.

Vegetable lubricants

Vegetable lubricants are based on soybean, corn, castor, canola, cotton seed and rape seed oils. These oils are triglyceride esters of higher fatty acids. Palm oil is triglyceride ester of palmitic acid ($C_{15}H_{31}COOH$) Vegetable oils are environmentally friendly alternative to mineral oils since they are biodegradable. Lubrication properties of vegetable base oils are identical to those of mineral oils. The main disadvantages of vegetable lubricants are their low oxidation and temperature stabilities.

Animal lubricants

Animal lubricants are produced from the animals fat. There are two main animal fats: hard fats (stearin) and soft fats (lard). Animal fats are mainly used for manufacturing greases.

Aniaml and vegetable oils have good oiliness ,hence these are sticked to the surface of machine parts even under high load & temperatures. These oils have limited uses due to high cost and low resistance to oxidation.

Blended Oils

Generally liquid lubricant is not pure single liquid, instead of it is blended oil. Desirable characteristics in the liquid lubricant can be developed by adding small amount of specific additives. Ana additive is a material which imparts desired or new property to the lubricating oil.

Additives used in lubricants—

A large number of additives are used to impart performance characteristics to the lubricants. The main families of additives with example are:

- **Antioxidants**—They retard oxidation e.g. aromatic amines,phenols
- **Anti-wear**—They reduce friction and wear e.g.organic phosphates
- **Metal deactivators**—They decrease catalytic effect of metals, e.g. amines,
- **Corrosion inhibitors**—They decrease corrosion of metals e.g. metal phenolates
- **Friction modifiers**—They change coefficient of friction e.g. organic fatty acid, ester
- **Extreme Pressure**—they are used under high pressure, e.g. organic phosphates,organic chlorides, organic sulphonates.
- **Anti-foaming agents**—They prevent fam formation, e.g. silicon polymers
- **Viscosity index improvers**—They increase V.I.. e.g. alkylated styrene
- Stickiness improver, provide adhesive property towards tool surface (in metalworking)—Poly vinyl alcohol.
- **Detergents**—They keep surfaces deposit free. E.g. Magnesium phenolates and sulphonates

Note that many of the basic chemical compounds used as detergents (example: calcium sulfonate) serve the purpose of the first seven items in the list as well. Usually it is not economically or technically feasible to use a single do-it-all additive compound. Oils for hypoid gear lubrication will contain high content of EP additives. Grease lubricants may contain large amount of solid particle friction modifiers, such as graphite, molybdenum sulfide, etc.

Complexing agent (in case of greases)-Metal alloys, composites and pure metals can be used as grease additives or the sole constituents of sliding surfaces and bearings. Cadmium and Gold are used for plating surfaces which gives them good corrosion resistance and sliding properties, Lead, Tin, Zinc alloys and various Bronze alloys are used as sliding bearings, or their powder can be used to lubricate sliding surfaces alone, or as additives to greases.

A further phenomenon that has undergone investigation in relation to high temperature wear prevention and lubrication, is that of 'glaze' formation. Glaze formation is the high temperature wearing property. This is the generation of a compacted oxide layer which sinters together to form a crystalline 'glaze' (not the amorphous layer seen in pottery) generally at high temperatures, from metallic surfaces sliding against each other (or a metallic surface against a ceramic surface). Due to the elimination of metallic contact and adhesion by the generation of oxide, friction and wear is reduced. Effectively, such a surface is self-lubricating.As the 'glaze' is already an oxide, it can survive to very high temperatures in air or oxidising environments. However, it is disadvantaged by it being necessary for the base metal (or ceramic) having to undergo some wear first to generate sufficient oxide debris.

Used liquid lubricants can be recycled or burned as a fuel source. Burning liquid lubricants is heavily regulated and requires specially built facilities to prevent air pollution. Burning liquid lubricants at home is never recommended: Not only is it illegal in most areas, the resulting smoke is often toxic and can cause serious medical emergencies.

SEMI-SOLID LUBRICANTS (GREASES)

Semi-fluid lubricants (greases) are produced by emulsifying oils or fats with metallic soap and water at 400-600°F (204-316°C).

TYPICAL MINERAL OIL BASE GREASE IS VASELINE

Grease properties are determined by a type of oil (mineral, synthetic, vegetable, animal fat), type of soap (lithium, sodium, calcium, etc. salts of long-chained fatty acids) and additives (extra pressure, corrosion protection, anti-oxidation, etc.).

If Lithium salt of fatty acid is mixed with oil (e.g. $C_{15}H_{31}COOLi$ + Palm Oil) then grease is known as Lithium based grease .These greases are stable upto 150°C. Similarly sodium based grease is prepared by mixing sodium salt of fatty acid with oil, as the sodium salt of fatty acid is water soluble so this grease is not water resistant.This grease is stable upto 175°C.Calcium based greases are the cheapest grease and stable upto 80°C only. Semi-fluid lubricants (greases) are used in variety applications where fluid oil is not applicable and where thick lubrication film is required: lubrication of roller bearings in railway car wheels, rolling mill bearings, steam turbines, spindles, jet engine bearings and other various machinery bearings.

EMULSION LUBRICANT

Emulsion lubricants are of two types viz oil in water and water in oil.they are prepared as emulsion colloids are prepared by proper stirring the mixture of oil and water along with some emulsifying agent (soaps). Emulsifying agents are mixed in about 3-10%. Soap has both ends polar and non polar ends. Carboxylate end is polar(Which is shown in the figure) ,which is soluble in water phase while non polar end (Carbon end) is soluble in oil phase, in this way soap holds both phases oil as well as water phase and behaves like emulsifying agent. Emulsion lubricants are used in 2-stroke engine oils and machines.

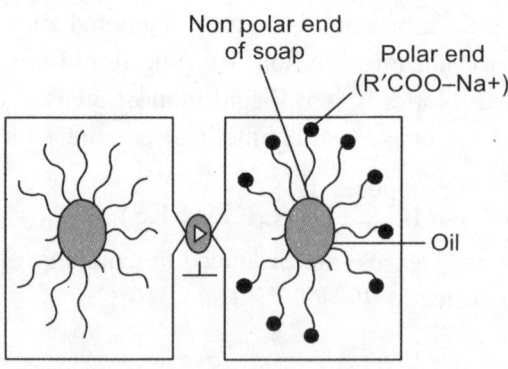

Fig. 10.3

SYNTHETIC LUBRICANTS

They are prepared in the lab by synthetic methods under mechanical and chemical action. They are designed as per requirement of properties in the lubricant, so they are not economical and almost non-biodegradable.

Poly alpha oleins are the most popular synthetic lubticant. PAO's chemical structure and properties are identical to those of mineral oils.

Polyalphaoleins (synthetic hydrocarbons) are manufactured by polymerization of hydrocarbon molecules (alphaoleins). The process occurs in reaction of ethylene gas in presence of a metallic catalyst.

▪ Polyglycols (PAG)

Polyglycols are produced by oxidation of ethylene and propylene. The oxides are then polymerized resulting in formation of polyglycol.

Polyglycols are water soluble

Polyglycols are characterized by very low coefficient of friction. They are also able to withstand high pressures without EP (extreme pressure) additives.

▪ Ester oils

Ester oils are produced by reaction of acids and alcohols with water.

Ester oils are characterized by very good high temperature and low temperature resistance.

▪ Silicones

Silicones are a group of inorganic polymers, molecules of which represent a backbone structure built from repeated chemical units (monomers) containing $Si = O$ moieties. Two organic groups are attached to each $Si = O$ moiety: eg. methyl + methyl $((CH_3)_2)$, methyl + phenyl $(CH_3 + C_6H_5)$, phenyl + phenyl $((C_6H_5)_2)$.

The most popular silicone is polydimethylsiloxane (PDMS). Its monomer is $(CH_3)_2SiO$. PDMS is produced from silicon and methylchloride.

Other examples of silicones are polymethylphenylsiloxane and polydiphenylsiloxane.

Viscosity of silicones depends on the length of the polymer molecules and on the degere of their cross linking. Short non-cross-linked molecules make fluid silicone. Long cross-linked molecules result in elastomer silicone.

Silicone lubricants (oils and greases) are characterized by broad temperature range: $-100°F$ to $+ 570°F$ ($-73°C$ to $300°C$).

Disposal and environmental issues related to lubricant :

It is estimated that 40% of all lubricants are released into the environment.

Disposal: Recycling, burning, landfill and discharge into water may achieve disposal of used lubricant. There are typically strict regulations in most countries regarding disposal in landfill and discharge into water as even small amount of lubricant can contaminate a large amount of water. Most regulations permit a threshold level of lubricant that may be present in waste streams and companies spend hundreds of millions of dollars annually in treating their waste waters to get to acceptable levels. Burning the lubricant as fuel, typically to generate electricity, is also governed by regulations mainly on account of the relatively high level of additives present. Burning generates both airborne pollutants and ash rich in toxic materials, mainly heavy metal compounds. Thus lubricant burning takes place in specialized facilities that have incorporated special scrubbers to remove airborne pollutants and have access to landfill sites with permits to handle the toxic ash. Unfortunately, most lubricant that ends up directly in the environment is due to general public discharging it onto the ground, into drains and directly into landfills as trash. Other direct contamination sources include runoff from roadways, accidental spillages, natural or man-made disasters and pipeline leakages. Improvement in filtration technologies and processes has now made recycling a viable option (with rising price of base stock and crude oil). Typically various filtration systems remove particulates, additives and oxidation products and recover the base oil. The oil may get refined during the process. This base oil is then treated much the same as virgin base oil however there is considerable reluctance to use recycled oils as they are generally considered inferior. Base stock fractionally vacuum distilled from used lubricants has superior properties to all natural oils, but cost effectiveness depends on many factors. Used lubricant may also be used as refinery feedstock to become part of crude oil. Again there is considerable reluctance to this use as the additives, soot and wear metals will seriously poison/deactivate the critical catalysts in the process. Cost prohibits carrying out both filtration (soot, additives removal) and re-refining (distilling, isomerisation, hydrocrack, etc.) however the primary hindrance to recycling still remains the collection of fluids as refineries need continuous supply in amounts measured in cisterns, rail tanks. Occasionally, unused lubricant requires disposal. The best course of action in such situations is to return it to the manufacturer where it can be processed as a part of fresh batches.

Lubricants both fresh and used can cause considerable damage to the environment mainly due to their high potential of serious water pollution. Further the additives typically contained in lubricant can be toxic to flora and fauna. In used fluids the oxidation products can be toxic as well. Lubricant persistence in the environment largely depends upon the base fluid, however if very toxic additives are used they may negatively affect the persistence. Lanolin lubricants are non-toxic making them the environmental alternative which is safe for both users and the environment.

LUBRICATION MECHANISM

Mechanism for Lubrication

Lubrication mechanism can be classified into three types viz Thin Film Lubrication, Thick Film Lubrication and Extreme High Pressure Lubrication.

Thin Film Lubrication

Thin film or boundary lubrication involves a thin film of lubricant adsorbed on the surface at by van der Waals' forces , in this type of lubrication , the lubricant film becomes too thin to completely separate two surfaces in contact.This involves a thin film of lubricant adsorbed on the surface by van der Waals' forces. A thin layer of lubricant (less than 100 A°) is adsorbed on both the metallic surfaces which avoids almost direct metal to metal contact. The thickness may be only of two or three molecular layers and the lubricant is enough viscous to produce a film of sufficient thickness to separate the surfaces under heavy loads, such type of lubrication is also known as boundry lubrication. In this lubrication, the coefficient of friction is decreased to about 0.05. The bodies come into closer contact at their asperities; the heat developed by the local pressures causes a condition which is called stick-slip and some asperities break off. At the elevated temperature and pressure conditions chemically reactive constituents of the lubricant react with the contact surface forming a highly resistant tenacious layer, or film on the moving solid surfaces (boundary film) which is capable of supporting the load and major wear or breakdown is avoided. Boundary lubrication is also defined as that regime in which the load is carried by the surface asperities rather than by the lubricant.

Boundry lubrication depends on the oiliness of the lubricant mainly instead of viscosity of oil. This can happen due to increased machine speed or pressure.

Boundary lubrication occurs whenever a continuous fluid film of lubricant cannot be maintained. Such type of condition arises at the starting and stopping of machines, at low speed and high load, lubricant with low shear strength can reduce the friction under such conditions. It is well known that vegetable and animal oils have more oiliness than petroleum oils. This difference in oiliness has been attributed to the chemical constitution. Solid lubricants such as Graphite and MoS_2 are also useful under boundary lubrication conditions.

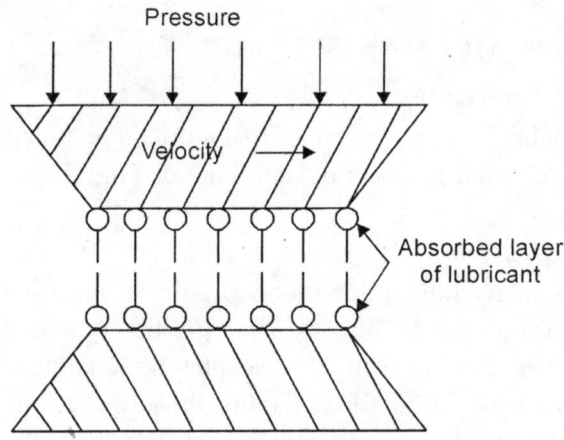

Fig. 10.4: Thin Film Lubrication

Thick film or fluid film or hydrodynamic lubrication

In Fluid film or hydrodynamic lubrication, a thick film of the lubricant (at least 1000A° thick is spread on the sliding surfaces so that there is no direct contact between the sliding surfaces and reduces the coefficient of friction to an extremely low value about 0.001-0.002. Normal finished metal

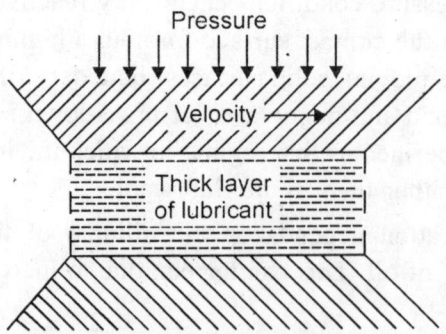

Fig. 10.5: Thick Film Lubrication

surface has coefficient of friction about 0.5 to 1.5. In this type of lubrication, friction reduction is maximum. This condition is also known as fluid film lubrication. The resistance to movement of sliding moving parts is only due to the internal resistance between the particles of the lubricants moving over each other. Therefore lubricant chosen should have the minimum sufficient viscosity under working conditions and at the same time, it should remain in place and separate the surfaces. This type of lubrication is commonly encountered in the well lubricated bearing (Journal bearing), delicate instruments, sewing machines, guns, scientific equipment, etc. Hydrocarbon oils blended with long chain polymers are suitable for fluid f i l m lubrication.

Extreme High Pressure Lubrication

Extreme high pressure lubrication i.e. lubrication which is required for the machines working under extreme conditions of pressure and temperature,it involves chemical action on the part of the lubricant. Under high speed load conditions resulting in high local temperatures the lubricant film melts and breaks down easily. Hence special additives called extreme pressure additives are blended with lubricating oil.When these additives are added in the lubricant then they form more durable film to withstand the high temperatures and pressures. Organic compounds containing phosphorus, sulphur and chlorine provide lubrication through chemical action by reacting metallic surfaces to form metallic phosphides, suiphides and chlorides. These additives along with lubricant molecules are adhered to the metal surface with chemical bonding not physical bonding(Thin film or thick film lubrication)actually reduce the friction but prevent the welding between the surfaces by providing an easily shear. These additives are not effective with chemically inert metal surfaces such as silver, chromum ritanium.

In heavy duty industrial gears, automotive hypoid gears, metal cutting and allied operations where high pressures and rubbing action are encountered, hydrodynamic lubrication cannot be maintained; so Extreme Pressure (EP) additives must be added to the lubricant for satisfactory performance. It has been shown, however that in the presence of chlorinated EP additives, a chloride film is formed on the metal surface. This film has a lower shear strength than that of the metal itself, so the friction between the metals in sliding contact is reduced. This low shear strength, low friction film thus prevents surface damage in gears and gives improved surface finish and increased tool life in metal cutting operations. In this lubrication thickness of lubricant between 100 to 1000A° and reduction in coefficient of friction is more than that of thin film lubrication but less than thick film lubrication.

Properties of Lubricant

Viscosity

The resistance to flow of liquid is known as viscosity. The unit of viscosity is poise. A smaller unit of viscosity is centipoise (1/100 of poise). OR the force in dyne, required to move one square centimetre layer of the liquid with a velocity 1 cm/sec. to another parallel layer of the liquid.

Viscosity of the lubricant determines its operating characteristics. Oil with a low viscosity cannot maintain the lubricating oil film between moving surfaces resulting in excessive wear of the surfaces. In contrast if the viscosity of the oil is too high, excessive friction will be resulted. Viscosity measurement is done by determining the time required for a given volume of oil to flow from a given height through a calibrated capillary tube under its own weight at a given temperature. The viscosity thus determined is

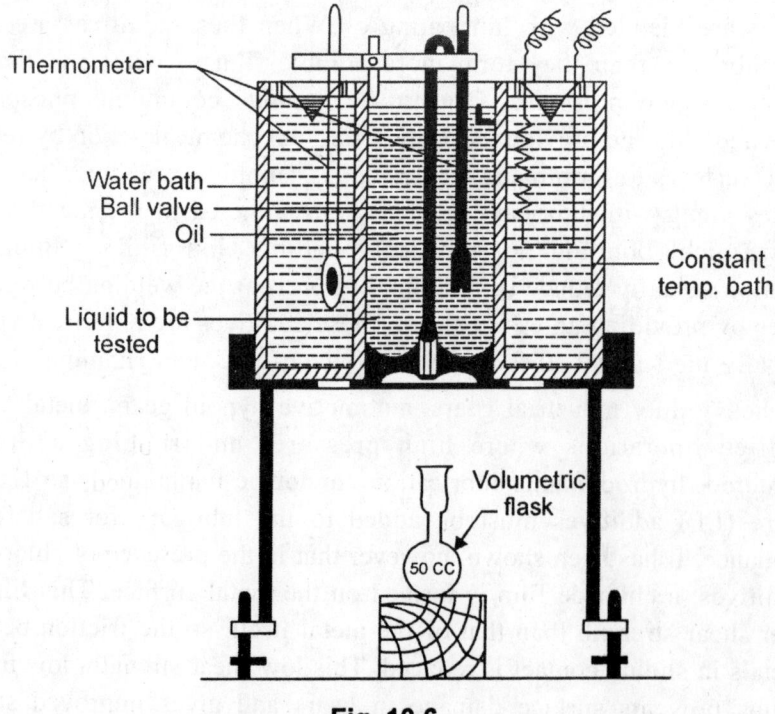

Fig. 10.6

known as **kinematic viscosity** and is equal to the absolute viscosity divided by the density of the oil.

kinematic viscosity = Absolute viscosity/density of oil

Unit (centistokes) = (centipoise/density in g/cc)

Practically, kinematic viscosity is determined by measuring the time taken in seconds for a given quantity of oil passing through a standard orifice under a given set of conditions. In UK and most other countries, the time in seconds, is measured for 50 ml of the oil to flow out of the orifice (at 140°F) in a Redwood viscometer is known as Redwood seconds. Diagram for Redwood viscometer is shown in the figure 10.6.

Formula used in the redwood viscometer is given as-

Kinematic viscosity (cst) = $0.26t - 171/t$,

where time (t) in seconds for 50 ml oil.

Redwood viscometer is of two types :

1. **Redwood viscometer No. 1**—This is used for thin or low viscous oils and length of orfice is 10mm, diameter is 1.6 mm. Oils having viscosity less than 2000 redwood seconds are generally treated as thin oil.

2. **Redwood viscometer No.2.**—This is used for thick or high viscous oils and length of orfice is 50mm, diameter is 3.8 mm.

Viscosity Index: The rate of change of viscosity with change in temperature is called viscosity index. A good lubricant is one whose viscosity does not change much with change in temperature.

Viscosity index (VI) is an arbitrary measure for the change of viscosity with temperature. It is used to characterize lubricating oil in the automotive industry.

The viscosity of liquids decreases as temperature increases. The viscosity of a lubricant is closely related to its ability to reduce friction. Generally, the least viscous lubricant which still forces the two moving surfaces apart is desired. If the lubricant is too viscous, it will require a large amount of energy to move (as in honey); if it is too thin, the surfaces will rub and friction will increase.

As stated above, the Viscosity Index highlights how a lubricant's viscosity changes with variations in temperature. Many lubricant applications require the lubricant to perform across a wide range of conditions: for example, in an engine. Automotive lubricants must reduce friction between engine components when it is started from cold (relative to engine operating temperatures) as well as when it is running (up to 200 °C/392 °F). The best oils (with the highest VI) will not vary much in viscosity over such a temperature range and therefore will perform well throughout.

The VI scale was set up by the Society of Automotive Engineers (SAE). The temperatures chosen arbitrarily for reference are 100 and 210 °F (37.8 and 98.9 °C). The original scale only stretched between VI = 0 (worst oil, naphthalene) and VI = 100 (best oil, paraffin) but since the conception of the scale better oils have also been produced, leading to VIs greater than 100.

VI improving additives and higher quality base oils are widely used nowadays which increase the VIs attainable beyond the value of 100. The Viscosity Index of synthetic oils ranges from 80 to over 400.

The viscosity index can be calculated using the following formula:

$$V = 100\frac{(L-U)}{(L-H)}$$

where V indicates the viscosity index, U the kinematic viscosity for sample under testing, L viscosity of lower standard oil(having V.I.–zero like gulf oil) and H viscosity of high viscosity standard oil (having V.I.–100 like pensulvanian oil) at 100°F.

Oilness

The power of an oil to maintain a continuous film under pressure while it is used as lubricants. A lubricant which does not squeeze out from the sliding surface and maintain a continuous film is known as lubricant having high degree of oiliness.

Volatility

Volatility of a lubricant is its tendency to vaporise with the increase of temperature. If the lubricant is highly volatile, it will vaporise readily even at low temperature. A good lubricant should have low volatility.

Flash Point

The minimum temperature at which a lubricant gives momentary (for less than a seconds) flash of light when a flame is applied to it, but it does not continue to burn. Lubricants with higher flash point are preferred. Flash and fire points are determined by using Pensky Marten apparatus (Fig. 10.7)

Fire Point

This is the minimum temperature at which sufficient vapours of the oils are produced which burns for about 5 seconds when test flame is brought to near it.i.e at this temperature lubricant catches fire and burns continuously when the flame is applied to it. Fire point of oil is always greater than its flash point.

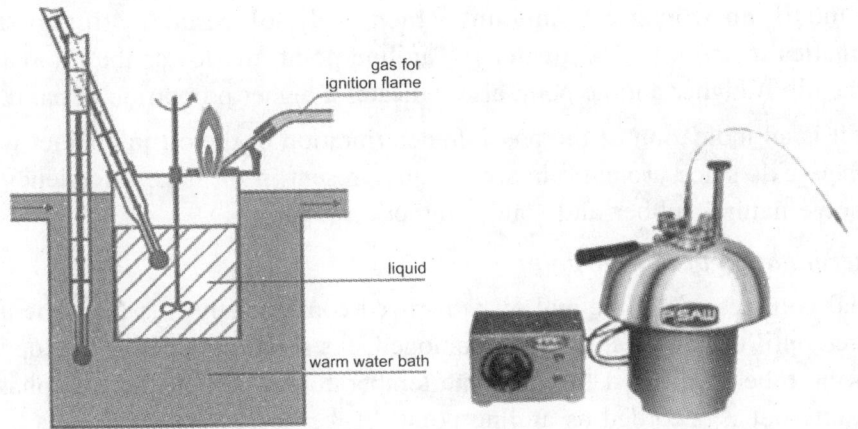

Fig. 10.7: Pensky-Marten flash point apparatus for flash and fire point

Pour Point

It is the lowest temperature at which the oil ceased to flow when cooled under prescribed conditions. If oil is used at a temperature below the pour point, the lubrication action will stop.

Cloud Point

The cloud point of lubricating oil is the temperature at which cloudiness develops due to separation of wax on cooling.

Neutralization Number or Acid Value

It is defined as "The number of milligrams of KOH required to neutalise one gram of the oil."

Saponification Number

It is defined as the number of milligram of KOH required to saponify onegram of oil or fats.

Emulsification

When oil is mixed with water or water is mixed with oil, emulsion is formed. A good lubricant is one which does not form emulsion and even if it forms, the emulsion should break quickly.

Aniline Point

The **aniline point** of an oil is defined as the minimum temperature at which equal volumes of aniline ($C_6H_5NH_2$) and the desired oil are completely miscible.

The value gives an indication of the aromatic content of the oil, since aniline is an aromatic compound which is dissolved on heating by the aromatics in the oil. The greater the aniline point, the lower the aromatics in the oil. A higher aniline point also indicates a higher proportion of paraffin.

It is an indication of the possible deterioration of the oil in contact with rubber seals since aromatic hydrocarbons present in oil have a tendency to dissolve natural rubber and some synthetic rubber.

Determination of aniline point

Equal volumes of aniline and oil are stirred continuously in a test tube and heated until the two merge into a homogeneous solution. Heating is stopped and the tube is allowed to cool. The temperature at which the two phases separate out is recorded as aniline point.

Copper strip test for Corrosion

In this test, a smooth and polished copper strip is immersed in the lubricating oil for a particular length of time at a specific temperature. Copper strip is taken out after specified time. If some pitting or furnished spots are observed, it means the lubricating oil contain some corrosive material. The presence of corrosive material reduces the quality of lubricants.

Carbon Residue Test

The deposit ion of carbon by a lubricating oil, when it is subjected to heat under working conditions is called carbon residue test. Deposition of carbon is harmful.

The gears are generally subjected to high pressures so, it must have following properties.

(1) It should possess good oiliness.

(2) It should not be removed by centrifugal force from the place of application.

(3) It should be highly resistant to oxidation.

(4) It should have high load carrying capacity. Selection of lubricants for Cutting Tools.

Cutting metal tools when used for performing any machining operating such as cutting sawing, turning, boring, drilling etc. required the use of certain oil known as cutting oils must have following properties.

(1) The oil must have both lubricating and cooling properties.

(2) It should be chemically stable.

(3) It should have high conductance to thermal

Selection of lubricants for Steam Turbines

In steam turbines, lubricating oil is exposed to high temperature and oxidizing conditions hands it should have following properties.

(1) It should have emulsification properties.

(2) It should have antifoaming properties.

(3) It should have corrosion resistance properties.

(4) It should have high oxidation properties

QUESTIONS FOR EXAMINATION

Q.1. Explain boundary lubrication. (with diagram).

Q.2. Classify lubricants with examples. Explain liquid lubricants in detail.

Q.3. Define flash point and fire point, viscosity, saponification number.

Q.4. Explain Extreme pressure lubrication.

Q.5. What type of lubricants you will select for cutting tools?

Q.6. What is importance of copper strip test of a lubricant?

Q.7. Write primary aims of lubrication.

Q.8. Which type of lubricants will you select for gears?

Q.9. Explain fluid film lubrication.

Q.10. Write at least five functions of lubricants.

Q.11. Explain 5 important properties of lubricant.

Q.12. Differentiate between thin film and thick film lubrication.

Chapter 11
PETROLEUM CHEMISTRY: FUELS

> ➤ **Fuel-Introduction and types**
> ➤ **Solid fuel:Coal**
> ➤ **Liquid fuel:Petroleum**
> ➤ **Gaseous Fuels**
> ➤ **Calorific values: Bomb Calorimeter**
> ➤ **Biofuels**
> ➤ **Numerical problems**

FUEL

In general, fuels can be defined as any material or substance which yield a large amount of energy on combustion fossil fuel-coal, wood, petroleum compounds, all are fuels. The main element responsible for undergoing energy yielding combustion is carbon. During combustion carbon is oxidised to CO_2 hydrogen to water with the simultaneous release of energy, which is used for different purposes.

Fossil Fuels

The term fossil fuel is used exclusively for coal and crude petroleum, which are formed from the fossilized remains of plants and animals. The organic matter of plants and animals are partially consumed by bacteria as food and the major portion is converted into cellulose which in turn is converted into coal over a period of several millions of years..

Classification of Fuels

On the basis of occurrence fuels can be classified as primary or naturals fuel and secondary or artificial fuels. Fuels which are found in nature as such are clled as primary fuels e.g. wood, coal, natural gas.

Fuels which are obtained by some chemical and mechanical action from primary fuels are called as secondary fuels.

Fuels are classified on the basis of the physical state of their natural existence into solid fuel, liquid fuel or gaseous fuels. Each of these classes consists of primary fuels and secondary fuels.

Type of fuel	Primary or natural fuel	Secondary fuel
Solid	Wood, coal	Coke, charcoal
Liquid	Crude oil	Petrol, diesel
Gaseous	Natural gas	Coal gas, bio gas, water gas

Fuels can be divided into three groups:

- **Biomass Fuels:** These depend directly on the photosynthetic conversion of sunlight into plant matter.
  Examples: Food-stuffs, animal wastes, wood
  These may be used directly as fuels or converted into more usable forms such as biogas or alcohols.
- **Fossil Fuels:** These derive their energy from photosynthesis in the long distant past, the living matter having been modified by geological activity such as high temperature and pressure over a long period of time.
  Examples: Coal, oil, natural gas
- **Nuclear Fuels:** Depend on the nuclear forces within atoms.
  Examples: Uranium-235, plutonium-239

Fuels can be classed as renewable or non-renewable

- **Renewable fuels:** are those derived from biomass sources (plants) or from the conversion of solar energy into chemical energy
- **Non-renewable fuels:** are those derived from fossil sources (coal, oil, natural gas) or minerals (nuclear fuels)

Factors to consider when choosing a fuel

Energy or calorific Value

Energy Value is the heat of combustion of a fuel given per gram of fuel.

The higher the energy value, the more energy is released, the better the fuel.

Heat of combustion of hydrogen is 285kJ/mole

1 mole of hydrogen gas (H_2) has a mass equal to its molecular mass (molecular weight)

$$= 2 \times 1.008 = 2.016$$

The heat produced per gram of hydrogen gas $= 285 \div 2.016$

$$= 141.4 kJ/g$$

The energy value for hydrogen gas is 141.4kJ/g

Ignition Temperature

Ignition Temperature is the minimum temperature to which the fuel-oxidiser mixture (or a portion of it) must be heated in order for the combustion reaction to occur.

High ignition temperature means the fuel is difficult to ignite, low ignition temperature means the fuel ignites easily making the fuel potentially hazardous.

The greater the activation energy of a reaction, the higher the ignition temperature will be.

A match and its striking surface contain a fuel and its oxidiser with a low activation energy and therefore low ignition temperature, so low that the friction of striking the match generates enough heat to raise the temperature sufficiently for ignition to occur.

Petrol and oxygen in a car engine have a higher activation energy and therefore a higher ignition temperature. A spark is needed to raise the temperature of the mixture sufficiently near the spark for the mixture to ignite. The heat of reaction generated heats up more of the mixture so the reaction becomes self-sustaining.

Volatility

Fuels function by releasing combustible gases (vapours)

Boiling Point is an indicator of volatility: the higher the boiling point, the less volatile the fuel.

Vapour pressure is an indicator of volatility: the higher the vapour pressure, the more volatile the fuel. Vapour pressure increases with temperature, so the volatility of a fuel can be increased by raising the temperature.

A highly volatile fuel is more likely to form a flammable or explosive mixture with air than a non-volatile fuel. By definition, gases are volatile.

Liquid fuels are either sufficiently volatile at room temperature to produce combustible vapour (ethanol, petrol) or produce sufficient combustible vapours when heated (kerosene).

Solid fuels decompose above the vapourisation temperature to produce combustible vapours. Solid fuels will have a higher ignition temperature than liquid or gaseous fuels.

Flashpoint

Flashpoint is the minimum temperature to which the pure liquid fuel must be heated so that the vapour pressure is sufficiently high for an explosive mixture to be formed with air when then the liquid is allowed to evaporate and is brought into contact with a flame, spark or hot filament. Flashpoints are lower than Ignition temperatures.

A fuel with a flashpoint well above room temperature (kerosene) means that it can safely be handled at room temperature since exposure to flames, sparks or hot filaments will not cause an explosion.

A fuel with a flashpoint below room temperature (petrol, alcohol) is a safety hazard since exposure to flames, sparks or hot filaments will cause an explosion. These fuels need to be stored in a cool place to prevent the increased temperature raising the vapour pressure of the fuel and in a well-ventilated place so that any vapours that escape do not accumulate, and preferably in robust metal containers with narrow mouths and tightly sealing lids to prevent vapours escaping.

Moisture content and ash content should be as low as possible, higher the moisture and ash content, lower will be the calorific value.

Transportation and availability are also other factors to select the fuel.

Ease of liquefaction

Gases occupy large volumes, whereas liquids of the same mass occupy much less volume making them easier to transport. Critical temperature is the temperature below which a gas can be liquified (condensed) by increasing the pressure.

Liquid Petroleum Gas (LPG) is made up of propane (critical temperature 97°C) and butane (critical temperature 152°C) both of which are gases at room temperature and pressure but can be easily condensed to the liquid at room temperature by increasing the pressure since their critical temperatures are above room temperature.

Products of Combustion

- Complete combustion of carbon-based fuels produce carbon dioxide and water vapour. Carbon dioxide gas is the main contributor to the greenhouse effect.

- Incomplete combustion of carbon-based fuels produces toxic carbon monoxide and solid carbon (soot).
- Sulfur and nitrogen are present in fossil fuels. The sulfur burns to produce oxides which contribute to acid rain, while the nitrogen burns to produce oxides that contribute not only to acid rain but also to photochemical smog.
- Solid fuels such as coal contain incombusitible minerals leading to ash. The ash can damage machinery and can cause lung disease.
- Uncombusted fuel can also be released. Unburnt hydrocarbons from cars contribute to photochemical smog and some are carcinogenic.
- Some fuels contain additives (such as the lead in leaded petrol) which can be harmful

COMPARISON OF MERITS AND DEMERITS OF SOLID, LIQUID AND GASEOUS FUELS

Solid fuels have moderate ignition temperature and also have the advantages of less space, easy transportation, safety against spontaneous explosion and convenience of storage. However value and thermal efficiency of solid fuels are low due to the constituent moisture and ash content. Solid fuels require a large excess of air for complete combustion The combustion of solid fuels cannot be controlled easily. The products of combustion are associated with dust and soot.

Liquid fuels have higher calorific value per unit mass of fuel compared to solid fuels. They require less amount of air for complete combustion than solid fuels. They can be easily fired and be easily extinguished. The combustion process can be easily controlled by regulating the liquid fuel. The products of combustion are relatively clean, free from dust and soot. it can be used in internal combustion engines unlike solid fuels. However the liquid fuels have disadvantages such as high cost of production and storage, risk of fire hazard and bad odour etc.

Gaseous fuels have greater advantages compared to solid and liquid fuels in that they have higher calorific value. They bum completely with a slight excess of air without any smoke or ash formation and hence they are more environmentally clean.

Solid Fuels

Coals and their Characteristics

It is commonly adopted view that coal is a mineral substance of vegetable origin. The large deposits of coal in India are in Bengal, Bihar and Madhya Pradesh.

Indian coal is of low grade variety and coal washing to obtain low ash metallurgical coal is unavoidable. Over 30% of coal output is consumed by railways, another similar proportion is used by industry including iron and steel works. This leaves barely 40% of coal mined for use of the power supply undertakings.

Classification of coal

Coal is a readily combustible rock containing more than *50 percent* by weight of carbonaceous material formed from compaction and indurations of variously altered plant remains similar to those in peat.

After a considerable amount of time, heat, and burial pressure, it is etamorphosed from peat to lignite. Lignite is considered to be "immature" coal at this stage of development because it is still somewhat light in color and it remains soft.

- **Lignite** increases in maturity by becoming darker and harder and is then classified as sub-bituminous coal. After a continuous process of burial and alteration, chemical and physical changes occur until the coal is classified as bituminous - dark and hard coal.
- **Bituminous coal** ignites easily and burns long with a relatively long flame. If improperly fired bituminous coal is characterized with excess smoke and soot.
- **Anthracite coal** is the last classification, the ultimate maturation. Anthracite coal is very hard and shiny.

Secondary solid fuel (Coke)

- Coke and its Characteristics -It is obtained from destructive distillation of coal, being left in the shape of solid esidue. Coke can be classified into two categories: soft coke and hard coke. Soft coke is obtained as the solid residue from the destructive distillation of coal in the temperature range of 600-650°C. It contains 5 to 10% volatile matter. It burns without smoke. It is extensively used as domestic fuel. Hard coke is obtained as solid residue from the destructive distillation of coal in the temperature range of 1200-1400°C. It burns with smoke and is a useful fuel for metallurgical process

Analysis of Coal

To ascertain the commercial value of coal certain tests regarding its burning properties are performed before it is commercially marketed. Two commonly used tests are: Proximate analysis and Ultimate analysis of coal. Calorific value of coal is defined as the quantity of heat given out by burning one unit weight of coal in a calorimeter.

Proximate Analysis of Coal

This analysis of coal gives good indication about heating and burning properties of coal. The test gives the composition of coal in respect of moisture, volatile matter, ash and fixed carbon.

Moisture: The moisture test is performed by heating 1 gm of coal sample at 104°C to 110°C for 1 hour in an oven and finding the loss in weight.

Volatile matter: The volatile matter is determined by heating 1 gm of coal sample in a covered crucible at 950°C for 7 minutes and determining loss in weight, from which the moisture content as found from moisture test is deducted.

Ash content: It is found by completely burning the sample of coal in a muffled furnace at 700°C to 750°C and weighing the residue.

Fixed Carbon: The percentage of fixed carbon is determined by difference when moisture, volatile matter and ash have been accounted for. The results of proximate analysis of most coals indicate the following broad ranges of various constituents by weight

% Fixed carbon = 100–(%Moisture + % Ash content +

% volatile matter)

In a coal sample: Moisture 3-30%, Volatile matter 3-50%, Ash 2-30%, Fixed Carbon 16-92%.

The importance of volatile matter in coal is due to the fact that it largely governs the combustion which in turn governs the design of grate an combustions space used. High volatile matter is desirable in gas making, while low volatile matter for manufacturing of metallurgical coke.

The Ultimate Analysis of Coal

This analysis of coal is more precise way to find the chemical composition of coal with respect to the elements like carbon, hydrogen, oxygen, nitrogen, sulphur and ash. Sine the content of carbon and hydrogen that is already combined with oxygen to form carbondioxide and water is of no value for combustion, the chemical analysis of coal alone is not enough to predict the suitability of coal for purpose of heating. However, the chemical composition is very useful in combustion calculations and in finding the composition of flue gases. For most purposes the proximate analysis of coal is quite sufficient.

The broad range in which the constituents of coal vary by weight as determined by ultimate analysis are given below :

Carbon 50-95%, Hydrogen 2.5-5%, Oxygen 2-4%, Sulphur 0.5-7%, Nitrogen 0.5-3%, Ash 2-30%

Liquid Fuel

Petroleum and its Characteristics

Petroleum is a basic natural fuel. It is a dark greenish brown, viscous mineral oil, found deep in earth's crust. It is mainly composed of various hydrocarbons (like straight chain paraffins, cycloparaffins or napthenes, olefins, and aromatics) together with small amount of organic compounds containing oxygen nitrogen and sulphur. The average composition of crude petroleum is : C = 79.5 to 87.1%; H = 11.5 to 14.8%; S = 0.1 to 3.5%, N and O = 0.1 to 0.5%.

Petroleums are graded according to the following phsio-chemical properties :

(a) Specific gravity,

(b) Calorific value,

(c) Fish point or ignition point,

(d) Viscosity,

(e) Sulphur contents,

(f) Moisture and sediment content, and

(g) Specific heat and coefficient of expansion.

Classification of Petroleum

The chemical nature of crude petroleum varies with the part of the world in which it is found. They appear, however, to be three principal verities.

Paraffinic Base Type Crude Petroleum: This type of petroleum is mainly composed of the saturated hydrocarbons from CH_4 to $C_{35} H_{72}$ and a little of the napthenes and aromatics. The hydrocarbons from $C_{18} H_{38}$ to $C_{35} H_{72}$ are sometimes called waxes.

Asphalitc Base Type Crude Petroleum: It contains mainly cycloparaffins and or napthenes with smaller amount of parffins and aromatic hydrocarbons.

Mixed Base Type Crude Petroleum: It contains both paraffinic and asphaltic hydrocarbons and are generally rich in semi-solid waxes.

Synthetic or Manufactured Liquid Fuels and their Characteristics

Manufactured liquid fuels include Gasoline, Diesel oil, Kerosene, Heavy oil, Naptha, Lubricating oils, etc. These are obtained mostly by fractional distillation of crude petroleum or liquefaction of coal.

Gasoline or Petrol and its Characteristics: The straight run gasoline is obtained either from distillation of crude petroleum or by synthesis. It contains some undesirable unsaturated straight chain hydrocarbons and sulphur compounds. It has boiling range of 40-120°C. The, unsaturated hydrocarbons get oxidized and polymerized, thereby causing gum and sludge formation on storing. On the other hand, sulphur compounds lead to corrosion of internal combustion engine and at the same time they adversely affect tetraethyl lead, which is generally added to gasoline for better ignition properties.

The sulphur compounds from gasoline are generally removed by treating it with an alkaline solution sodium plumbite. Olefins and colouring matter of gasoline are usually removed by percolating through 'Fuller's earth' which absorbs preferentially only the colours and olefine. It is used in air-crafts. It is also used as motor fuel, in dry-cleaning and as a solvent.

Some of the characteristics of an ideal gasoline are the following :

(a) It must be cheap and readily available.

(b) It must burn clean and produce no corrosion, etc. on combustion.

(c) It should mix readily with air and afford uniform manifold distribution, i.e. should easily vaporize.

(d) It must be knock resistant.

(e) It should be pre-ignite easily.

(f) It must have a high calorific value.

Diesel Fuel and its Characteristics

The diesel fuel or gas oil is obtained between 250-320°C during the fractional distillation of crude petroleum. This oil generally contains 85% C. 12% H. Its calorific value is about 11,000 kcal/kg. The suitability of a diesel fuel is determined by its cetane value. Diesel fuels consist of longer hydrocarbons and have low values of ash, sediment, water and sulphalt contents.

The main characteristics of a diesel fuel is that it should easily ignite below compression temperature. The hydrocarbon molecules in a diesel fuel should be, as far as possible, the straight-chain ones, with a minimum admixture of aromatic and side-chain hydrocarbon molecules.

It is used in diesel engines as heating oil and for cracking to get gasoline.

Kerosene Oil and its Characteristics-Kerosene oil is obtained between 180-250°C during fractional distillation of crude petroleum. It is used as an illuminant, jet engine fuel, tractor fuel, and for preparing laboratory gas. With the development of jet engine, kerosene has become a material of far greater importance than it is used to be. When kerosene is used in domestic appliances, it is always vaporized before combustion. By using a fair excess of air it burns with a smokeless blue flame.

Heavy Oil and its Characteristics -It is a fraction obtained between 320-400°C during fractional distillation of crude petroleum. This oil on refractionation gives :

(a) Lubricating oils which are used as lubricants.

(b) Petroleum-jelly (Vaseline) which is used as lubricants in medicines and in cosmetics.

(c) Greases which are used as lubricants.

(d) Paraffin wax which is used in candles, boot polishes, wax paper, tarpolin cloth and for electrical insulation purposes

Gaseous fuel

Natural Gas and its Characteristics -Natural gas is generally associated with petroleum deposits and is obtained from wells dug in the oil-bearing regions. The approximate composition of natural gas is :

$$CH_4 = 70.9\%, \; C_2H_6 = 5.10\%, \; H_2 = 3\%, \; CO + CO_2 = 22\%$$

The calorific value varies from 12,000 to 14,000 kcal/m^3. It is an excellent domestic fuel and is conveyed in pipelines over very large distances. In America, it is available to a great extent, and so, is quite popular as a domestic fuel. It is now used in manufacture of chemicals by synthetic process. It is a colourless gas and is non-poisonous. Its specific gravity is usually between 0.57 to 0.7.

Synthetic or Manufactured Gases and their Characteristics —Synthetic gases are obtained form solid and liquid fuels. Some of the important manufactured gaseous fuels whose characteristics are discussed in the following sections are coal gas, blast furnace gas, water gas, producer gas and oil gas.

Coal Gas its Characteristics

Coal gas is obtained when it is carbonized or heated in absence of air at about 1300°C in either coke ovens or gas-making retorts. In gas making retort process coal is fed in closed silica retorts, which are then heated to about 1300 °C by burning producer gas and air mixture.

$$C + O \rightarrow CO + 29.5 \text{ kcal}$$

Coal gas is a colourless gas having a characteristic odour. It is lighter than air and burns with a long smoky flame. Its average composition is:

$H_2 = 47\%$, $CH_4 = 32\%$, $CO = \cdot7\%$, $C_2H_2 = 2\%$, $C_2H_4 = 3\%$, $N_2 = 4\%$, $CO_2 = 1\%$ and rest = 4%. Its calorific value is about 4,900 kcal/m^3 ..

It is used as (a) illuminant in cities and town, (b) a fuel, and (c) in metallurgical operations for providing reducing atmosphere.

Blast Furnace Gas and its Characteristics

It is a by product flue gas obtained during the reduction of ion ore by coke in the blast furnace. Its calorific value is about 1,000 kcal/m.

Water Gas and its Characteristics

Water gas is essentially a mixture of combustible gases CO and H^2 with a little fraction of non-combustible gases. It is made by passing alternatively steam and little air through a bed of red hot coal or coke maintained at about 900 to 1000°C in a rector, which consists of a steel vessel about 3 m wide and 4 m in height. It is lined inside with fire-bricks. It has a cup and cone feeder at the top and an opening at the top for the exit of water gas. At the base, it is provided with inlet pipes for passing air and steam.

Reactions

Supplied steam reacts with red hot coke (or coal) at 900-1000°C to form CO and H_2.

$$C + H_2O \rightarrow CO + H_2 - 29 \text{ kcal}$$
$$C + O_2 \rightarrow CO_2 + 97 \text{ kcal}$$

Composition

The average composition of water gas is : $H_2 = 51\%$; $CO = 41\%$; $N_2 = 4\%$; $CO_2 = 4\%$. Its calorific value is about 2,800 kcal/m^3.

Uses

It is used as (a) a source of hydrogen gas, (b) an illuminating gas, and (c) a fuel gas

Producer Gas and its Characteristics

Producer gas is essentially a mixture of combustible gases carbon monoxide and hydrogen associated with non-combustible gases N_2, CO_2, etc. It is prepared by passing air mixed with little steam (about 0.35 kg/kg of coal)

over a red hot coal or coke bed maintained at about 1100°C in a special reactor called gas producer. It consists of a steel vessel about 3 m in diameter and 4 m in height. The vessel is lined inside with fire bricks. It is provided with a cup and cone feeder at the top and a side opening for the exit of producer gas. At the base it has an inlet for passing air and steam. The producer at the base is also provided with an exit for the ash formed.

Reactions

The gas production reactions can be divided into four zones as follows :

Ash Zone: The lowest zone consists of mainly of ash, and therefore, it is known as ash zone.

Combustion Zone: The zone next to the ash zone is known as oxidation or combustion zone. Here the carbon burns and forms CO and CO_2. The temperature of this zone is about 1100°C. The following reactions take place.

$$C + O2 \rightarrow CO2 + 94 \text{ kcal}$$
$$C + O \rightarrow CO + 29.5 \text{ kcal}$$

Reduction Zone: Here carbon dioxide and steam combines with red hot carbon and liberates free hydrogen and carbon monoxide. The reactions are :

$$CO_2 + C \rightarrow 2CO - 94 \text{ kcal}$$
$$C + H_2O \rightarrow CO + H_2 \rightarrow 29 \text{ kcal}$$
$$C + 2H_2O \rightarrow CO_2 + 2H_2 - 19 \text{ kcal}$$

All these reduction reactions are endothermic, so, the temperature in the reduction zone falls to 1000°C..

Distillation Zone: In this zone (400 – 800°C) the incoming coal is heated by outgoing gases by giving sensible heat to the coal. The heat given by the gases and heat radiated from the reduction zone helps to distillate the fuel thereby volatile matter of coal is added to the outgoing gas.

Composition

The average composition of producer gas is CO = 22.3%, H_2 = 8.12%; N_2 = 52.55%; CO_2 = 3%. Its calorific value is about 1,300 kcal/m³.

Uses: It is cheap, clean and easily preparable gas and is used (i) for heating open-hearth furnaces (in steel and glass manufacture), muffle furnaces, retorts (used in coke and coal gas manufacture), etc. and (iii) as a reducing agent in metallurgical operations.

Oil Gas and its Characteristics

Oil gas is obtained by cracking kerosene oil. Oil in a thin steam is allowed to fall on a stout red hot cast iron retort, which is heated in coal fired furnace. Theresulting gaseous mixture passes out through a bonet cover to a hydraulic main, a tank containing water. Here tar gets condensed. Then at the testing cap, the proper cracking of oil is estimated from the colour of the gas produced. A good oil gas should have a golden colour. By proper adjusting the supply of air, gas of required colour can be obtained. The gas is finally stored over water in gas holders.

Composition

The average composition of oil gas is: $CH_4 = 25.30\%$; $H_2 = 50\text{-}55\%$; $CO = 10.12\%$; $CO_2 = 3\%$. Its calorific value is about 6,600 kcal/m^3.

Uses: It is used as laboratory gas

Calorific Value : GCV and NCV

The total amount of heat produced by combustion of unit mass of fuel sample in the presence of air is known as calorific value.

Units of calorific value: Common units are calorie/gm or Kcal/Kg, BTU, etc.

Calorie 1: Calorie is the amount of heat required to increase the temperature of 1g of water by 1°C.

BTU: This is the quantity of heat required to increase the temperature of one pund of water by 1°F.

$$1 \text{ BTU} = 252 \text{ calories}$$

Calorific values are of two types- Gross calorific vale(GCV)and Net calorifc value (NCV).

GCV: Gross calorific value is the quantity of heat produced by combustion when the water produced by combustion is allowed to return to the liquid state.

NCV (net calorific value) is the quantity of heat produced by combustion when the water produced by combustion remains gaseous. Since water releases heat when it condenses, GCV is clearly bigger than NCV. GCV is also called HHV (higher heating value); NCV is also called LHV (lower heating value.)

Relationship between GCV and NCV

The difference between the two heating values depends on the chemical composition of the fuel. In the case of pure carbon or carbon monoxide, the two heating values are almost identical, but for the compounds having different hydrogen, values of NCV will be lower than GCV, difference is due to heat of vaporization For hydrocarbons the difference depends on the hydrogen content of the fuel. For gasoline and diesel the higher heating value exceeds the lower heating value by about 10% and 7% respectively, and for natural gas about 11%.

A common method of relating GCV to NCV is(by definition)

$$NCV = GCV - \text{latent heat of water vapours} \quad ...(1)$$

Since 1 gm of Hydrogen produces 9 gm of water

$$(H_2 + 1/2\ O_2 \rightarrow H_2O)$$

If Hydrogen is H% in the given compound/fuel then 1 gm of fuel will have H/100 gm of Hydrogen

Then H/100 gm of Hydrogen will produce water = 9 H/100

And let latent heat of vaporization is L calorie/gm, then total latent heat produced due to total hydrogen present is latent heat of water vapours

$$\text{Latent heat of water vapours} = 9H.L/100 \quad ... (2)$$

Put the value from (2) into (1)

$$NCV = GCV - 9H\ .L/100$$

If

$$L = 587\ cal/gm\ then$$

$$NCV = GCV - 9H \times 587/100$$

Determination of calorific value

Calorific value of a fuel can be determined by using different types of

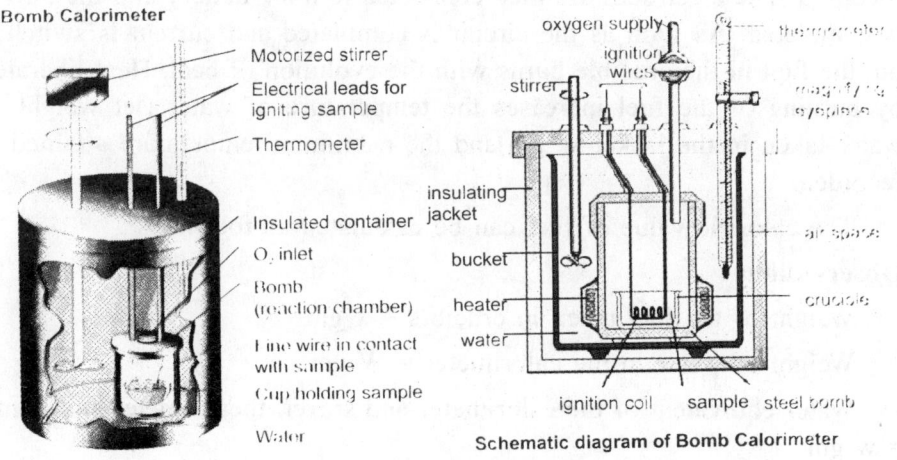

Fig.11.1: Bomb calorimeter

calorimeter.It can be determined by Bomb Calorimeter and Boy's Calorimeter. Bomb calorimeter is used to determine the calorific value of solid fuels and non-volatile liquid fuels. Boy's calorimeter is used to determine the calorific value of gaseous fuels and liquid fuels which get vaporized easily.

Principle: A known unit mass of the fuel is brunt and the quantity of heat produced is h water and measured. Then the quantity of heat produced by burning a unit mass of the fuel is calculated.

Construction: As shown in the above Fig. 11.1 is bomb calorimeter consists of a cylindrical bomb made up of chromium nickel-molybdenum steel, resistant to corrosion and capable of withstanding high pressures in the range of 40-50 atmospheres. It is provided with a lid which can be screwed firmly on the bomb. The lid in turn is provided with two electrodes and an oxygen inlet valve. A small ring is attached to one of the electrode which acts as a support for the crucible.

A copper calorimeter vessel with a known weight of water and in which the bomb stands. The calorimeter is surrounded by an air jacket and a water jacket to prevent the loss of heat due to radiation. The calorimeter is provided with an electrical stirrer for stirring water and a Beckmann thermometer which can read accurately temperature difference up to 0.01° C. The crucible used is made up of nickel, stainless steel or fused silica.

Working: A known amount of fuel (let × gm) is placed in the crucible. The crucible is then placed over a ring and a fine Magnesium wire touching the fuel sample is stretched across the electrodes. The lid is tightly screwed and the bomb is filled with O_2 upto 25atm pressure. The initial temp. is recorded. The electrodes are then connected to a 6V battery and the circuit is completed. As soon as the circuit is completed and current is switched on, the fuel in the crucible burns with the evolution of heat. Heat liberated by burning of the fuel increases the temperature of water (let weight of water taken in the jacket-W gm)and the maximum temperature attained is recorded.

The calorific value of fuel can be calculated as follows

Observations

Weight of the fuel taken in crucible = x gm

Weight of water in the calorimeter = W gm

Water equivalent of the calorimeter and stirrer, thermometer and bomb = w gm

Initial temperature of water in calorimeter = t_1°C

Final temperature of water in calorimeter = $t_2°C$

Let the higher or gross calorific value of the fuel = G cal/g

Then heat liberated by x gm of fuel= x.G cal/gm

Heat gained by water= $(W+w) \times (t_2 — t_1)$ calories

Now, by principle of calorimetry,

Heat liberated by fuel = Heat gained by water and calorimeter

$$x.G = (W + w) \times (t_2 - t_1)$$

or $\qquad\qquad G(GCV) = (W + w) \times (t_2 - t_1)/x \qquad\qquad$ ... (1)

This GCV is in the ideal conditions, but for more accurate results, the following corrections should be incorporated in the above formula(1) of GCV.

(i) **Cooling correction (t_c).** It is due to time taken for the water in the calorimeter from maximum temperature attained to room temperature with rate of cooling is dt°/minute and the actual time taken for cooling is t mins then the cooling correction = dTXt , it should be added to the observed raise in temperature.

(ii) **Acid correction (t_a).** During ignition, if sulphur and nitrogen are present in the fuel sample then they oxidized and forms corresponding acids along with the evolution of heat.

$$S + H_2 + 2O_2 = H_2SO_4$$

$$2N + H_2 + 3O_2 = 2HNO_3$$

Since heat is evolved So, this heat is also included in the measured heat and hence it must be subtracted.

(iii) **Fuse wire correction (t_f):** The heat liberated includes the heat due to ignition of Mg fuse wire, it should be subtracted from total heat eveloved.

(iv) **Cotton thread correction (t_t):** When cotton thread is used in the packing of bomb calorimeter, then during ignition, it is also ignited and produces some heat, that should be subtracted from total heat.

Now after incorporation of all corrections,

$$GCV = [(W+w) \times (t_2 - t_1 + \text{cooling correction}) - $$
$$(\text{Acid} + \text{fuse wire} + \text{cotton thread})]/ \times$$

If H be the percentage of Hydrogen in the fuel sample then

$$NCV = GCV - 0.09H. \text{ Latent heat}$$

Biofuel

A **biofuel** is a type of fuel whose energy is derived from biological carbon fixation. Biofuels include fuels derived from biomass conversion, as well as solid biomass, liquid fuels and various biogases. Although fossil fuels have their origin in ancient carbon fixation, they are not considered biofuels because they contain carbon that has been "out" of the carbon cycle for a very long time. Biofuels are gaining increased public and scientific attention, driven by factors such as oil price hikes, the need for increased energy security, concern over greenhouse gas emissions from fossil fuels, and support from government subsidies.

Bioethanol is an alcohol made by fermentation, mostly from carbohydrates produced in sugar or starch crops such as corn or sugarcane. Cellulosic biomass, derived from non-food sources such as trees and grasses, is also being developed as a feedstock for ethanol production. Ethanol can be used as a fuel for vehicles in its pure form, but it is usually used as a gasoline additive to increase octane and improve vehicle emissions. Bioethanol is widely used in the USA and in Brazil. Current plant design does not provide for converting the lignin portion of plant raw materials to fuel components by fermentation. Biofuels contribute 2.7% of the world's fuels for road transport, a contribution largely made up of ethanol and biodiesel.

Biodiesel is made from vegetable oils and animal fats. Biodiesel can be used as a fuel for vehicles in its pure form, but it is usually used as a diesel additive to reduce levels of particulates, carbon monoxide, and hydrocarbons from diesel-powered vehicles. Biodiesel is produced from oils or fats using **transesterification and esterification** process.

Biofuels may be classified as 1st generation and second generation biofuels.

First generation biofuels

'First-generation' or conventional biofuels are biofuels made from sugar, starch, and vegetable oil.

Second generation biofuels (advanced biofuels)

Second generation biofuels are produced from sustainable feedstock such as Cellulosic ethanol, Algae fuel., biohydrogen, biomethanol, DMF, BioDME, Fischer-Tropsch diesel, biohydrogen diesel, mixed alcohols and wood diesel.

Cellulosic ethanol production uses non-food crops or inedible waste products and does not divert food away from the animal or human food chain. Lignocellulose is the "woody" structural material of plants. This feedstock is abundant and diverse. Producing ethanol from cellulose is a difficult technical problem to solve. In nature, ruminant livestock (like cattle) eat grass and then use slow enzymatic digestive processes to break it intoglucose (sugar). The use of high temperatures, has been identified as an important factor in improving the overall economic feasibility of the biofuel industry and the identification of enzymes that are stable and can operate efficiently at extreme temperatures is an area of active research.

The recent discovery of the fungus *Gliocladium roseum* points toward the production of so-called myco-diesel from cellulose. This organism (recently discovered in rainforests of northern Patagonia has the unique capability of converting cellulose into medium length hydrocarbons typically found in diesel fuel.

Bioalcohols

Alcohols, most commonly ethanol, and less commonly propanol and butanol, are produced by the action of microorganisms andenzymes through the fermentation of sugars or starches (easiest), or cellulose (which is more difficult). Biobutanol (also called biogasoline) is often claimed to provide a direct replacement for gasoline, because it can be used directly in a gasoline engine (in a similar way to biodiesel in diesel engines).

Ethanol fuel is the most common biofuel worldwide, particularly in Brazil. Alcohol fuels are produced by fermentation of sugars derived from wheat, corn, sugar beets, sugar cane, molasses and any sugar or starch that alcoholic beverages can be made from (like potato and fruit waste, etc.). The ethanol production methods used are enzyme digestion (to release sugars from stored starches), fermentation of the sugars, distillation and drying. The distillation process requires significant energy input for heat.

Ethanol can be used in petrol engines as a replacement for gasoline; it can be mixed with gasoline to any percentage. Most existing car petrol engines can run on blends of up to 15% bioethanol with petroleum/gasoline. Ethanol has a smaller energy density than does gasoline; this fact means that it takes more fuel (volume and mass) to produce the same amount of work. An advantage of ethanol (CH_3CH_2OH) is that it has a higher octane rating than ethanol-free gasoline available at roadside gas stations which allows an increase of an engine's compression ratio for increased thermal efficiency.

Biodiesel: It is produced from oils or fats using transesterification and is a liquid similar in composition to fossil/mineral diesel. Chemically, it consists mostly of fatty acid methyl (or ethyl) esters (FAMEs).Biodiesel is the most common biofuel in Europe. In some countries biodiesel is less expensive than conventional diesel. Feedstocks for biodiesel include animal fats, vegetable oils, soy, rapeseed, jatropha, mahua, mustard, flax, sunflower, palm oil and algae. Pure biodiesel (B100) is the lowest emission diesel fuel. Although liquefied petroleum gas and hydrogen have cleaner combustion, they are used to fuel much less efficient petrol engines and are not as widely available.

Biodiesel is also safe to handle and transport because it is as biodegradable as sugar, 10 times less toxic than table salt, and has a high flash point of about 300 F (148 C) compared to petroleum diesel fuel, which has a flash point of 125 F (52°C). Biodiesel can be used in any diesel engine when mixed with mineral diesel.

Esterification and transesterification

Esterification & transesterification are important steps which are used for the production of biodiesel.

Esterification is the process of ester formation. Esters are produced when carboxylic acids are heated with alcohols in the presence of an acid catalyst. The catalyst is usually concentrated sulphuric acid or dry HCl.

The esterification reaction is both slow and reversible. The equation for the reaction between an acid RCOOH and an alcohol R'OH (where R and R' can be the same or different) is:

$$R-C\overset{O}{\underset{O-H}{<}} \; + \; R'OH \; \rightleftharpoons \; R-C\overset{O}{\underset{O-R'}{<}} \; + \; H_2O$$

So, for example, if we want ethyl ethanoate from ethanoic acid and ethanol, the equation would be:

$$CH_3-C\overset{O}{\underset{O-H}{<}} \; + \; CH_3CH_2OH \; \rightleftharpoons \; CH_3-C\overset{O}{\underset{O-CH_2CH_3}{<}} \; + \; H_2O$$

In organic chemistry, transesterification is the process of exchanging the organic group of an ester with the organic group of an alcohol. These reactions are often catalyzed by the addition of an acid or base catalyst. The reaction can also be accomplished with the help of enzymes (biocatalysts) particularly lipases. The reverse reaction, methanolysis, is also an example of transesterification. This process has been used to recycle polyesters into individual monomers. It is also used to convert fats (triglycerides) into biodiesel.

Transesterification: alcohol + ester → different alcohol + different ester

$$R'OH \; + \; \underset{R''O}{\overset{O}{\|}}{\diagdown}R \; \longrightarrow \; R''OH \; + \; \underset{R''O}{\overset{O}{\|}}{\diagdown}R$$

Biomass

Biomass is biological material from living, or recently living organisms like plant waste, crop waste, animal dung, etc. As an energy source, biomass can either be used directly, or converted into other energy products such as biofuel. Biomass is a renewable energy source.

Biomass is plant matter than can be used to generate electricity with steam turbines and gasifiers or produce heat, usually by direct combustion. Examples include forest residues such as dead trees, branches wood chips and even municipal solid waste etc. biomass includes plant or animal matter that can be converted into fibers or other industrial chemicals, including biofuels.

Biomass is carbon, hydrogen and oxygen based. Biomass energy is derived from five distinct energy sources: garbage, wood, waste, landfill gases, and alcohol fuels. Wood energy is derived by using lignocellulosic biomass (second generation biofuels) as fuel. This is either using harvested wood directly as a fuel, or collecting from wood waste streams. The largest source of energy from wood is pulping liquor or "black liquor," a waste product from processes of the pulp, paper and paperboard industry. Waste energy is the second-largest source of biomass energy. The main contributors of waste energy are municipal solid waste (first generation biofuels), such as sugarcane and corn, are used to produce bioethanol, an alcohol fuel. Alcohol fuels can be used directly, like other fuels, or as an additive to gasoline. Biomass can be converted to other usable forms of energy like methane gas or transportation fuels like ethanol and biodiesel. Rotting garbage, and agricultural and human waste, all release methane gas—also called "landfill gas" or "biogas." Crops such as corn and sugar cane can be fermented to produce the transportation fuel, ethanol. Biodiesel, another transportation fuel, can be produced from left-over food products like vegetable oils and animal fats.

The biomass used for electricity generation varies by region. Forest by-products, such as wood residues, are common in the United States.

Agricultural waste is common in Mauritius (sugar cane residue) and Southeast Asia (rice husks). Animal husbandry residues, such as poultry litter, are common in the UK.

There are a number of technological options available to make use of a wide variety of biomass types as a renewable energy source. Conversion technologies may release the energy directly, in the form of heat or electricity, or may convert it to another form, such as liquid biofuel or combustible biogas.

Thermal conversion

These are processes in which heat is the dominant mechanism to convert the biomass into another chemical form. (mainly controlled by the availability of oxygen and conversion temperature).

Chemical conversion

A range of chemical processes may be used to convert biomass into other forms, such as to produce a fuel that is more conveniently used, transported or stored.

Biochemical conversion

Biochemical conversion makes use of the enzymes of bacteria and other micro-organisms to break down biomass. In most cases micro-organisms are used to perform the conversion process: anaerobic digestion, fermentation and composting. Other chemical processes such as converting straight and waste vegetable oils into biodiesel is transesterification.

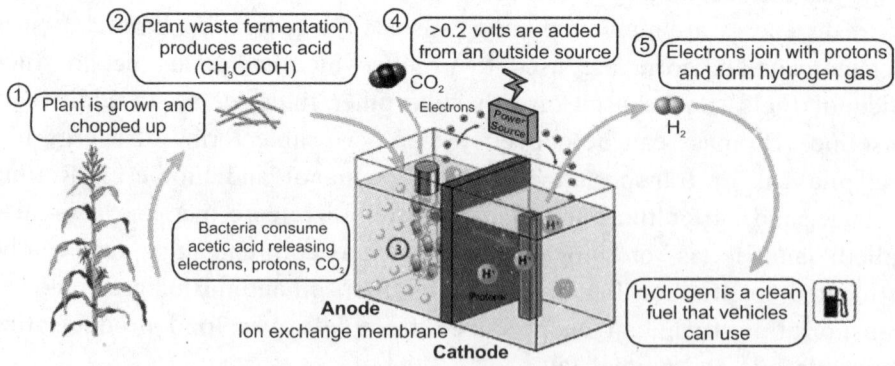

Fig. 11. 2: Microbial Electrolysis Cell

Algal biofuels

by utilizing algae biofuel is generated that have a natural oil content greater than 50%, Algae can be grown on algae ponds at wastewater treatment plants. This oil-rich algae can then be extracted from the system and processed into biofuels, with the dried remainder further reprocessed to create ethanol.

Jatropha biofuels

Several groups in various sectors are conducting research on Jatropha curcas, a poisonous shrub-like tree that produces seeds considered by many to be a viable source of biofuels feedstock oil. Much of this research focuses on improving the overall per acre oil yield of Jatropha through advancements in genetics, soil science, and horticultural practices. SG Biofuels, a San Diego-based Jatropha developer, has used molecular breeding and biotechnology to produce elite hybrid seeds of Jatropha that show significant yield improvements over first generation varieties. Successful exploration of these disciplines is projected to increase Jatropha farm production yields by 200-300% in the next ten years.

Fungi *Cunninghamella japonica, Gliocladium roseum* are being processed to get biofuel in an economically efficient manner.

Biogas

Biogas typically refers to a gas produced by the biological breakdown of organic matter in the absence of oxygen. Organic waste such as dead plant and animal material, animal feces, and kitchen waste can be converted into a gaseous fuel called biogas. Biogas originates from biogenic material and is a type of bio fuel.

Biogas is produced by the anaerobic digestion or fermentation of biodegradable materials such as biomass, manure, sewage, municipal waste, green waste, plant material, and crops. Biogas comprises primarily methane (CH_4) and carbon dioxide (CO_2) and may have small amounts of hydrogen sulphide (H_2S), moisture and siloxanes.

The gases methane, hydrogen, and carbon monoxide (CO) can be combusted or oxidized with oxygen. This energy release allows biogas to be used as a fuel. Biogas can be used as a fuel in any country for any heating purpose, such as cooking. It can also be used in anaerobic digesters where it is typically used in a gas engine to convert the energy in the gas into electricity and heat. Biogas can be compressed, much like natural gas, and used to power motor vehicles. Biogas is a renewable fuel, A *biogas plant* is the name often given to an anaerobic digester that treats farm wastes or energy crops. Biogas can be produced using anaerobic digesters. Animal /plant / crops waste along with water are taken . Landfill gas is produced by wet organic waste decomposing under anaerobic conditions in a landfill. Biogas is practically produced as landfill gas (LFG) or digester gas. The waste is covered and mechanically compressed by the weight of the material that is deposited from above. This material prevents oxygen exposure thus allowing anaerobic microbes to thrive. Anaerobic microbes breaks complex organic molecule in to simple gaseous molecules like CH_4, CO_2, H_2S, N_2 etc This gas builds up and collected and when sufficient pressure is developed then it is used.It takes about 2-3 days to develop sufficient pressure for use as fuel for cooking. This gas is generally used at

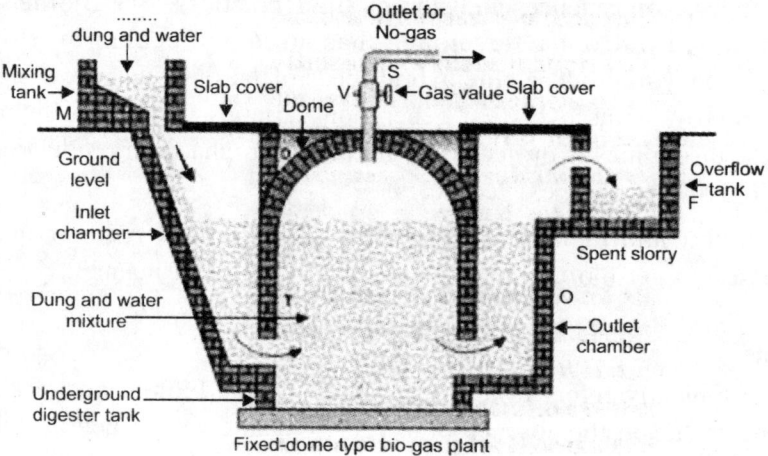

Fixed-dome type bio-gas plant

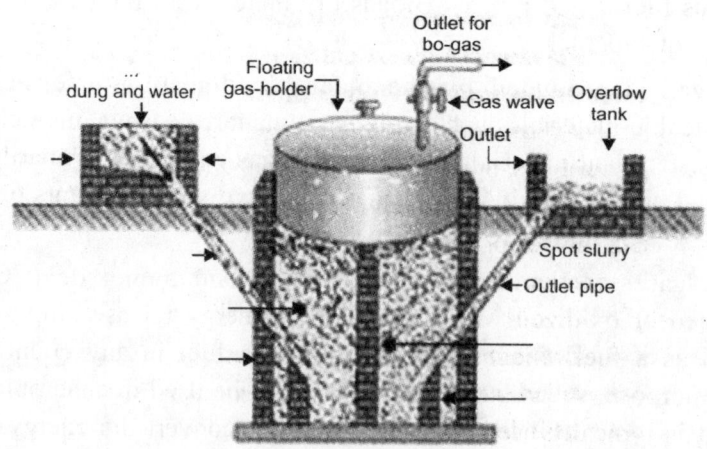

Fig. 11.3: Bio gas Plant

the distance of 10 meter circle. Fixed dome type and floating type bio gas plants are constructed, which are shown in the Fig. 11.3.

Typical Biogas composition is given in the table.

Compound Name	Molecular formula	%
Methane	CH_4	50–75
Carbon dioxide	CO_2	25–50
Nitrogen	N_2	0–10
Hydrogen	H_2	0–1
Hydrogen sulfide	H_2S	0–3

NUMERICAL PROBLEMS

Q.1. Calculate the GCV and NCV of the coal sample containing 90%C, 8% H and 2% ash. Other data for bomb calorimeter is given below: Weight of coal- 0.75 gm, weight of water taken-750 gm, water equivalent of calorimeter-2200gm, increase in temperature-2.5°C, fuse wire correction- 10 cal, cooling correction 0.5°C, acid correction-50 cal, cotton thread correction-2 cal

Solution: We know the formula that

$$GCV = [(W + w) \times (t_2 - t_1 + \text{cooling correction})$$
$$- (\text{Acid} + \text{fuse wire} + \text{cotton thread})]/\times$$
$$= [(750 + 2200)(2.5 + 0.5) -$$
$$(50 + 10 + 2)]/0.75$$
$$= 11717.3 \text{ cal/gm}$$

Now for NCV let Latent heat of vaporization- 587 cal/gm

If H(8%) be the percentage of Hydrogen in the fuel sample then

$$NCV = GCV - 0.09H.\text{Latent heat}$$
$$NCV = 11717.3 - 0.09 \times 8 \times 587$$
$$= 11294.7 \text{ cal/gm}$$

Q.2. Calculate the GCV and NCV of the coal sample containing 88%C, 7% H,3%O and 2% ash. Other data for bomb calorimeter is given below-

Weight of coal- 0.92 gm, weight of water taken-800 gm, water equivalent of calorimeter-1.8kg, increase in temperature-2.2°C, fuse wire correction- 15 cal, cooling correction 0.3°C, acid correction- 30 cal, latent heat- 580 cal/gm

Solution: We know the formula that

$$GCV = [(W + w) \times (t_2 - t_1 + \text{cooling correction}) -$$
(Acid + fuse wire + cotton thread)]/×

$$= [(800 + 1800)(2.2 + 0.3)$$
$$- (30 + 15 + 0)]/0.92 = 7016.3 \text{ cal/gm}$$

Now for NCV let Latent heat of vaporization- 580 cal/gm

If H(7%) be the percentage of Hydrogen in the fuel sample then

$$NCV = GCV - 0.09 \text{ H.Latent heat}$$
$$NCV = 7016.3 - 0.09 \times 7 \times 580 = 6650.9 \text{ cal/gm}$$

Calculation of air quantities-

Calculation for Requirement of Theoretical Amount of Air

First the combustion reaction is written for individual combustible elements/constituents in the presence of oxygen ,then amount of required oxygen is calculated, and finally air is calculated by using the concept that Air has 23% oxygen by weight and 21% by volume

Q.3. Calculate the amount of air required for a sample of 100 kg of oil sample, which is having the chemical composition as C-85.9%, H- 12%, S-0.5%

Solution: Reactions are

$$C + O_2 - CO_2$$
$$H_2 + 1/2O_2 - H_2O$$
$$S + O_2 - SO_2$$

In the sample oxygen present = 100 − (85.9 + 12 + 0.5) = 1.6

Constituents of fuel

$$C + O_2 - CO_2$$
$$12 + 32 = 44$$

12 kg of carbon requires 32 kg of oxygen to form 44 kg of carbon dioxide therefore 1 kg of carbon requires 32/12 kg i.e 2.67 kg of oxygen

$$(85.9)C + (85.9 \times 2.67) O_2 - 315.25CO_2$$
$$2H_2 + O_2 - 2H_2O$$
$$4 + 32 = 36$$

4 kg of hydrogen requires 32 kg of oxygen to form 36 kg of water, therefore 1 kg of hydrogen requires 32/4 kg i.e 8 kg of oxygen

$$(12) H_2 + (12 \times 8) O_2 - (12 \times 9) H_2O$$
$$S + O_2 - SO_2$$
$$32 + 32 = 64$$

32 kg of sulphur requires 32 kg of oxygen to form 64 kg of sulphur dioxide, therefore 1 kg of sulphur requires 32/32 kg i.e 1 kg of oxygen

$$(0.5) \ S + (0.5 \times 1) \ \text{——} \ (O2 \times 1.0) \ SO_2$$

Total Oxygen required = 325.57 kg for 100 kg sample

$$(229.07 + 96 + 0.5)$$

Oxygen already present in

100 kg fuel (given) = 1.6 kg

Additional Oxygen Required = 325.57 – 1.6 = 324.27 kg

Therefore quantity of dry air reqd. = (324.87)/0.23

(air contains 23% oxygen by wt.)

$$= 1412.45 \ \text{kg of air}$$

THEORETICAL QUESTIONS

(a) What is the difference between natural and manufactured fuels?

(b) What are the merits and demerits of solid fuels?

(c) What are the main constituents of wood?

(d) What is the difference between ultimate analysis and proximate analysis of coal?

(e) Mention the uses of different types of coal.

(f) What is GCV and NCV and find a relationship between them

(g) Mention the composition of crude petroleum.

(h) Mention the uses of different types of manufactured liquid fuels.

(i) Mention the origin and composition of natural gas.

(j) Mention the characteristics of the following gaseous fuels :
  (i) Coal gas,
  (ii) Water gas,
  (iii) Producer gas, and

(k) Define calorific value and explain the Bomb Calorimeter method for the determination of calorific value.

(l) Write short note on Biofuel and biodiesel.

(m) Explain working of Bio-gas plan with its composition.

(n) Write a note on Esterification and transesterification with reaction and application .

(o) Explain Bio-mass and its uses.

Chapter 12
BONDING IN THE MOLECULES

➢ **Chemical bonding: Ionic and Covalent**
➢ **Hybridisation**
➢ **Metallic bonding**
➢ **Hydrogen Bonding**
➢ **VSEPR**
➢ **MOT**
➢ **Homo Atomic Molecules**
➢ **Hetero atomic Molecules**
➢ **Numerical Problems**

CHEMICAL BONDING

Though the periodic table has only 118 or so elements, there are obviously more substances in nature than 118 pure elements. This is because atoms can react with one another to form new substances called compounds which are formed when two or more atoms chemically bond together, the resulting compound is unique both chemically and physically from its parent atoms. Let's take an example, The element sodium is a silver-coloured metal that reacts so violently with water that flames are produced when sodium gets wet. The element chlorine is a greenish-coloured gas that is so poisonous that it was used as a weapon in World War I. When chemically bonded together, these two dangerous substances form the compound sodium chloride, a compound so safe that we eat it every day - common table salt. So, over all there is type of bonding which alters the properties of the molecule.This bonding is chemical bonding like ionic or covalent bonding or coordinate bonding or in combination of these. Sometimes there are other types of bonding like Hydrogen bonding, metallic bonding which explain the specific properties of the compound.

Atoms are the building blocks of all substances. They are held together by **CHEMICAL BONDS**, strong attractive forces between atoms. Without these ties that bind, the universe would be nothing more than a mass chaos of individual atoms.A bond is formed when electrons from two atoms interact with each other and their atoms become joined. The electrons that interact with each other are **VALENCE ELECTRONS,** the ones that reside in the outermost electron shell of an atom. A **COVALENTBOND** results when two atoms "share" valence electrons between them. An **IONIC BOND** occurs when one atom gains a valence electron from a different atom, forming a negative ion (**ANION**) and a positive ion (**CATION**), respectively. These oppositely charged ions are attracted to each other, forming an ionic bond. The chemical bonding that takes place in NaCl is different than that in HCl. This gives NaCl and HCl very different structures, appearances, and properties.

The bonds that hold the carbon and hydrogen atoms in rubber together, on the other hand, are not ionic but covalent. Each carbon atom shares four of its outermost electrons with its immediate neighbours. Under stress, the bonds stretch, then snap back as each atom pulls on the shared electrons. And that's the way the ball bounces.

Types of bonding: Traditional types of bonding are ionic and covalent. Some other types are coordinate bonding, metallic bonding, hydrogen bonding.

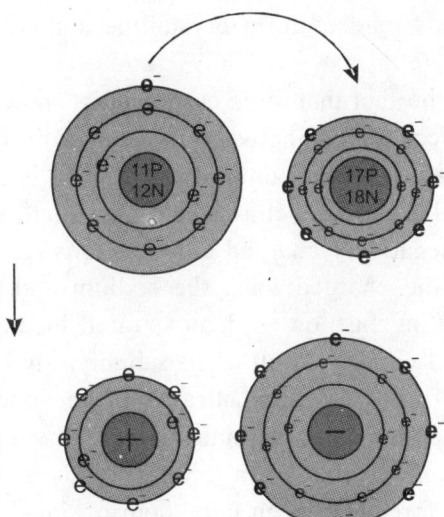

Fig. 12.1: Sodium (on the left) loses its one valence electron to chlorine (on the right), resul-ting in a positively charged sodium ion (left) and a negatively charged chlorine ion (right).

Ionic Bonding

In ionic bonding, electrons are completely transferred from one atom to another. In the process of either losing or gaining negatively charged electrons, the reacting atoms form ions. The oppositely charged ions are attracted to each other by electrostatic forces, which are the basis of theionic bond.

For example (Fig. 12.1), during the reaction of sodium with chlorine:

The Reaction of Sodium with Chlorine

Notice that when sodium loses its one valence electron it gets smaller in size, while chlorine grows larger when it gains an additional valence electron. This is typical of the relative sizes of ions to atoms. Positive ions tend to be smaller than their parent atoms while negative ions tend to be larger than their parent. After the reaction takes place, the charged Na^+ and Cl^- ions are held together by electrostatic forces, thus forming an ionic bond. Ionic compounds share many features in common:

- Ionic bonds are formed between metals and nonmetals, n naming simple ionic compounds, the metal is always first, the nonmetal second (e.g., sodium chloride).
- Ionic compounds are dissolved easily in water and other polar solvents.
- In solution, ionic compounds easily conduct electricity.
- Ionic compounds tend to form crystalline solids with high melting temperatures.

This last feature, the fact that ionic compounds are solids, results from the intermolecular forces (forces between molecules) in ionic solids. If we consider a solid crystal of sodium chloride, the solid is made up of many positively charged sodium ions (pictured below as small gray spheres) and an equal number of negatively charged chlorine ions (green spheres). Due to the interaction of the charged ions, the sodium and chlorine ions are arranged in an alternating fashion as demonstrated in the schematic. Each sodium ion is attracted equally to all of its neighboring chlorine ions, and likewise for the chlorine to sodium attraction. The concept of a single molecule does not apply to ionic crystals because the solid exists as one continuous system. Ionic solids form crystals with high melting points because of the strong forces between neighbouring ions.

Covalent bonding

The second major type of atomic bonding occurs when atoms share electrons.

As opposed to ionic bonding in which a complete transfer of electrons occurs, covalent bonding occurs when two (or more) elements share electrons. Covalent bonding occurs because the atoms in the compound have a similar tendency for electrons (generally to gain electrons). This most commonly occurs when two nonmetals bond together. Because both of the non metals will want to gain electrons, the elements involved will share electrons in an effort to fill their valence shells. A good example of a covalent bond is that which occurs between two hydrogen atoms. Atoms of hydrogen (H) have one valence electron in their first electron shell. Since the capacity of this shell is two electrons, each hydrogen atom will "want" to pick up a second electron. In an effort to pick up a second electron, hydrogen atoms will react with nearby hydrogen (H) atoms to form the compound H_2. Because the hydrogen compound is a combination of equally matched atoms, the atoms will share each other's single electron, forming one covalent bond. In this way, both atoms share the stability of a full valence shell.

Unlike ionic compounds, covalent molecules exist as true molecules. Because electrons are shared in covalent molecules, no full ionic charges are formed. Thus covalent molecules are not strongly attracted to one another. As a result, covalent molecules move about freely and tend to exist as liquids or gases at room temperature.

Multiple Bonds

For every pair of electrons shared between two atoms, a single covalent bond is formed. Some atoms can share multiple pairs of electrons, forming multiple covalent bonds. For example, oxygen (which has six valence electrons) needs two electrons to complete its valence shell. When two oxygen atoms form the compound O_2, they share two pairs of electrons, forming two covalent bonds.

Lewis Dot Structures

Lewis dot structures are a shorthand to represent the valence electrons of an atom. The structures are written as the element symbol surrounded by dots that represent the valence electrons. The Lewis structures for the elements in the first two periods of the periodic table are shown in Fig. 12.2 and 12.3.

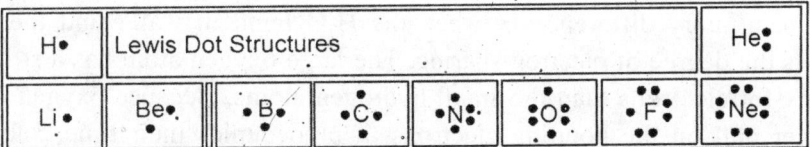

Fig. 12.2

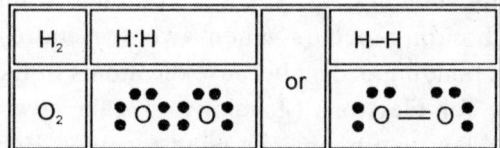

Fig. 12.3

Lewis structures can also be used to show bonding between atoms. The bonding electrons are placed between the atoms and can be represented by a pair of dots or a dash (each dash represents one pair of electrons, or one bond). Lewis structures for H_2 and O_2 are shown above.

Polar and nonpolar covalent bonding

There are, in fact, two subtypes of covalent bonds. The H_2 molecule is a good example of the first type of covalent bond, the nonpolar bond. Because both atoms in the H_2 molecule have an equal attraction (or affinity) for electrons, the bonding electrons are equally shared by the two atoms, and a nonpolar covalent bond is formed. Whenever two atoms of the same element bond together, a nonpolar bond is formed.

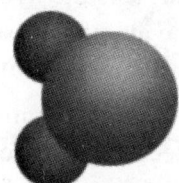

Fig.12.4. : H_2O: a water molecule

A polar bond is formed when electrons are unequally shared between two atoms. Polar covalent bonding occurs because one atom has a stronger affinity for electrons than the other (yet not enough to pull the electrons away completely and form an ion). In a polar covalent bond, the bonding electrons will spend a greater amount of time around the atom that has the stronger affinity for electrons. A good example of a polar covalent bond is the hydrogen-oxygen bond in the water molecule.

Water molecules contain two hydrogen atoms bonded to one oxygen atom (blue). Oxygen, with six valence electrons, needs two additional electrons to complete its valence shell. Each hydrogen contains one electron. Thus oxygen shares the electrons from two hydrogen atoms to complete its own valence shell, and in return shares two of its own electrons with each hydrogen, completing the H valence shells.

The primary difference between the H-O bond in water and the H-H bond is the degree of electron sharing. The large oxygen atom has a stronger affinity for electrons than the small hydrogen atoms. Because oxygen has a stronger pull on the bonding electrons, it preoccupies their time, and this leads to unequal sharing and the formation of a polar covalent bond.

METALLIC BONDING

There is a third type of bonding, called **Metallic bonding.**

As the name implies, metallic bonding usually occurs in metals, such as copper. A piece of copper metal has a certain arrangement of copper atoms. The valence electrons of these atoms are free to move about the piece of metal and are attracted to the positive cores of copper, thus holding the atoms together.

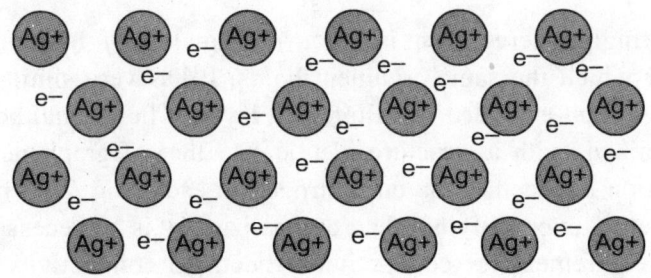

Fig. 12.5: These silver atoms are joined by metallic bonds

Metallic bonding is the electrostatic attractive forces between the delocalized electrons, called conduction electrons, gathered in an "electron sea", and the positively charged metal ions. Understood as the sharing of "free" electrons among a lattice of positively charged ions (cations), metallic bonding is sometimes compared with that of molten salts; however, this simplistic view holds true for very few metals. In a more quantum-mechanical view, the conduction electrons divide their density equally over all atoms that function as neutral (non-charged) entities. Metallic bonding accounts for many physical properties of metals, such as strength, malleability, ductility, thermal and electrical conductivity, opacity, and luster.

Although the term "metallic bond" is often used in contrast to the term "covalent bond", it is preferable to use the term *metallic bonding*, because this type of bonding is collective in nature and a single "metallic bond" does not exist. Not all metals exhibit metallic bonding: one such example is the mercurous ion (H_{g2}^{++}) which forms covalent metal-metal bonds.

The nature of metallic bonding

The combination of two phenomena gives rise to metallic bonding: *delocalization of electrons* and the availability of a far larger number of delocalized energy states than of delocalized electrons. The latter could be called *electron deficiency*.

Delocalization

Bonding that involves more than one pair of atoms held together by one pair of electrons—is most familiar from the example of benzene C_6H_6, where six electrons from six carbon atoms are engaged in joint aromatic bonding. The principle can easily be extended over larger aromatic molecules like naphthalene, anthracene, ovalene, and so on; if the process is taken to its extreme:graphene. The latter is an example of a system delocalized in two dimensions(2D).

Interestingly, there is an isoelectronic analog of benzene, borazine $B_3N_3H_6$ for which the same argument holds. It has very similar properties to benzene. When extended indefinitely, a layer of hexagonal boron nitride, BN, is obtained, with a structure identical to that of graphene apart from the alternation between boron and nitrogen in each ring. This material is a semiconductor, exemplifying that delocalization is a necessary but not sufficient requirement for conductivity. Electrical conductivity does occur in graphene, because the π and π^*-like bands overlap, making it a semimetal, with *partly filled bands*, fulfilling the other requirement for conductivity.

Delocalization(3D)-Metal aromaticity in metal clusters is another example of delocalization, this time often in three-dimensional entities. Metals take the delocalization principle to its extreme and one could say that a crystal of a metal represents a single molecule over which all conduction electrons are delocalized in all three dimensions. This means that inside the metal one can generally not distinguish molecules so that the metallic bonding is neither intra- nor intermolecular. 'Nonmolecular' would perhaps be a better term. Metallic bonding is mostly non-polar, because even in alloys there is little difference among the electronegativities of the atoms participating in the bonding interaction (and in pure elemental metals, none at all). Thus metallic bonding is an extremely delocalized communal form of covalent bonding. In a sense metallic bonding is not a 'new' type of bonding at all therefore and it only describes the bonding as present in a chunk of condensed matter, be it crystalline solid, liquid or even glass. Metallic vapours by contrast are often atomic (Hg) or at times contain molecules like Na_2 held together by a more conventional covalent bond. This is why it is not correct to speak of a single 'metallic bond'. The delocalization is most pronounced for s- and p-electrons. For caesium it is so strong that the electrons are virtually free from the caesium atoms to form a gas only constrained by the surface of the metal. For caesium therefore the picture of Cs^+-ions held together by a negatively charged electron gas is not too inaccurate. For other elements the electrons are less free, in that they still experience the potential of the metal atoms, sometimes quite strongly. They require a more intricate quantum mechanical treatment (e.g. tight binding) in which the atoms are viewed as neutral much like the carbon atoms in benzene. For d- and especially f-electrons the delocalization is not strong at all and this explains why these electrons are able to continue behaving as unpaired electrons that retain their spin, adding interesting magnetic properties to these metals.

Electron deficiency and mobility

Metal atoms contain few electrons in their valence shells relative to their periods or energy levels. They are electron deficient elements and the communal sharing does not change that. There remain far more available energy states than there are shared electrons. Both requirements for conductivity are therefore fulfilled: strong delocalization and partly filled energy bands. Such electrons can therefore easily change from one energy state into a slightly different one. Thus, not only do they become delocalized, forming a sea of electrons permeating the lattice, but they are also able to migrate through the lattice when an external electrical field is imposed, leading to electrical conductivity. Without the field there are electrons moving equally in all directions. Under the field some will adjust their state slightly, adopting a different wave vector. Consequently, there will be more moving one way than the other and a net current will result.

The freedom of conduction electrons to migrate also give metal atoms, or layers of them, the capacity to slide past each other. Locally bonds can easily be broken and replaced by new ones after the deformation. This process does not affect the communal metallic bonding very much. This gives rise to metals' typical characteristic phenomena of malleability and ductility. This is particularly true for pure elements. In the presence of dissolved impurities the defects in the lattice that function as cleavage points may get blocked and the material becomes harder. Gold for example is very soft in pure form (24 kt), which is why for jewellery alloys of 18 kt or lower are preferred.

Metals are typically also good conductors of heat, but the conduction electrons only contribute partly to this phenomenon. Collective (i.e. delocalized) vibrations of the atoms known as phonons that travel through the solid as a wave, contribute strongly.

However, the latter also holds for a substance like diamond. It conducts heat quite well but *not* electricity. The latter is *not* a consequence of the fact that delocalization is absent in diamond, but simply that carbon is not electron deficient. The position of carbon in the middle of its period in the Periodic Table makes that there are precisely enough electrons to fill the energy states. Under a field electrons are not able to adopt a different wave vector because there are no empty states to move into. This makes a current impossible in this wide band gap semiconductor. However, as soon as charge carriers are introduced by doping the crystal with a suitable impurity the resulting charge carriers are as mobile as in a metal, though far fewer in number. Even without doping the vibrational motions (the phonons) are delocalized over the crystal explaining the heat conduction. Still the bonding in diamond is better described as covalent than as metallic if only because there is a very strong directional preference for tetrahedral stacking, producing a structure that is extremely hard to deform and by no means close packed.

Clearly, the electron deficiency is an important point in distinguishing metallic from more conventional covalent bonding. Thus, we should amend the expression given above into: *Metallic bonding is an extremely delocalized communal form of electron deficient covalent bonding.*

Metallic Radius

Metallic radius is defined as one half of the distance between neighbouring atoms in the metal solid. This radius depends on the nature of the atom as well as its environment, specifically on the coordination number (CN) which in turn depends on the temperature and applied pressure.

When comparing periodic trends in the size of atoms it is often desirable to apply so-called Goldschmidt correction which converts the radii to the values the atoms would have if they were 12-coordinated. Since metallic radii are always biggest for the highest coordination number, correction for less dense coordinations involves dividing by x, where $0 < x < 1$. Specifically, for CN = 4, x = 0.88; for CN = 6, x = 0.96, and for CN = 8, x = 0.97. The correction is named after Victor Goldschmidt who obtained the numerical values quoted above.

The radii follow general periodic trends: they decrease across the period due to increase in the effective nuclear charge which is not offset by the increased number of valence electrons. The radii also decrease down the group due to increase in principal quantum number. Between rows 3 and 4 the lanthanide contraction is observed–there is very little increase of the radius down the group due to the presence of poorly shielding f orbitals.

Strength of the bond

The atoms in metals have a strong attractive force between them. Much energy is required to overcome it. Therefore, metals often have high boiling points, with tungsten (5828 K) being extremely high. A remarkable exception are the elements of the zinc group: Zn, Cd and Hg. Their electron configuration ends in $...ns^2$ and this comes to resemble a noble gas configuration like that of helium more and more when going down in the periodic table because the energy distance to the empty np orbitals becomes larger. These metals are therefore relatively volatile, and are avoided in ultra-high vacuum systems. Otherwise, metallic bonding can be very strong, even in the melt. Gallium is a good example of that. Even though it melts by the heat of one's hand just above room temperature, its boiling point is not far from that of copper. Molten gallium is therefore a very nonvolatile liquid thanks to its strong metallic bonding. The presence of an ocean of mobile charge carriers has profound effects on the optical properties of metals. They can only be understood by considering the electrons as a *collective* rather than considering the states of individual electrons involved in more conventional covalent bonds.

HYDROGEN BOND

A **hydrogen bond** is the attractive interaction of a hydrogen atom with an electronegative atom, such as nitrogen, oxygen or fluorine, that comes from another molecule or chemical group. The hydrogen must be covalently bonded to another electronegative atom to create the bond. These bonds can occur between molecules (*intermolecular H bonding*), or within different parts of a single molecule (*intramolecular H bonding*). The hydrogen bond (5 to 30 kJ/mole) is stronger than a vander Waals interaction, but weaker than covalent or ionic bonds. This type of bond occurs in both inorganic molecules such as water and organic molecules such as DNA.

Intermolecular hydrogen bonding is responsible for the high boiling point of water (100°C) compared to the other group 16 hydrides that have no hydrogen bonds. Intramolecular hydrogen bonding is partly responsible for the secondary, tertiary, and quaternary structures of proteins and nucleic acids. It also plays an important role in the structure of polymers, both synthetic and natural.

The bond lengths give some indication of the bond strength. A normal covalent bond is 0.96 Angstroms, while the hydrogen bond length is 1.97 A.

The most ubiquitous, and perhaps simplest, example of a hydrogen bond is found between water molecules. In a discrete water molecule, there are two hydrogen atoms and one oxygen atom. Two molecules of water can form a hydrogen bond between them; the simplest case, when only two molecules are present, is called the water dimer and is often used as a model system. When more molecules are present, as is the case of liquid water, more bonds are possible because the oxygen of one water molecule has two lone pairs of electrons, each of which can form a hydrogen bond with a hydrogen on another water molecule. This can repeat such that every water molecule is H-bonded with up to four other molecules, as shown in the figure (two through its two lone pairs, and two through its two hydrogen atoms). Hydrogen bonding strongly affects the crystal structure of ice, helping to create an open hexagonal lattice. The density of ice is less than water at the same temperature; thus, the solid phase of water floats on the liquid, unlike most other substances.

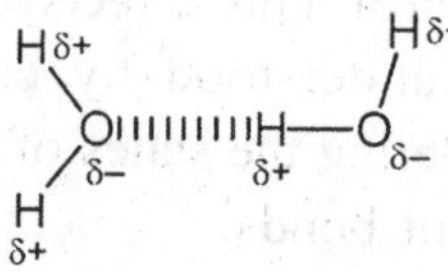

Fig. 12.6: Types of Hydrogen Bonding

Hydrogen bond can be classified into two types:

(a) **Inter molecular hydrogen bond:** This type of bond is formed between two different molecules of the same or different substances. Like in water, HF, Ammonia, amines, alcohols etc.

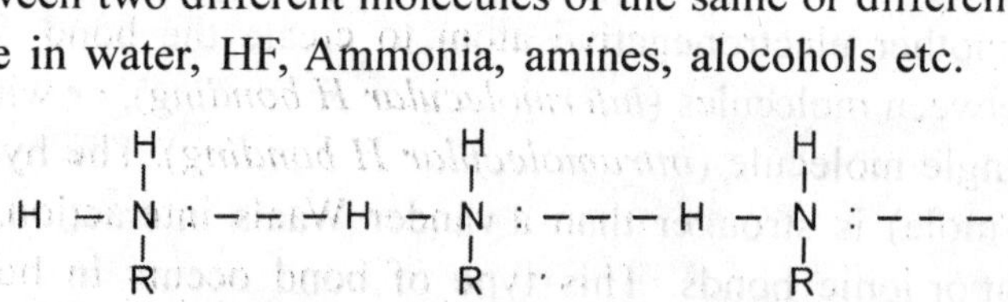

Hydrogen bonding in amines

Intermolecular H bonding increases the boiling point, melting point and solubility in water. This bonding This bonding also increases the observed molecular weight.This type of bonding increases the association of molecules hence higher energy (high temp) is required to break the bonding so that molecules are free to escape, consequently boiling point increases. Liquid water's high boiling point is due to the high number of hydrogen bonds each molecule can form relative to its low molecular mass. Owing to the difficulty of breaking these bonds, water has a very high boiling point, melting point, and viscosity compared to otherwise similar liquids not conjoined by hydrogen bonds. Water is unique because its oxygen atom has two lone pairs and two hydrogen atoms, meaning that the total number of bonds of a water molecule is up to four.

For another example, carboxylic acid exist as a dimer. hydrogen fluoride—which has three lone pairs on the F atom but only one H atom—can form only two bonds; (ammonia has the opposite problem: three hydrogen atoms but only one lone pair). Hyrdogen Bonding in HF is more stronger than H-Cl and H-Br due to high electronegativity of fluorine, hence HF is viscous liquid at room temperature while HCl and HI are gas. H-F···H-F···H-F .

Hydrogen bonding is directly affected by electro negativity and size of atom, indirectly upon the inter atomic distance and charges present on H atom and other electronegative atom. Since the nature of bonding is electrostatic hence its magnitude ($F = k.q_1q_2/r^2$) is directly proportional to the charges (q) and inversely proportional to the square of distance between the hydrogen atom and other atom (r^2).

Lower alcohols are soluble in water but higher alcohols (containing more number of C atoms) are insouluble, this is also attributed due to inter molecular hydrogen bonding between water (H-O-H) and alcohol (R-O-H) molecule. As the size of alkyl group (R) increases in the alcohol, distance between the water and alcohol molecules increases, electrostatic force of attraction (H bonding) decreases, consequently solubility decreases.

(b) **Intra molecular hydrogen bond:** This type of bond is formed between the hydrogen atom and the highly electronegative atom (F, O or N) present in the same molecule. This bonding causes the shrinkage in the molecule, consequently molecule is volatile at lower temperature, i.e. it decreases the B.P and M.P. Due to this bonding o-nitrophenol or o-salicylaldehyde is volatile in nature as compared to their para isomers. In the para form distance between the Some other examples are given below.

O–Chlorophenol

Salicylaldehyde

Acetylacelone

Ethyl acetoacetate

With the help of hydrogen bonding we can also explain the acidic and basic nature in the compounds forming Hydrogen bonding. Acidic strength of o-nitrophenol is less than its para isomer. This is due to the presence of intramolecular H-bonding in the ortho isomer because of this release of H^+ becomes more difficult from the ortho form as compared to para form and we know that acidic strength depends up on the easy availability of H^+ ions.

Valence Bond Theory and Molecular Orbital Theory

Valence bond theory

In chemistry, valence bond (VB) theory is one of two basic theories, along with molecular orbital (MO) theory, that were developed to use the methods of quantum mechanics to explain chemical bonding. It focuses on how the atomic orbitals of the dissociated atoms combine to give individual chemical bonds when a molecule is formed. In contrast, molecular orbital theory has orbitals that cover the whole molecule.

In 1916, G.N. Lewis proposed that a chemical bond forms by the interaction of two shared bonding electrons, with the representation of molecules as Lewis structures.

According to this theory a covalent bond is formed between the two atoms by the overlap of half filled valence atomic orbitals of each atom containing one unpaired electron. A valence bond structure is similar to a Lewis structure, but where a single Lewis structure cannot be written, several valence bond structures are used. Each of these VB structures represents a specific Lewis structure. This combination of valence bond structures is the main point of resonance theory. Valence bond theory considers that the overlapping atomic orbitals of the participating atoms form a chemical bond. Because of the overlapping, it is most probable that electrons should be in the bond region. Valence bond theory views bonds as weakly coupled orbitals (small overlap). Valence bond theory is typically easier to employ in ground state molecules.

The overlapping atomic orbitals can differ. The two types of overlapping orbitals are sigma and pi. Sigma bonds occur when the orbitals of two shared electrons overlap head-to-head. Pi bonds occur when two orbitals overlap when they are parallel. For example, a bond between two s-orbital electrons is a sigma bond, because two spheres are always coaxial. In terms of bond order, single bonds have one sigma bond, double bonds consist of one sigma bond and one pi bond, and triple bonds contain one sigma bond and two pi bonds. However, the atomic orbitals for bonding may be hybrids. Often, the bonding atomic orbitals have a character of several possible types of orbitals. The methods to get an atomic orbital with the proper character for the bonding is called hybridization.

An important aspect of the VB theory is the condition of maximum overlap which leads to the formation of the strongest possible bonds. This theory is used to explain the covalent bond formation in many molecules.

For Example in the case of the F_2 molecule the F - F bond is formed by the overlap of p_z orbitals of the two F atoms, each containing an unpaired electron. Since the natures of the overlapping orbitals are different in H_2 and F_2 molecules, the bond strength and bond lengths differ between H_2 and F_2 molecules. Bonding arises from the overlap of orbitals. Sigma (σ) bonds arise from the 'end-to end ' overlapping between adjacent orbitals. This leads to a region of high electron density along the inter-nuclear axis. In an HF molecule the covalent bond is formed by the overlap of the 1s orbital of H and the $2p_z$ orbital of F, each containing an unpaired electron. Mutual sharing of electrons between H and F results in a covalent bond in HF. Pi (π) bonds arise from the 'side-on' overlap between adjacent orbitals. This leads to two regions of high electron density on opposite sides of the inter-nuclear axis (not cylindrically symmetrical). Bonding involves the overlap of valence orbitals on the central atom with those of the surrounding atoms. Hybridization of pure atomic orbitals to form a special set of orbitals for use in bonding.

VALENCE SHELL ELECTRON PAIR REPULSION (VSEPR) THEORY

Valence shell electron pair repulsion (VSEPR) theory is a model in chemistry used to predict the shape of individual molecules based upon the extent of electron-pair electrostatic repulsion. It is also named Gillespie–Nyholm theory after its two main developers. The acronym "VSEPR" is sometimes pronounced "vesper" for ease of pronunciation; however, the phonetic pronunciation is technically more correct.The premise of VSEPR is that the valence electron pairs surrounding an atom mutually repel each other, and will therefore adopt an arrangement that minimizes this repulsion, thus determining themolecular geometry. The number of electron pairs surrounding an atom, both bonding and nonbonding, is called its steric number. VSEPR theory is usually compared and contrasted with valence bond theory, which addresses molecular shape through orbitals that are energetically accessible for bonding. Valence bond theory concerns itself with the formation of sigma and pi bonds

VSEPR theory mainly involves predicting the layout of electron pairs surrounding one or more central atoms in a molecule, which are bonded to two or more other atoms. The geometry of these central atoms in turn determines the geometry of the larger whole.

The number of electron pairs in the valence shell of a central atom is determined by drawing the Lewis structure of the molecule, expanded to show all lone pairs of electrons, alongside protruding and projecting bonds. Where two or more resonance structures can depict a molecule, the VSEPR model is applicable to any such structure. For the purposes of VSEPR theory, the multiple electron pairs in a multiple bond are treated as though they were a single "pair".

These electron pairs are assumed to lie on the surface of a sphere centered on the central atom, and since they are negatively charged, tend to occupy positions that minimizes their mutual electrostatic repulsions by maximising the distance between them. The number of electron pairs therefore determine the overall geometry that they will adopt.

For example, when there are two electron pairs surrounding the central atom, their mutual repulsion is minimal when they lie at opposite poles of the sphere. Therefore, the central atom is predicted to adopt a linear geometry. If there are 3 electron pairs surrounding the central atom, their repulsion is minimized by placing them at the vertices of a triangle centered on the atom. Therefore, the predicted geometry is trigonal. Similarly, for 4 electron pairs, the optimal arrangement is tetrahedral.

This overall geometry is further refined by distinguishing between bonding and nonbonding electron pairs. A bonding electron pair is involved in a sigma bond with an adjacent atom, and, being shared with that other atom, lies farther away from the central atom than does a nonbonding pair (lone pair), which is held close to the central atom by its positively-charged nucleus. Therefore, the repulsion caused by the lone pair is greater than the repulsion caused by the bonding pair. As such, when the overall geometry has two sets of positions that experience different degrees of repulsion, the lone pair(s) will tend to occupy the positions that experience less repulsion. In other words, the lone pair-lone pair (lp-lp) repulsion is considered to be stronger than the lone pair-bonding pair (lp-bp) repulsion, which in turn is stronger than the bonding pair-bonding pair (bp-bp) repulsion. Hence, the weaker bp-bp repulsion is preferred over the lp-lp or lp-bp repulsion.

When there are 5 electron pairs surrounding the central atom, the optimal arrangement is a trigonal bipyramid. In this geometry, two positions lie at 180° angles to each other and 90° angles to the other 3 adjacent positions, whereas the other 3 positions lie at 120° to each other and at 90° to the first two positions. The first two positions therefore experience more repulsion than the last three positions. Hence, when there are one or more lone pairs, the lone pairs will tend to occupy the last three positions first. The difference between lone pairs and bonding pairs may also be used to rationalize deviations from idealized geometries. For example, the H_2O molecule has four electron pairs in its valence shell: two lone pairs and two bond pairs. The four electron pairs are spread so as to point roughly towards the apices of a tetrahedron. However, the bond angle between the two O-H bonds is only 104.5°, rather than the 109.5° of a regular tetrahedron, because the two lone pairs (whose density or probability envelopes lie closer to the oxygen nucleus) exert a greater mutual repulsion than the two bond pairs.

AXE Method

The "AXE method" of electron counting is commonly used when applying the VSEPR theory. The A represents the central atom and always has an implied subscript one. The X represents the number of sigma bonds between the central atoms and outside atoms. Multiple covalent bonds (double, triple, etc) count as one X. The E represents the number of lone electron pairs surrounding the central atom. The sum of X and E, known as the steric number, is also associated with the total number of hybridized orbitals used by valence bond theory.

Based on the steric number and distribution of X's and E's, VSEPR theory makes the predictions in the following tables 12.1 and 12.2. Note that the geometries are named according to the atomic positions only and not the electron arrangement. For example the description of AX_2E_1 as bent means that AX_2 is a bent molecule without reference to the lone pair, although the lone pair helps to determine the geometry.

Tables 12.1: Lone pairs and Geometry

Steric No.	Basic geometry			
	0 lone pair	1 lone pair	2 lone pairs	3 lone pairs
2.	X—A—X Linear			
3.	Trigonal planar	Bent		
4.	Tetrahedral	Trigonal pyramid	Bent	
5.	Trigonal bipyramid	Seesaw	T-shaped	Linear
6.	Octahedral	Square pyramid	Square planar	
7.	Pentagonal bipyramid	Pentagonal pyramid		
8.	Square antiprismatic			

Table 12.2: Molecule type and Geometry

Molecule Type	Shape arrangement[†]	Electron	Geometry[‡]	Examples
AX_1E_n	Diatomic			HF, O_2
AX_2E_0	Linear			$BeCl_2$, $HgCl_2$, CO_2
AX_2E_1	Bent			NO_2^-, SO_2, O_3
AX_2E_2	Bent			H_2O, OF_2
AX_2E_3	Linear			XeF_2, I_3^-
AX_3E_0	Trigonal planar			BF_3, CO_3^{2-}, NO_3^-, SO_3
AX_3E_1	Trigonal pyramidal			NH_3, PCl_3
AX_3E_2	T-shaped			ClF_3, BrF_3
AX_4E_0	Tetrahedral			CH_4, PO_4^{3-}, SO_4^{2-}, ClO_4^-

AX$_4$E$_1$	Seesaw	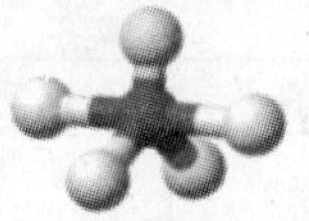	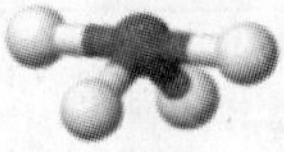	SF$_4$
AX$_4$E$_2$	Square planar	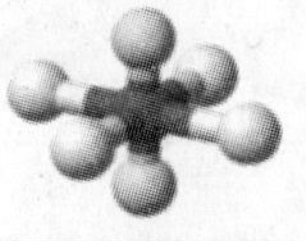	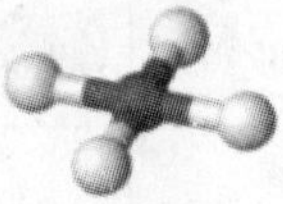	XeF$_4$
AX$_5$E$_0$	Trigonal bipyramidal	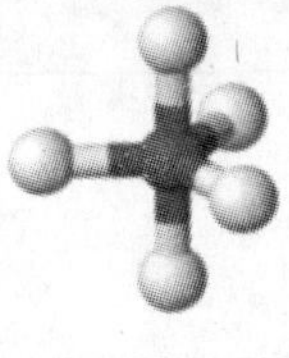	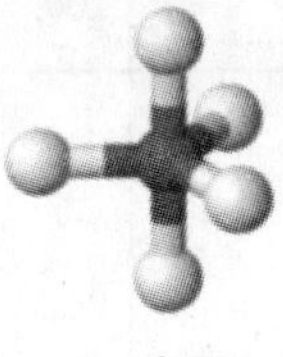	PCl$_5$
AX$_5$E$_1$	Square pyramidal	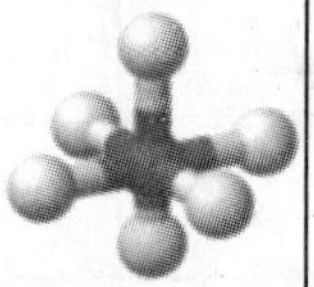	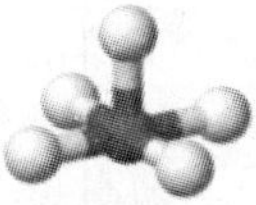	ClF$_5$, BrF$_5$
AX$_6$E$_0$	Octahedral	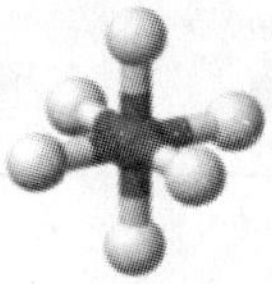	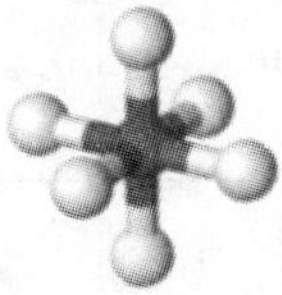	SF$_6$
AX$_6$E$_1$	Pentagonal pyramidal	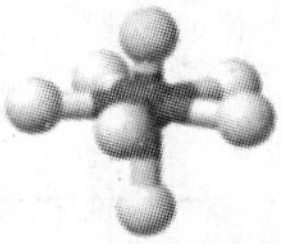	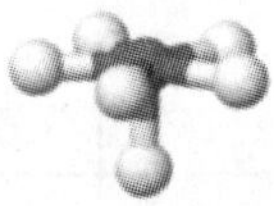	XeOF$_5^-$, IOF$_5^{2-}$ [7]
AX$_7$E$_0$	Pentagonal bipyramidal	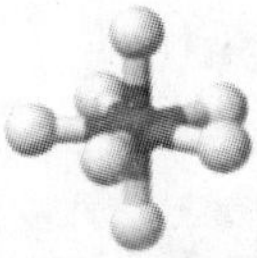	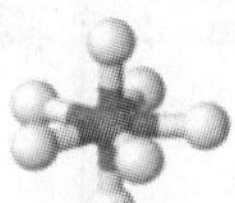	IF$_7$
AX$_8$E$_0$	Square antiprismatic			XeF2$^-$8

- Assumes that each atom in a molecule will be positioned so that there is **minimal repulsion** between the valence electrons of that atom.

In simple molecules in which there are no nonbonding electrons, there are five basic shapes:

1. LINEAR – Bond angle = 180

    o All diatomic molecules are linear.

    o Molecules with two atoms around a central atom such as BF_2 are linear because positioning the two attachments at opposite ends of the central atom minimizes electron repulsion.

    o Generic Formula: MX or MX_2 (where M is the central atom and X is are the bonding atoms).

2. TRIGONAL PLANAR – Bond angle = 120

    o Molecules with three atoms around a central atom such as BF_3 are trigonal planar because electron repulsion is minimized by positioning the three attachments toward the corners of an equilateral triangle.

    o Generic Formula: MX_3 (where M is the central atom and X is are the bonding atoms).

3. TETRAHEDRAL – Bond angle = 109.5

    o Molecules with four atoms around a central atom such as CH_4 are tetrahedral because electron repulsion is minimized by position the four attachments toward the corners of a tetrahedron.

    o Generic Formula: MX_4 (where M is the central atom and X is are the bonding atoms).

4. TRIGONAL BIPYRAMIDAL

    o Bond angle within the equatorial plane = 120

    o Bond angle between equatorial and axial plane = 90

    o Molecules with five atoms around a central atom such as PF_5 are trigonal bipyramidal. Three of the attachments are positioned in a trigonal plane with 120 bond angles. The remaining two attachments are positioned perpendicular (90) to the trigonal plane at opposite ends of the central atom. This arrangement of atoms minimizes electron repulsion.

    o Generic Formula: MX_5 (where M is the central atom and X is are the bonding atoms).

5. OCTAHEDRAL – Bond angle = 90

    o Molecules with six atoms around a central atom such as SF_6 are octahedral. Four of the attachments are positioned in a square plane with 90 bond angles. The remaining two attachments are positioned perpendicular (90) to the square plane at opposite ends of the central atom. This arrangement of atoms minimizes repulsion.

   o Generic Formula: MX_6 (where M is the central atom and X is are the bonding atoms)

There are seven shapes for molecules with one or more pairs of nonbonding electrons.

  1. BENT (ANGULAR or V-SHAPED)

    o Molecules with two atoms and one or two pairs of nonbonding electrons around a central atom such as H_2O are bent. It can be imagined that a linear molecule with two atoms attached to a central atom is altered when electrons are added to the top of the central atom. The repulsion caused by the addition of these extra electrons causes the molecule to become bent. The angle of bent molecules is less than 120 if there is one pair of nonbonding electrons and is less than 109.5 if there are two pairs of nonbonding electrons.

    o Some molecules, such as NO_2 have two atoms and a single unpaired electron around a central atom. These molecules are also bent due to the repulsion of the single atom added to the central atom.

    o Generic Formula: MX_2E or MXE_2 (where M is the central atom, X is are the bonding atoms, and E are nonbonding pairs of electrons)

  2. TRIGONAL PYRAMIDAL

    o Molecules with three atoms and one pair of nonbonding electrons around a central atom such as NH_3 are trigonal pyramidal. These molecules are essentially tetrahedral molecules with one of the attached atoms replaced by a pair of nonbonding electrons. The force of repulsion of these electrons makes the bond angle between the attached atoms less than 109.5. For example, in NH_3, the H-N-H bond is 107.5.

    o Generic Formula: MX_3E (where M is the central atom, X is are the bonding atoms, and E are nonbonding pairs of electrons).

  3. SEESAW-SHAPED (DISTORTED TETRAHEDRAL)

    o Molecules with four atoms and one pair of nonbonding electrons around a central atom such as SF_4 are seesaw-shaped. These molecules are essentially trigonal bipyramidal molecules with one of the equatorial-positioned atoms (in the trigonal plane) replaced by a pair of nonbonding electrons. This leaves the two axial-positioned atoms and two of the equatorial-positioned atoms in the shape of a seesaw or a teeter-totter.

o Generic Formula: MX_4E (where M is the central atom, X is are the bonding atoms, and E are nonbonding pairs of electrons).

4. T-SHAPED

o Molecules with three atoms and two pairs of nonbonding electrons around a central atom such as ClF_3 are T-shaped. These molecules are essentially trigonal bipyramidal molecules with two of the equatorial-positioned atoms (in the trigonal plane) each replaced by a pair of nonbonding electrons. This leaves the two axial-positioned atoms and one of the equatorial-positioned atoms in a T-shape.

o Generic Formula: MX_3E_2 (where M is the central atom, X is are the bonding atoms, and E are nonbonding pairs of electrons).

5. LINEAR

o Molecules with two atoms and three pairs of nonbonding electrons around a central atom such as XeF_2 are linear. These molecules are essential trigonal bipyramidal molecules with all three of the equatorial-positioned atoms (in the trigonal plane) each replaced by a pair of nonbonding electrons. This leaves only the two axial-positioned atoms which are still 180 from each other on opposite ends of the central atom.

o Generic Formula: MX_2E_3 (where M is the central atom, X is are the bonding atoms, and E are nonbonding pairs of electrons).

6. SQUARE PYRAMIDAL

o Molecules with five atoms and one pair of nonbonding electrons around a central atom such as BrF_5 are square pyramidal. These molecules are essentially octahedral molecules with one of the attached atoms replaced by a pair of nonbonding electrons. This leaves four atoms in a plane as a square base and one atom positioned perpendicular (90) to this plane.

o Generic Formula: MX_5E (where M is the central atom, X is are the bonding atoms, and E are nonbonding pairs of electrons).

7. SQUARE PLANAR-Molecules with four atoms and two pairs of nonbonding electrons around a central atom such as XeF_4 are square planar. These molecules are essentially octahedral molecules with two of the attached atoms opposite each other around the central atom each replaced by a pair of nonbonding electrons. This leaves four atoms in a square plane.

o Generic Formula: MX_4E_2 (where M is the central atom, X is are the bonding atoms, and E are nonbonding pairs of electrons)

Molecular Orbital Theory

Molecule orbital theory was given by Robert Mullikan. In VB theory, the overlapped orbitals are usually only two orbitals and they closely resemble the orbitals they are made from. No mention is made of anti- or non- bonding orbitals in VB theory, and no mathematical attempt is made to actually define the resultant orbitals. In MO theory, however, the MOs are calculated precisely to give new orbitals, usually in pairs of anti-bonding and bonding orbitals. Also several orbitals can be combined to form several MOs (think of the MOs for benzene... valence bond doesn't come close to that).because of that, MO theory can predict several things that VB theory can't, such as magnetism, precise bond order and aromaticity .

LCAO-Molecular orbital are formed by addition and subtraction of AO's, this is known as Linear Combination of Atomic Orbitals (LCAO).Like hybrid AO's but the MO involves the whole molecule.

All molecular orbitals (MOs) are made by combining atomic orbitals (AOs). These AOs are the general s and *p* orbitals. When atoms combine to make molecules, atomic orbitals must combine to make molecular orbitals. The total number or orbitals does not change. 10 atomic orbitals will combine to give 10 molecular orbitals. When two atomic orbitals combine to make a bond, the result will be two molecular orbitals; one with lower energy (bonding orbital) and one with higher energy (antibonding orbital). The electrons in the bond will be in the lower energy bonding orbital and the system is lower in energy with a bond than without. This more stable combination of orbitals is the reason for the existence covalent bonds.

A general rule is that n AO = n MO's

Interaction of 2 AO = 2 MO's

Drawing representations of AO's

- Need to be able to draw AO's when considering their interactions in MO's

— So far diagrams have been to help visualise the 3D nature of AO's

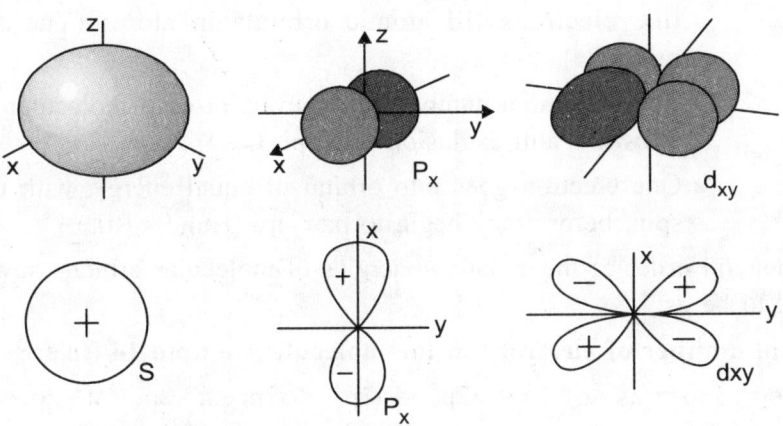

Fig. 12.7

Rules for Orbital Combinations

To have atomic orbitals interact to create molecular orbitals we must be able to mathematically combine them. In order for the combination to be possible we must obey the following rules.

1. The orbitals must be physically close enough to interact. The magnitude of the combination is inversely proportional to the distance between the .atoms.

2. The orbitals must combine along an axis of mutual symmetry. The magnitude of the combination will be proportional to the cosine of the angle between the orbitals if they are not perfectly aligned.

3. The orbitals must be similar in size and energy. The magnitude of the combination is inversely proportional to the difference in size or energy.

   • Molecular orbital are formed by addition and subtraction of AO's., which is known as Linear combination of atomic orbitals– like hybrid AO's but the MO involves the whole molecule.

     ▪ In atoms, electrons occupy atomic orbitals, but in molecules they occupy similar molecular orbitals which surround the molecule.

     ▪ The two 1s atomic orbitals combine to form two molecular orbitals, one bonding (s) and one antibonding (s*).

- Electrons go into the lowest energy orbital available to form lowest potential energy for the molecule.

- Molecular orbitals are filled in the order of increasing energy, like electrons fill atomic orbitals in atoms (The Aufbau principle)

- The maximum number of electrons in each molecular orbital is two. (Pauli exclusion principle)

- One electron goes into orbital of equal energy, with parallel spin, before they begin to pair up. (Hund's Rule.)

General order of the relative energies of molecular orbitals have been found to be as:

If total number of electrons in the molecule are upto 14-(like H_2 to N_2)

σ 1s $<\sigma^*$ 1s $<\sigma$ 2s $<\sigma^*$ 2s $< \pi 2p_x = \pi 2p_y <\sigma 2p_z <\pi^*$ $2p_x = \pi^*$ $2p_y <\sigma^*$ $2p_z$

If total number of electrons in the molecule are above 14- (like O_2 to Ne_2)

σ 1s $< \sigma^*$ 1s $< \sigma$ 2s $< \sigma^*$ 2s $< \sigma$ $2p_z < \pi$ $2p_x = \pi$ $2p_y < \pi^*$ $2p_x = \pi^*$ $2p_y < \sigma^*$ $2p_z$

(To remember, σ $2p_z$ has lower energy than corresponding π MO for having above 14 total electrons, this is confirmed by Spectroscopic methods)

Bond Order = (No of electrons present in the BMO- No of electrons present in the ABMO*) **/2**

Bond Energy is directly proportional to the bond order, but bond length is inversely proportional to the bond order.

M agnetic B eh av iour

if unpaired electrons are present in the molecular orbitals then, molecule in paramagnetic, if all electrons are paired then diamagnetic.

Molecular Orbital configuration and Diagram for Homonuclear diatomic molecules:

Molecular Orbital formation for H_2

H_2 configuration:

σ $1s^2 < \sigma^*$ 1s (Diamagnetic since all electrons are paired)

Bond Order = (Bonding e – Antibonding e)/2 i.e. $(2 - 0)/2 = 1$

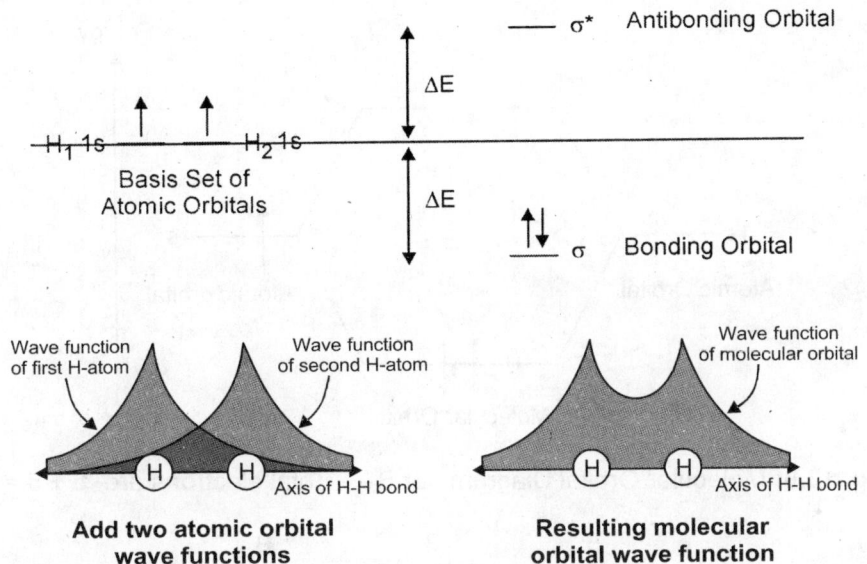

In the above diagrams, 2 atomic orbitals of Hydrogen or overlapping for giving bonding and antibonding molecular orbitals. Bonding molecular orbital (σ BMO) has lower energy than antibonding molecular orbital (σ * ABMO). σ Is (BMO) and σ 1s* (ABMO) are formed.

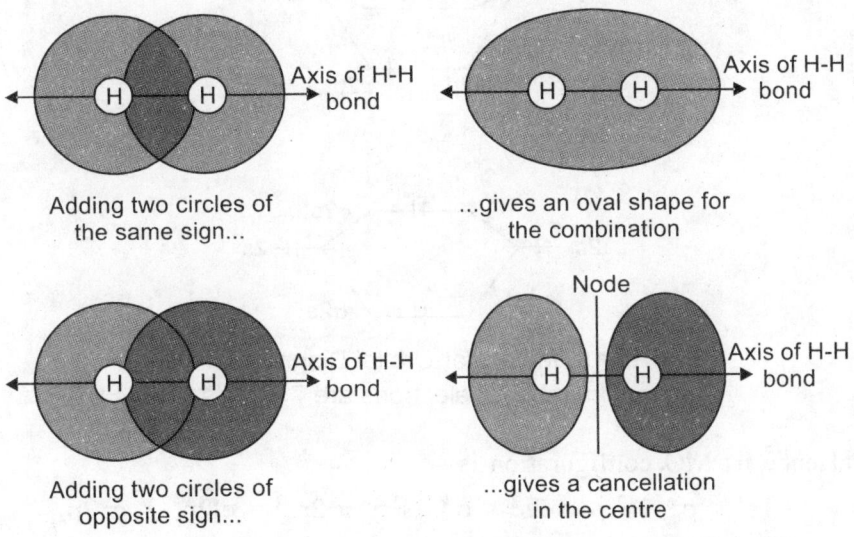

Fig. 12.8: Molecular Orbital for H_2

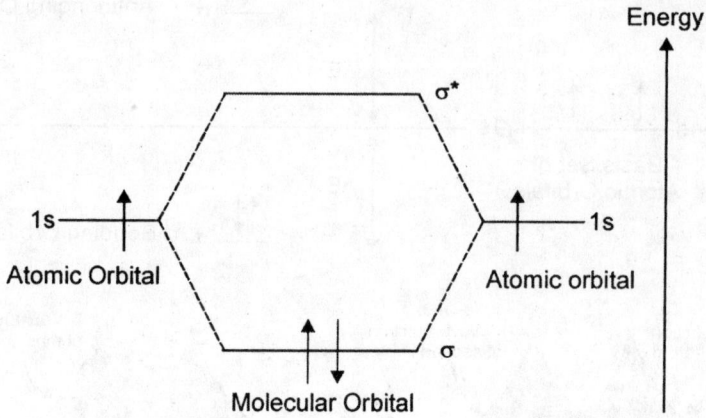

Fig. 12.9: Molecular Orbital Diagram for B_2- Total electrons are- 5 + 5 = 10

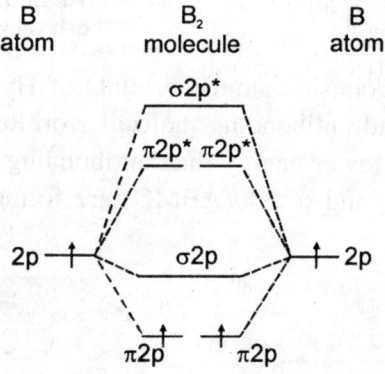

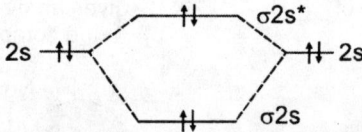

Fig. 12.10: Molecular Orbital Diagram for N_2—
Total number of electrons are 7 + 7 = 14

Hence its MO configuration is—

$$\sigma\ 1s^2 < \sigma^*\ 1s^2 < \sigma\ 2s^2 < \sigma^*\ 2s^2 < \pi\ 2p_x^2 = \pi\ 2p_y^2 < \sigma\ 2p_z^2$$

Since all electrons are paired hence diamagnetic behavior and bond order is 3

Bond order = (10 − 4)/2 = 3

In the Nitrogen molecule

$\pi\ 2p_x^2 = \pi\ 2p_y^2$ orbitals have lower energy hence are filled first then $\sigma\ 2p_z^2$.

MO Diagram for O_2 – Total number of electrons are $8 + 8 = 16$ (above 14)

Hence its MO configuration is-

$$\sigma\ 1s^2 < \sigma^*\ 1s^2 < \sigma\ 2s^2 < \sigma^*\ 2s^2 < \sigma\ 2p_z^2 < \pi\ 2p_x^2 = \pi\ 2p_y^2 < \pi^*\ 2p_x^1$$
$$= \pi^*\ 2p_y^1 < \sigma\ ^*\ 2p_z$$

Since unpaired electrons are present hence paramagnetic behavoiur and bond order is 2

$$\text{Bond order} = (10 - 6)/2 = 2$$

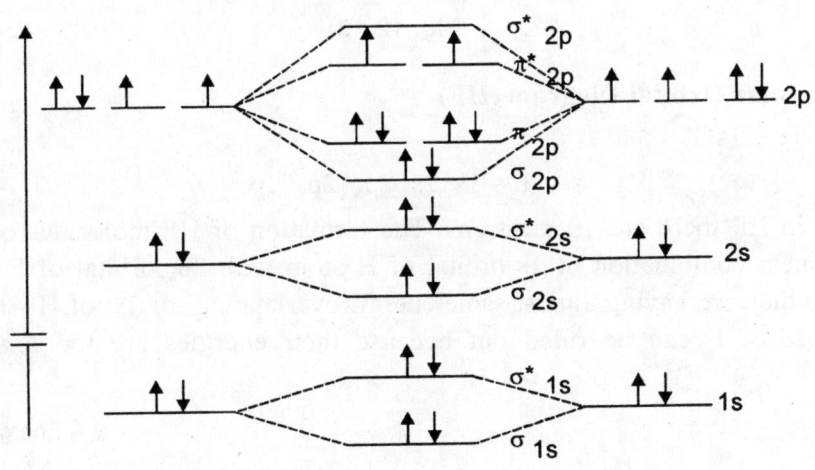

Fig. 12.11

Molecular Orbital configuration and Diagram for Heteronuclear diatomic molecules-

Nitric Oxide(NO) – total electrons are $7 + 8 = 15$

$$\sigma\ 1s^2 < \sigma^*\ 1s^2 < \sigma\ 2s^2 < \sigma^*\ 2s^2 < \pi\ 2p_x^2 = \pi\ 2p_y^2 < \pi^*\ 2p_x^1 = \pi^*\ 2p_y$$
$$\text{Bond Order} = (10 - 5)/2 = 2.5$$

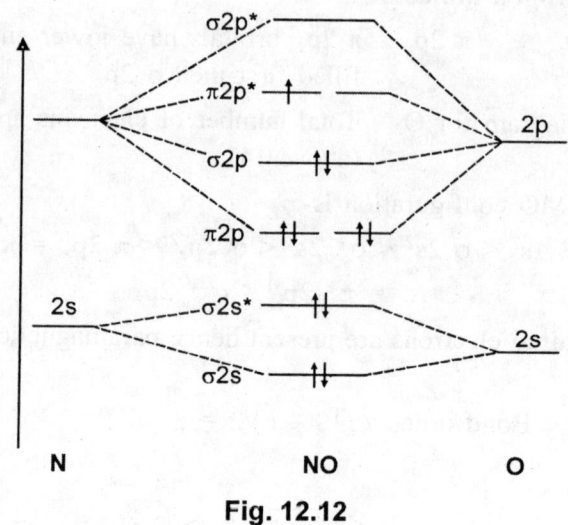

Fig. 12.12

Molecular Orbital Diagram (HF)

For   H – 1s^1

$$F - 1s^2\, 2s^2\, 2p_x^{\,2}\, 2p_y^{\,2}\, 2p_z^{\,1}$$

thus in HF there are 10 electrons. The formation of HF molecules occurs by linear combination of 1s orbital of H atom with $2p_x$ orbital of F atom since they are having almost same energy, overlapping of 1s^1 of H with 1s and 2s of F can be ruled out because their energies are too low. The

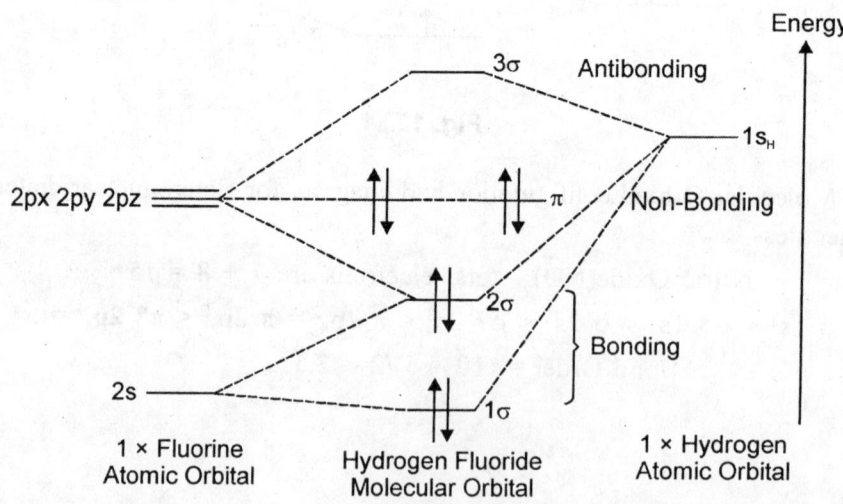

Fig. 12.13

combination of $1s^1$ of H and $2p_x^1$ of F gives 2 MOs i.e one is σ sp_x (BMO) and σ^* sp_x (ABMO), moreover 2 electrons occupy the BMO leaving the ABMO (σ^* sp_x) empty. Thus Bond order becomes $(2 - 0)/2 = 1$ (one)

In the similar mannar for HCl, $1s^1$ of H combines with $3 p_x^1$ orbital (having nearly equal energy) of Chlorine to form σ sp_x (BMO) and σ^* sp_x (ABMO), moreover 2 electrons occupy the BMO leaving the ABMO(σ^* sp_x) empty. Thus Bond order becomes $(2 - 0)/2 = 1$ (one)

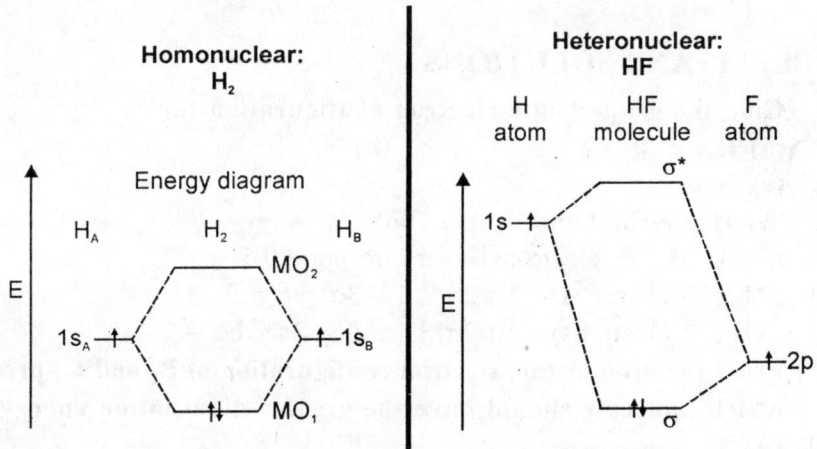

Fig. 12.14: Comparison between homonuclear (H_2) and heteronuclear (HF)

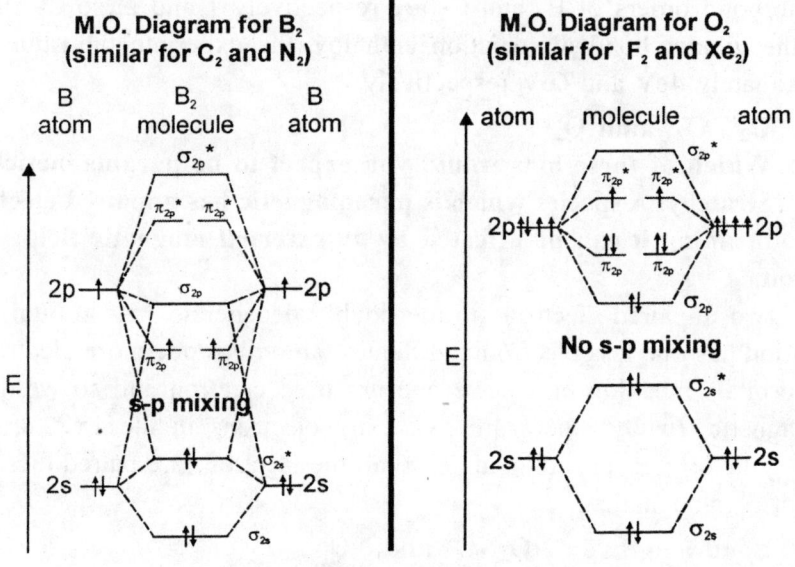

Fig. 12.15

Mixing of s-p orbitals – Ordering of σ2p and π2p molecular orbitals depends upon s-p mixing. In some cases like B, C, N have mixing of orbitals in their MO configuration. These B, C, N all have ≤ half filled 2p orbitals. Having more than half filled orbitals raises the energies of orbitals due to e- e- repulsion. Electron repel each other due to negative charge.if 2 electrons are forced to be in the same orbital, their energies go up.

s-p mixing only occurs when the s and p atomic orbitals are close in energy (≤ half filled 2p orbitals)

PROBLEMS AND SOLUTIONS

1. **Give the groundstate electron configuration for**
   (a) H_2,   **(b) N_2**
   (c) O_2
   What are the bond orders (bo)

Solution: (a) : H^-_2 (3 electrons) : $1\sigma^2 2\sigma^*$ bo = 0.5
   (b) : N_2 (10 electrons) : $1\sigma^2 2\sigma^{*2} 1\pi^4 3\sigma^2$ bo = 3
   (c) : O_2 (12 electrons) : $1\sigma^2 2\sigma^{*2} 1\pi^4 3\sigma^2 2\pi^{*2}$ bo = 2

2. **From the groundstate electron configuration of B_2 and C_2 predict**
   which molecule should have the greater dissociation energy.

Solution :
   B_2 (6 electrons) : $1\sigma^2 2\sigma^{*2} 1\pi^2$ b = 1
   B_2 (6 electrons) : $1\sigma^2 2\sigma^{*2} 1\pi^2$ b = 1

The bond orders of B_2 and C_2 are respectively 1 and 2; so C_2 should have the greater bond dissociation enthalpy, the experimental values are approximately 4eV and 6eV respectively.

3. **O_2^+, O_2^- amd O_2^{2-}**
   Which of these ions would you expect to be paramagnetic?
   Strategy: A species which is paramagnetic has unpaired electrons
   meaning it can be affected by an external magnetic field.

Solution

O_2 has two unpaired electrons in the doubly degenerate $1\pi_2^*$ orbital. The O_2^+ cation has one less electron and the O_2^- anion has one more electron in these orbitals meaning both have one unpaired electron and so would be paramagnetic. In O_2^{2-} there are two extra electrons in the $1\pi_g^*$ orbitals meaning the orbitals are full and hence all the electrons are paired therefore it is not paramagnetic.

4. **Bond lengths in NO_2NO^+ and NO^-**
   What common anion is isolectronic with NO^+?
   Strategy: Species are described as isoelectronic when they have

the same number of electrons. To solve this problem, write down the electronic configuration of both species involved in the heteronuclear diatomic. As the species is a monovalent cation, remove one electron from the total and compare with similar species in the same period of the Perodic Table.

Solution: Nitrogen has 5 valence electrons and oxygen has 6. Therefore the neutral species has 11 electrons. Removal of one electron to form the cation gives 10 electrons.

NO^+ is isoelectronic with N_2, CO and CN^-.

4. **Consider the following data for these homonuclear diatomic species:**

	N_2	N_2^+	O_2	O_2^+
Bond energy (kJ/mol)	945	841	498	623
Bond length (pm)	110	112	121	112
No. of valence electrons	10	9	12	11

Plan: We first draw the MO energy levels for the four species, recalling that they differ for N_2 and O_2. Then we determine the bond orders and compare them with the data: bond order is related directly to bond energy and inversely to bond length.

Solution: The MO energy levels are:

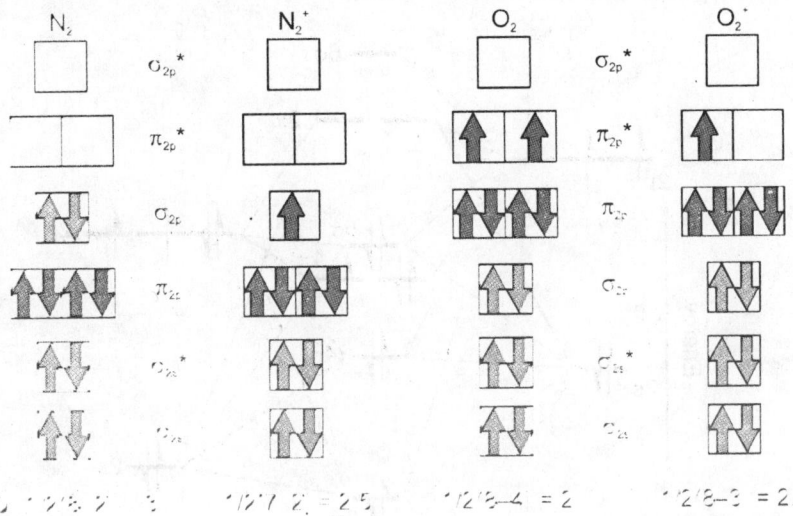

5. **Draw a labelled molecular orbital energy level diagram for the cyanide anion CN^-. What is the bond order in CN^-? How would**

the bond length and magnetic behaviour of neutral CN differ
from those observed for CN⁻?

**Strategy: Draw the molecular orbital diagram for CN,
remembering that a common pitfall in drawing heteronuclear
molecular orbital diagrams is to forget that the atomic orbitals
of C and N will be at different energies due to the difference in
electronegativity between the atoms. Consider the distribution
of electrons in the molecular orbitals of bonding and antibonding
character and then calculate the bond order. As the bond order
increase between the same pair of atoms, the bond becomes
stronger and shorter. Finally, in order for a molecule to show
magnetic behaviour (i.e. be affected by an external magnetic
field) it must have some unpaired electrons (paramagnetic)
rather than have all paired electrons (diamagnetic).**

Solution

The bond order for CN⁻ is 3. On going from CN⁻ to CN an electron is
removed from a bonding orbital. The bond order in CN is therefore 2.5 and
the bond length would be greater than in CN⁻. CN has an unpaired electron
so is paramagnetic, in contrast to CN⁻ which is dia,agmetic.

MO diagram for CN⁻

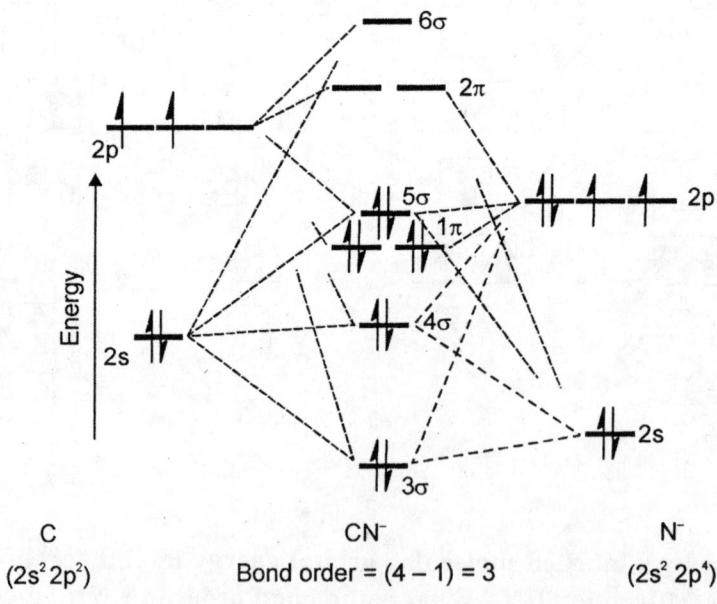

Sample Problem: Use the M.O. model to predict the changes in magnetism and bond order upon oxidation of NO to make NO^+.

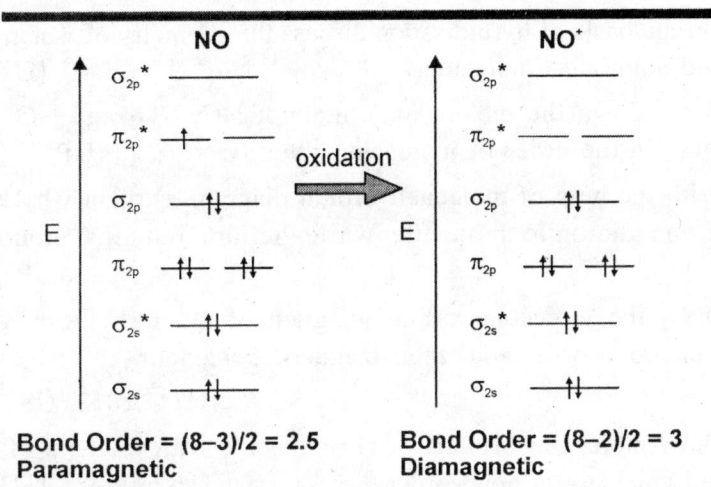

Bond Order = (8–3)/2 = 2.5
Paramagnetic

Bond Order = (8–2)/2 = 3
Diamagnetic

6. **Bond length of CO^+ is observed to be lesser or higher bond order than that of CO, why.**

Solution: The decrease in bond length or increase in bond order (CO to CO^+) indicates that the electron must have been removed from an anti bonding orbital. The most probable explanation is that the σ 2s and σ 2s MOs have wide gap in energy than expected, so energy of σ *2s (ABMO) is much higher than $\sigma 2p$ and $\pi 2p$ (BMO), in this way the configuration is as—

$$CO \mid \sigma 1s^2 < \sigma^* 1s^2 < \sigma 2s^2 < \pi\, 2p_x^2 = \pi\, 2p_y^2 < \sigma\, 2p_z^2 < \sigma^*\, 2s^2$$

(Bond order for CO = 10 – 4/2 = 3)

$$CO^+ - \sigma 1s^2 < \sigma^* 1s^2 < \sigma 2s^2 < \pi 2p_x^2 = \pi 2p_y^2 < \sigma 2p_z^2 < \sigma^*\, 2s^1$$

(Bond order for CO^+ = (10 – 3)/2 = 3.5 higher bonder order hence shorter bond length)

hence

(Bond order of CO^+ > Bond order of CO)

QUESTIONS FOR EXAMINATIONS

1. Why is bond energy of N_2 higher than that of O?

IUPTU. 2004, UTU-2005)

2. Draw the molecular orbital diagram of CO and also comment on the magnetic behaviour of the molecule. [UPTU-2010)

3. Explain why O_2, is paramagnetic and N_2 is diamagnetic in nature.
   (UPTU. 2003, UTU-2007)

4. Calculate the bond order of N_2CO, NO and O_2 .

5. On the basis of hyrbidisation discuss the geometry of water, methane and ammonia molecules.   [UTU-2010)

6. Write down the molecular orbitals of NO, NO^- and NO^+ Arrange them in the order of increasing stability.   (UPTU-2008-09)

7. With the help of molecualr orbital diagram, explain why hydrogen forms diatomic molecule while helium remains monoatomic?
   (UPTU-2011)

8. Draw the molecular orbital diagram of O_2, O_2^-, O_2 +. Calcultae their bond order and their magnetic behaviour.
   (UTU-2012, UPTU-2008)

9. Show molecular orbitals of HF molecule with the help of diagram and calculate is bond order.   (UPTU-2006-07, UTU-2011).

10. What is metallic bond? Explain conductor and insulators .

11. Discuss the electrical conductivity of solids based on band theory. Explain conductor, semiconductors and insulators.   (UTU-2011)

12. What is hydrogen bond? How does an intermolecular hydrogen bond differ from intramolecular hydrogen bond.

13. Explain, why o-Nitrophenol is volatile but p-Nitrophenol not.
    (UTU-2011)

14. Explain why lower alcohols are soluble in water but higher are insoluble.

Chapter 13
STATES OF MATTER

- ➤ **Basic concepts**
- ➤ **Crystallography**
- ➤ **Calculation of Density**
- ➤ **Bragg's Equation and Numericals**
- ➤ **Liquid Crystals**
- ➤ **Fullerenes**

BASIC CONCEPTS/TERMS

Crystalline solids: They have highly regular arrangement of atoms, ions, molecules - periodic (repeating) .They have sharp melting point. They show anisotropic behaviour i.e. different values of the property in different directions. (e.g. NaCl)

Amorphous solids: They have no repeating pattern of atoms or molecules, they may have only short range order, they show isotropic behaviour and no definite melting point. (e.g. glasses).

Crystallinity – have a repeating unit = **unit cell**

To define repeating unit, we use concept of **a lattice**

A lattice is "an infinite 1,2, or 3-D regular arrangement of points, each of which has identical surroundings". Any periodic pattern can be described by placing lattice points at equivalent positions within each unit of the pattern.

Space lattice: It is a periodical arrangement of atoms or ions in regular manner and having repeat distance in three(x,y or z) directions. If at these lattice points, we place atoms, molecule or ions which is called the basis, then we obtain a crystalline solid structure.

Crystal structure = Lattice + basis

Types of unit cell

The crystal structure of a material or the arrangement of atoms within a given type of crystal structure can be described in terms of its unit cell. The unit cell is a small box containing one or more atoms, a spatial arrangement of atoms. The unit cells stacked in three-dimensional space describe the bulk arrangement of atoms of the crystal. The crystal structure has a three dimensional shape. The unit cell is given by its lattice parameters which are the length of the cell edges and the angles between them, while the positions of the atoms inside the unit cell are described by the set of atomic positions (x_i, y_i, z_i) measured from a lattice point.

Unit cells are of three types: Primitive or simple cubic, Body centred and Face centred

Cubic Lattices

3 types; Simple cubic (also called primitive cubic), lattice points only at corners.

Body Centered Cubic (BCC), lattice points at corners and in middle of cube.

Face Centered Cubic (FCC) lattice points at the corners and in the middle of each face.

How many lattice points and/or atoms "belong" to a unit cell ?

Corners: The points at the corner of the cell are shared by the surrounding unit cells, therefore each one is shared by 8 in total and is only "worth" 1/8 to each cell.

Faces: These lattice points are shared by 2 cells, each one is "worth" 1/2 to each cell.

Body: This is the sole possesion of that cell, worth 1.

Total number lattice points

Primitive unit or simple cubic (SCC) = 8(1/8) = 1;

$$FCC = 6 \times 1/2 + 8(1/8) = 4;$$
$$BCC = 8(1/8) + 1 = 2.$$

Unit Cell : Seven Crystal System

There are 7 unique unit-cell shapes that can fill all 3-D space. These are the 7 **Crystal systems.**

We define the size of the unit cell using **lattice parameters** (sometimes called lattice constants, or cell parameters). These are 3 vectors, a, b, c. The angles between these vectors are given by a (angle between b and c), b (angle between a and c), and g (angle between a and b). Although there are only 7 crystal systems or shapes, there are 14 different crystal lattices, called **Bravais Lattices**. (3 different cubic types, 2 different tetragonal types, 4 different orthorhombic types, 2 different monoclinic types, 1 rhombohedral, 1 hexagonal, 1 triclinic). See below.

Real crystals always possess one of these lattice types, but different crystalline compounds that have the same lattice can have different motifs and different lattice parameters (these depend upon the chemical formula and the sizes of the atoms in the unit cell). We will only concern ourselves

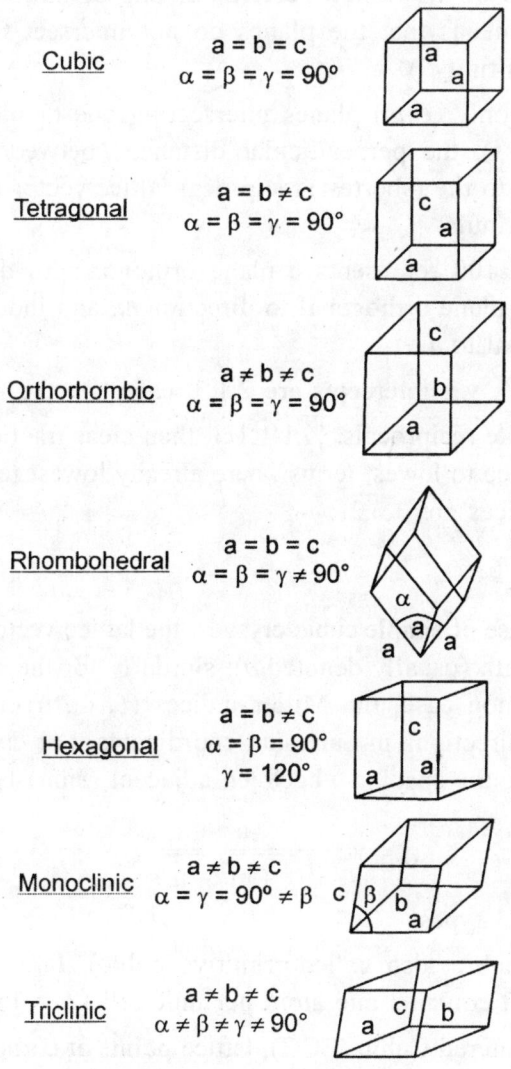

Cubic	$a = b = c$ $\alpha = \beta = \gamma = 90°$
Tetragonal	$a = b \neq c$ $\alpha = \beta = \gamma = 90°$
Orthorhombic	$a \neq b \neq c$ $\alpha = \beta = \gamma = 90°$
Rhombohedral	$a = b = c$ $\alpha = \beta = \gamma \neq 90°$
Hexagonal	$a = b \neq c$ $\alpha = \beta = 90°$ $\gamma = 120°$
Monoclinic	$a \neq b \neq c$ $\alpha = \gamma = 90° \neq \beta$
Triclinic	$a \neq b \neq c$ $\alpha \neq \beta \neq \gamma \neq 90°$

with the cubic lattices, though we will refer to the hexagonal lattice in passing.

Miller indices-Vectors and atomic planes in a crystal lattice can be described by a three-value Miller index notation (ℓmn). The ℓ, m and n directional indices are separated by 90°, and are thus orthogonal. In fact, the ℓ component is mutually perpendicular to the m and n indices.

By definition, (ℓmn) denotes a plane that intercepts the three points a_1/ℓ, a_2/m, and a_3/n, or some multiple thereof. That is, the Miller indices are proportional to the *inverses* of the intercepts of the plane with the unit cell (in the basis of the lattice vectors). If one or more of the indices is zero, it simply means that the planes do not intersect that axis (i.e. the intercept is "at infinity").

Considering only (ℓmn) planes intersecting one or more lattice points (the *lattice planes*), the perpendicular distance *d* between adjacent lattice planes is related to the (shortest) reciprocal lattice vector orthogonal to the planes by the formula:

Miller index 100 represents a plane orthogonal to direction ℓ; index 010 represents a plane orthogonal to direction m, and index 001 represents a plane orthogonal to n.

Problem: If x y z intercepts are 2,1,3, calculate the miller indices.

Solution: Take reciprocals, ½,1/1,1/3, then clear fractions (multiply by 6) i.e. 3,6,2. reduce to lowest terms , here already lowest terms are available hence miller indices are 3,6,2.

Cubic structures

For the special case of simple cubic crystals, the lattice vectors are orthogonal and of equal length (usually denoted *a*); similarly for the reciprocal lattice. So, in this common case, the Miller indices (ℓ, m, n) and both simply denote normals/directions in Cartesian coordinates. For cubic crystals with lattice constant *a*, the spacing *d* between adjacent (ℓmn) lattice planes is:

$$d_{\ell mn} = \frac{a}{\sqrt{\ell^2 + m^2 + n^2}}$$

Cubic Lattices: 3 types;

1. Simple cubic (also called primitive cubic), lattice points only at corners It contains one atom per unit cell (Z = 1).
2. Body Centered Cubic (BCC), lattice points at corners and in middle of cube. It contains two atom per unit cell (Z = 2).

3. Face Centered Cubic (FCC) lattice points at the corners and in the middle of each face. It contains four atom per unit cell (Z = 4).

CALCULATION INVOLVING DENSITY AND UNIT CELL DIMENSIONS

From the unit cell dimensions, it is possible to calculate the volume of the unit cell. Knowing the density of the metal. We can calculate the mass of the atoms in the unit cell. The determination of the mass of a single atom gives an accurate determination of Avogadro constant.

Suppose edge of unit cell of a cubic crystal determined by X–Ray diffraction is a, d is density of the solid substance and M is the molar mass, then in case of cubic crystal

Volume of a unit cell = a^3,

Mass of the unit cell = no. of atoms in the unit cell ×

mass of each atom = Z × m

Here   Z = no. of atoms present in one unit cell,

m = mass of a single atom

Mass of an atom present in the unit cell = m/N_A

∴ Density d = mass of unit cell/volume of unit cell

$$= Z.m/a^3$$

$$d = Z.M. / a^3 × N_A$$

(Density of the unit cell is same as the density of the substance)

Q.1. *An element having atomic mass 60 has face centred cubic unit cell. The edge length of the unit cell is 400 pm. Find out the density of the element?*

Solution: Unit cell edge length = 400 pm

$$= 400 × 10^{-10} \text{ cm}$$

Volume of unit cell = $(400 × 10^{-10})^3 = 64 × 10^{-24} \text{ cm}^3$

Mass of the unit cell = No. of atoms in the unit cell ×

mass of each atom

No. of atoms in fcc unit cell(z) = 8 × 1/8 + 6 × 1/2 = 4

∴ Mass of unit cell = $4 × 60 / 6.023 × 10^{23}$

Density of unit cell = mass of unit cell/

Volume of unit cell = $4 × 60 / 6.023 × 10^{23} × 64 × 10^{-24}$

$$= 6.2 \text{ g/cm}^3$$

Q.2. *An element has a body centred cubic (bcc) structure with a cell edge of 288 pm. The density of the element is 7.2 g/cm^3. How many atoms are present in 208 g of the element?*

Solution: Volume of unit cell = $(288 \times 10^{-10})^3 \text{cm}^3$

$$= 2.39 \times 10^{-23} \text{cm}^3$$

Volume of 208 g of the element = mass/volume

$$= 208/7.2 = 28.88 \text{cm}^3$$

No of unit cells in this volume = $28.88/2.39 \times 10^{-23}$

$$= 12.08 \times 10^{23}$$

Since each bcc unit cell contains 2 atoms

$\therefore$ no of atom in 208 g = $2 \times 12.08 \times 10^{23}$

$$= 24.16 \times 10^{23} \text{ atom}$$

Q.3. *The spacing between principal planes of NaCl crystal is 2.82A^0. It is found that 2nd order bragg reflection occurs at an angle of 15^0. What is the wavelength of X-rays.*

Solution: By using   **n λ = 2dsinθ – (1)**

Here n = 2, d = 2.82A^0 θ = 15^0 put in eq-1,

we get λ = **0.73 A^0.**

Radius Ratio rule—

The structure of an ionic solid depends on the relative size of the ions that form the solid. The relative size of these ions is given by the **radius ratio**, which is the radius of the positive ion divided by the radius of the negative ion.

$$\text{Radius ratio} = \frac{\text{radius of the positive ion}}{\text{radius of the negative ion}} = \frac{Y_+}{Y_-}$$

The relationship between the coordination number of the positive ions in ionic solids and the radius ratio of the ions is given in the table below. As the radius ratio increases, the number of negative ions that can pack around each positive ion increases. When the radius ratio is between 0.225 and 0.414, positive ions tend to pack in tetrahedral holes between planes of negative ions in a cubic or hexagonal closest-packed structure. When the radius ratio is between 0.414 and 0.732, the positive ions tend to pack in octahedral holes between planes of negative ions in a closest-packed structure.

Table 13.1: Radius Ratio Rules

Radius Ratio	Coordinatio Number	Holes in Which Positive Ions Pack
0.225 - 0.414	4	tetrahedral holes
0.414 - 0.732	6	octahedral holes
0.732 - 1	8	cubic holes
1	12	closest-packed structure

The table 13.1 above suggests that tetrahedral holes aren't used until the positive ion is large enough to touch all four of the negative ions that form this hole. As the radius ratio increases from 0.225 to 0.414, the positive ion distorts the structure of the negative ions toward a structure that purists might describe as *closely-packed*.

As soon as the positive ion is large enough to touch all six negative ions in an octahedral hole, the positive ions start to pack in octahedral holes. These holes are used until the positive ion is so large that it can't fit into even a distorted octahedral hole.

Eventually a point is reached at which the positive ion can no longer fit into either the tetrahedral or octahedral holes in a closest-packed crystal. When the radius ratio is between about 0.732 and 1, ionic solids tend to crystallize in a simple cubic array of negative ions with positive ions occupying some or all of the cubic holes between these planes. When the radius ratio is about 1, the positive ions can be incorporated directly into the positions of the closest-packed structure.

The Structure of Metals and Other Monatomic Solids: Packing

The structures of pure metals are easy to describe because the atoms that form these metals can be thought of as identical perfect spheres. The same can be said about the structure of the rare gases (He, Ne, Ar, and so on) at very low temperatures. These substances all crystallize in one of four basic structures: simple cubic (*SC*), body-centered cubic (*BCC*), hexagonal closest-packed (*HCP*), and cubic closest-packed (*CCP*).

Simple Cubic Packing

When a solid crystallizes, the particles that form the solid pack as tightly as possible. To illustrate this principle, let's try to imagine the best way of packing spheres, such as ping-pong balls, into an empty box.

One approach involves carefully packing the ping-pong balls to form a square packed plane of spheres, as shown in the Fig. 13.1.

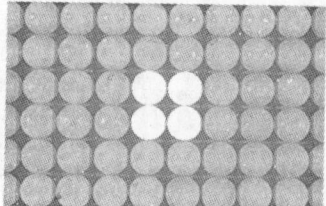

Fig. 13.1

By tilting the box to one side, we can stack a second plane of spheres directly on top of the first. The result is a regular structure in which the simplest repeating unit is a cube of eight spheres, as shown in the Fig. 13.2.

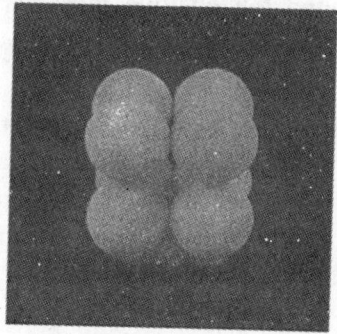

Fig. 13.2

This structure is called **simple cubic packing**. Each sphere in this structure touches four identical spheres in the same plane. It also touches one sphere in the plane above and one in the plane below. Each atom in this structure can form bonds to its six nearest neighbors. Each sphere is therefore said to have a **coordination number** of 6.

A simple cubic structure is not an efficient way of using space. Only 52% of the available space is actually occupied by the spheres in a simple cubic structure. The rest is empty space. Because this structure is inefficient, only one element—polonium—crystallizes in a simple cubic structure.

Body-Centered Cubic Packing

Another approach starts by separating the spheres to form a square-packed plane in which they do not quite touch each other, as shown in the Fig. 13.3.

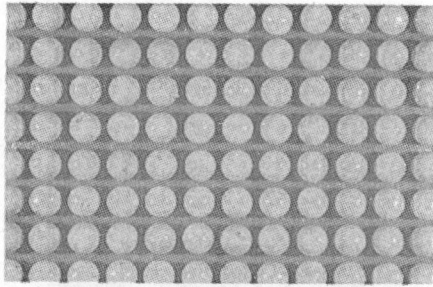

Fig. 13.3

The spheres in the second plane pack above the holes in the first plane, as shown in the Fig. 13.4.

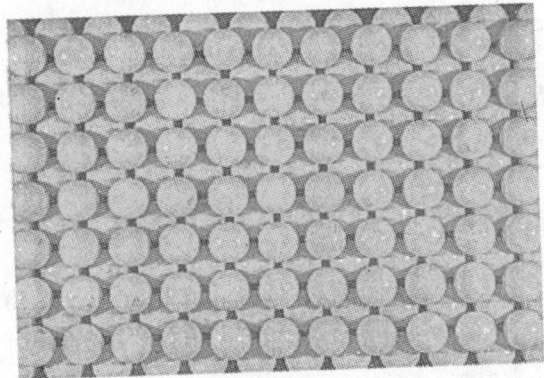

Fig. 13.4

Spheres in the third plane pack above holes in the second plane. Spheres in the fourth plane pack above holes in the third plane, and so on. The result is a structure in which the odd-numbered planes of atoms are identical and the even-numbered planes are identical. This *ABABABAB*. . . repeating structure is known as **body-centered cubic packing**.

This structure is called *body-centered cubic* because each sphere touches four spheres in the plane above and four more in the plane below, arranged toward the corners of a cube. Thus, the repeating unit in this structure is a cube of eight spheres with a ninth identical sphere in the center of the bodyin other words, a body-centered cube, as shown in the figure below. The coordination number in this structure is 8.

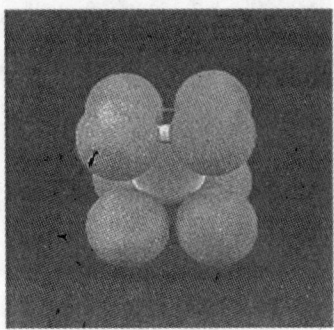

Fig. 13.5

Body-centered **cubic packing** is **a more effic**ient way of using space than simple cubic packing68% of the space in this structure is filled. All of the metals in Group IA (Li, Na, K, and so on), the heavier metals in Group IIA (Ca, Sr, and Ba), and a number of the early transition metals (such as Ti, V, Cr, Mo, W, and Fe) pack in a body-centered cubic structure.

Closest-Packed Structures

Two structures pack spheres so efficiently they are called **closest-packed structures**.

Both start by packing the spheres in planes in which each sphere touches six others oriented toward the **corners of a hexagon,** as shown in Fig. 13.6.

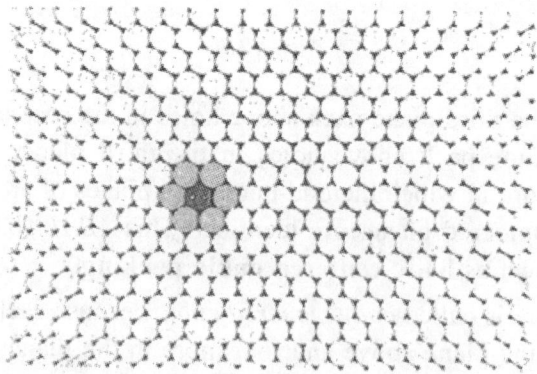

Fig. 13.6

A second plane is then formed by **packing spheres** above the triangular holes in the first plane, as shown in Fig. 13.7.

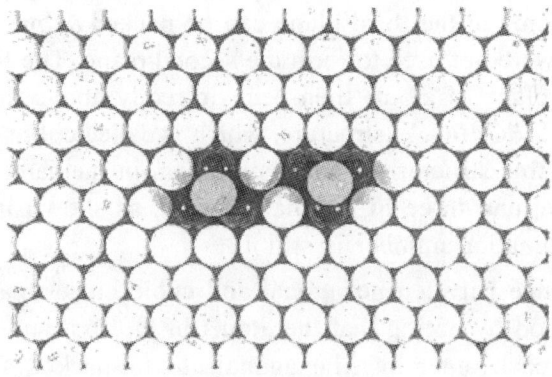

Fig. 13.7

The spheres **in the third plane could pack** directly *above the spheres* in the first plane to form an *ABABABAB. . .* repeating structure. Because this structure is composed of alternating planes of hexagonal closest-packed spheres, it is called a **hexagonal closest-packed structure**. Each sphere touches three spheres in the plane above, three spheres in the plane below, and six spheres in the same plane, as shown in the figure below. Thus, the coordination number in a hexagonal closest-packed structure is 12.

74% of the space in a hexagonal closest-packed structure is filled. No more efficient way of packing spheres is known, and the hexagonal closest-packed structure is important for metals such as Be, Co, Mg, and Zn, as well as the rare gas He at low temperatures.

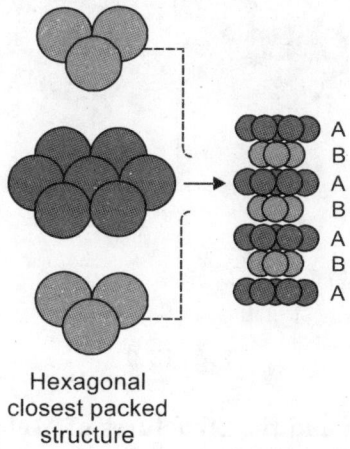

Hexagonal
closest packed
structure

Fig. 13.8

There is another way of stacking hexagonal closest-packed planes of spheres. The atoms in the third plane can be packed *above the holes* in the first plane that were not used to form the second plane. The fourth hexagonal closest-packed plane of atoms then packs directly above the first. The net result is an *ABCABCABC.* . . structure, which is called **cubic closest-packed**. Each sphere in this structure touches six others in the same plane, three in the plane above, and three in the plane below, as shown in the Fig. 13.9. Thus, the coordination number is still 12.

The difference between hexagonal and cubic closest-packed structures can be understood by noting that the atoms in the first and third planes lie directly above each other in a hexagonal closest-packed structure. In the cubic closest-packed structure, the atoms in these planes are oriented in different directions. The cubic closest-packed structure is just as efficient as the hexagonal closest packed structure. (Both use 74% of the available space.) Many metals, including Ag, Al, Au, Ca, Co, Cu, Ni, Pb, and Pt, crystallize in a cubic closest-packed structure. So do all the rare gases except helium when these gases are cooled to low enough temperatures to solidify. The face-centered cubic unit cell is the simplest repeating unit in a cubic closest-packed structure. In fact, the presence of face-centered cubic unit cells in this structure explains why the structure is known as *cubic* closest-packed.

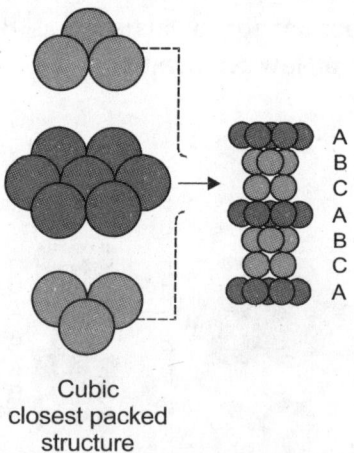

Cubic
closest packed
structure

Fig. 13.9

Coordination Numbers and the Structures of Metals

The coordination numbers of the four structures of metals are summarized in the table below. It is easy to understand why metals pack in hexagonal or cubic closest-packed structures. Not only do these structures use space as efficiently as possible, they also have the largest possible coordination numbers, which allows each metal atom to form bonds to the largest number of neighboring metal atoms.

Table 13.2: Coordination Numbers for Common Crystal Structures

Structure	CoordinationNumber	Stacking Pattern
simple cubic	6	*AAAAAAAA. . .*
body-centered cubic	8	*ABABABAB. . .*
hexagonal closest-packed	12	*ABABABAB. . .*
cubic closest-packed	12	*ABCABCABC. . .*

It is less obvious why one-third of the metals pack in a body-centered cubic structure, in which the coordination number is only 8. The popularity of this structure can be understood by referring to the Fig. 13.10.

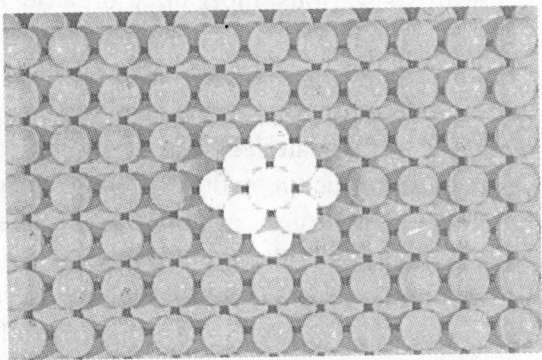

Fig. 13.10

The coordination **number for body-centered** cubic structures given in the table above counts only the atoms that actually touch a given atom in this structure. The figure above shows that each atom also *almost touches* four neighbors in the same plane, a fifth neighbor two planes above, and a sixth two planes below. The distance from each atom to the nuclei of these nearby atoms is only 15% larger than the distance to the nuclei of the atoms that it actually touches. Each atom in a body-centered cubic structure therefore can form a total of 14 bonds eight strong bonds to the atoms that it touches and six weaker bonds to the atoms it almost touches.

This makes it easier to understand why a metal might prefer the body-centered cubic structure to the hexagonal or cubic closest-packed structure.

Each metal atom in the closest-packed structures can form strong bonds to 12 neighboring atoms. In the body-centered cubic structure, each atom forms a total of 14 bonds to neighboring atoms, although six of these bonds are somewhat weaker than the other eight.

Method for the Structure Determination of Crystal Compound

X-ray crystallography

X-ray crystallography is a method of determining the arrangement of atoms within a crystal, in which a beam of X-rays strikes a crystal and diffracts into many specific directions. From the angles and intensities of these diffracted beams, a crystallographer can produce a three-dimensional picture of the density of electrons within the crystal. From this electron density, the mean positions of the atoms in the crystal can be determined, as well as their chemical bonds, their disorder and various other information.

Since many materials can form crystals—such as salts, metals, minerals, semiconductors, as well as various inorganic, organic and biological molecules—X-ray crystallography has been fundamental in the development of many scientific fields. In its first decades of use, this method determined the size of atoms, the lengths and types of chemical bonds, and the atomic-scale differences among various materials, especially minerals and alloys. The method also revealed the structure and functioning of many biological molecules, including vitamins, drugs, proteins and nucleic acids such as DNA. X-ray crystallography is still the chief method for characterizing the atomic structure of new materials and in discerning materials that appear similar by other experiments. X-ray crystal structures can also account for unusual electronic or elastic properties of a material, shed light on chemical interactions and processes, or serve as the basis for designing pharmaceuticals against diseases.

Bragg's Law

It is the result of experiments into the diffraction of X-rays or neutrons off crystal surfaces at certain angles, derived by physicist Sir William Lawrence Bragg in 1912.

Bragg's equation is **n λ = 2d sinλ**

Here d is the spacing between diffracting planes, θ is the incident angle, n is any integer, and λ is the wavelength of the beam. These specific directions appear as spots on the diffraction pattern called *reflections*. Thus, X-ray diffraction results from an electromagnetic wave (the X-ray) impinging on a regular array of scatterers (the repeating arrangement of atoms within the crystal). X-rays are used to produce the diffraction pattern because their wavelength λ is typically the same order of magnitude (1–100 angstroms) as the spacing *d* between planes in the crystal.

Deriving Bragg's equation **(n λ = 2d sin θ)**

Bragg's Law can easily be derived by considering the conditions necessary to make the phases of the beams coincide when the incident angle equals and reflecting angle. The rays of the incident beam are always in phase and parallel up to the point at which the top beam strikes the top layer at atom z (Fig. 1). The second beam continues to the next layer where it is scattered by atom B. The second beam must travel the extra distance AB + BC if the two beams are to continue traveling adjacent and parallel. This extra distance must be an integral (n) multiple of the wavelength (λ) for the phases of the two beams to be the same:

Following to Bragg law, path difference is integral multiple of wavelength of incident X-ray(λ).

Path difference = n λ (1),

From the Fig. 13.11, it is clear that

Path difference between the two parallel incident rays = AB + BC (2).

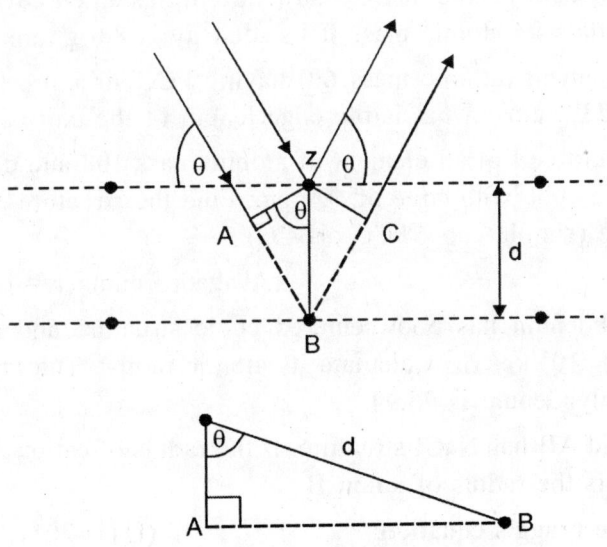

Fig. 13.11: X-ray reflection

Recognizing d as the hypotenuse of the right triangle Abz, we can use trigonometry to relate d and q to the distance (AB + BC). The distance AB is opposite angle θ so,

$$AB = d \sin \theta \ (3).$$

Because $AB = BC$ eq. (2) becomes,

$$n\lambda = 2AB \ (4)$$

Substituting eq. (3) in eq. (4) we have, $n\lambda = 2 \ d \sin \theta$. The location of the surface does not change the derivation of Bragg's Law. where n = 1,2,3.... (for 1st order reflection n = 1 and 2nd order n = 2).

QUESTIONS FOR EXAMINATIONS

1. X-rays of wavelength 1.54 A° is falling at an angle of 14°12′ on a crystal to show 2nd order reflection, calculate the separation between two parallel planes of the crystal.

2. The density of NaCI is 2.163 g/cc, calculate the edge of its cubic cell, assuming that four molecules of NaCI are associated per unit cell.

3. The edge length of NaCI unit cell is 564 pm. What is the density of NaCl in g /cc (atomic masses of Na = 23.0, Cl = 35.5).

4. An element occurs in BCC structure. It has a cell edge of 250 pin. Calculate its atomic mass if its density is 8.0 g /cm^{-3}.

5. An element (atomic mass 60) having FCC structure has a density of 6.23 g cm^{-3} .what is the edge length of the unit cell?

6. The unit cell of an element of atomic mass 108 and density 10.5g/cc is a cube with edge of 409 pm. Find the structure of the cyrstal lattice (simple cube, FCC orBCC).

    (Avagadro number = 6.023×10^{23})

7. Molybdenum has body.centered cubic structure and a density of 10.2×10^4 kg/ rn^3 Calculate its atomic radius. The atomic weight of molybdenum is 95.94.

8. A solid AB has NaCI structure. If the radius of cation A is 120 pm, what is the radius of anion B.

9. Derive bragg's equation.   (UTU-2011,UPTU-2005)

LIQUID CRYSTALS
General- Definition and History
Types, Thermotropic and Lyotropic
Nematic Schematic and Chiral/Cholesteric phase Applications

LIQUID CRYSTALS (LCs)

There are three common states of matter that most people know about: solid, liquid, and gas. Liquid crystal is a fourth "state" that certain kinds of matter can enter under the right conditions. The molecules in solids exhibit both positional and orientational order, in other words, the molecules are constrained to point only certain directions and to be only in certain positions with respect to each other. In liquids, the molecules do not have any positional or orientational order,the direction the molecules point and their positions are random. The liquid crystal also known as *mesophase* exists between the solid and the liquid phase,the molecules in liquid crystal do not exhibit any positional order, but they do possess a certain degree of orientational order. The molecules do not all point the same direction all the time. They merely tend to point more in one direction over time than other directions. This direction is referred to as the *director* of the liquid crystal. Figs. 13.12,13.13 and 13.14 show arrangement of molecules in solid state, liquid crystalline and liquid state respectively.

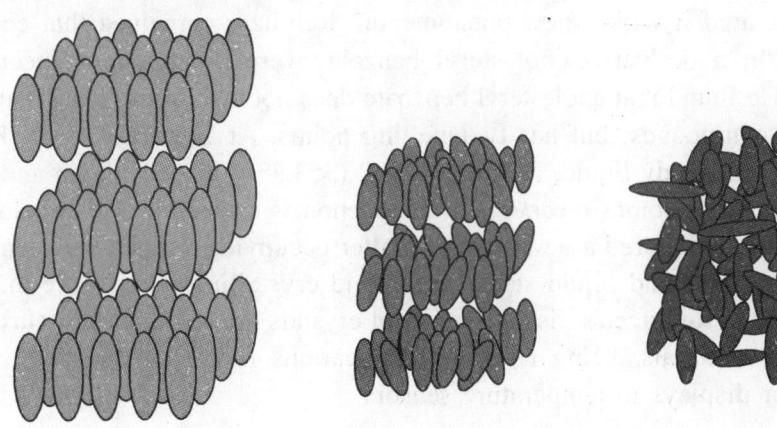

Fig .13.12: Solid)　　**Fig. 13.13:** Liquid Crystal　　**Fig. 13.14:** Liquid

Liquid crystals have properties between those of a conventional liquid and those of a solid crystal. For instance, an LC may flow like a liquid, but its molecules may be oriented in a crystal-like way. There are many different types of LC phases, which can be distinguished by their different optical properties. When viewed under a microscope using a polarized light source, different liquid crystal phases will appear to have distinct textures. LC materials may not always be in an LC phase (just as water may turn into ice or steam). Liquid crystal is an *anisotropic* material, meaning that the properties of the material differ in different directions. Liquid crystal behaves differently depending on what direction electric or magnetic fields are applied relative to the director.

Cholesterol myristate (a derivative of cholesterol) is a crystalline solid below 71°C, above this temperature it turns into a cloudy liquid. When the cloudy liquid is heated to 86°C, it becomes a clear liquid. The intermediate state between the crystalline solid state (71°C) and the liquid state (86°C), has been the liquid crystal state.

Cholesterol myristate (71°C)   above 71°C   Cloudy turbid state   above 86°C   Clear liquid
(Solid crystalline phase) ⟶   *(Liquid Crystal)* ⟶   (Liquid phase)

HISTORY

In 1888, Austrian botanical physiologist Friedrich Reinitzer, working at the Charles University in Prague, examined the physico-chemical properties of various derivatives of cholesterol, which are now known as cholesteric liquid crystals. Previously, other researchers had observed distinct color effects when cooling cholesterol derivatives just above the freezing point, but had not associated it with a new phenomenon. Reinitzer perceived that colour changes in a derivative cholesteryl benzoate were not the most peculiar feature. He found that cholesteryl benzoate does not melt in the same manner as other compounds, but has two melting points. At 145.5°C (293.9 °F) it melts into a cloudy liquid, and at 178.5°C (353.3°F) it melts again and the cloudy liquid becomes clear. The phenomenon is reversible. He concluded that he had discovered a new state of matter occupying a niche between the crystalline solid and liquid states: the liquid crystalline state. More than a century after Reinitzer's discovery, liquid crystals are an important class of advanced materials, being used for applications ranging from clock and calculator displays to temperature sensors.

TYPES OF LIQUID CRYSTALS

Liquid crystals can be broadly divided into types viz thermotropic and lyotropic. Thermotropic and lyotropic LCs consist of organic molecules. Thermotropic LCs exhibit a phase transition into the LC phase as temperature is changed. Lyotropic LCs exhibit phase transitions as a function of both temperature and concentration of the LC molecules in a solvent (typically water). There is one another phase in which LC may exist is known as metallotropic phase. Metallotropic LCs are composed of both organic and inorganic molecules; their LC transition depends not only on temperature and concentration, but also on the inorganic-organic composition ratio.

Thermotropic Liquid Crystals

Thermotropic phases are those that occur in a certain temperature range. If the temperature rise is too high, thermal motion will destroy the delicate cooperative ordering of the LC phase, pushing the material into a conventional isotropic liquid phase. At too low temperature, most LC materials will form a conventional crystal. Many thermotropic LCs exhibit a variety of phases as temperature is changed. A particular type of LC molecule may exhibit various phases like smectic and nematic (and finally isotropic) as temperature is increased. An example of a compound displaying thermotropic LC behavior is para-azoxyanisole.

Lyotropic Liquid Crystals

A lyotropic liquid crystal consists of two or more components that exhibit liquid-crystalline properties in certain concentration ranges. In the lyotropicphases, solvent molecules fill the space around the compounds to provide fluidity to the system. In contrast to thermotropic liquid crystals, these lyotropics have another degree of freedom of concentration that enables them to induce a variety of different phases.

A compound, which has two immiscible hydrophilic and hydrophobic parts within the same molecule, is called an amphiphilic molecule. Many amphiphilic molecules show lyotropic liquid-crystalline phase sequences depending on the volume balances between the hydrophilic part and hydrophobic part. These structures are formed through the micro-phase segregation of two incompatible components on a nanometer scale. Soap is an everyday example of a lyotropic liquid crystal.

The content of water or other solvent molecules changes the self-assembled structures. At very low amphiphile concentration, the molecules will be dispersed randomly without any ordering. At slightly higher (but still low) concentration, amphiphilic molecules will spontaneously assemble into micellesor vesicles. This is done so as to 'hide' the hydrophobic tail of the amphiphile inside the micelle core, exposing a hydrophilic (water-soluble) surface to aqueous solution. These spherical objects do not order themselves

in solution, however. At higher concentration, the assemblies will become
ordered. A typical phase is a hexagonal columnar phase, where the
amphiphiles form long cylinders (again with a hydrophilic surface) that
arrange themselves into a roughly hexagonal lattice. This is called the middle
soap phase. At still higher concentration, a lamellar phase (neat soap phase)
may form, wherein extended sheets of amphiphiles are separated by thin
layers of water. For some systems, a cubic (also called viscous isotropic)
phase may exist between the hexagonal and lamellar phases, wherein spheres
are formed that create a dense cubic lattice. These spheres may also be
connected to one another, forming a bicontinuous cubic phase. Sodium
stearate is an example of this type. These *lytropic* liquid crystal substances
are extremely important in display applications.

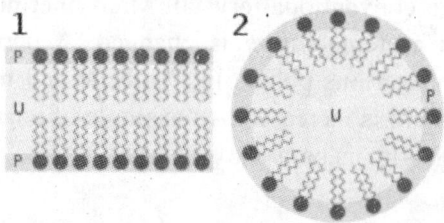

Fig. 13.15: Structure of lyotropic liquid crystal.
The circular heads of surfactant molecules are in contact with water,
whereas the tails are immersed in oil : bilayer (left) and micelle (right)

Nematic phase

One of the most common LC phases is the nematic. The word *nematic* is a
Greek word which means "thread". This term originates from the thread-
like structure observed in nematics.The least ordered liquid crystalline phase
for rodlike molecules is the nematic phase, in which the long axes of
individual molecules have an approximate direction (which is called the
director, n). A nematic phase material has a low viscosity and is therefore
very fluid. Thus, the molecules are free to flow and their center of mass
positions are randomly distributed as in a liquid, but still maintain their
long-range directional order. Most nematics are uniaxial: they have one axis
that is longer and preferred, with the other two being equivalent (can be
approximated as cylinders or rods). However, some liquid crystals are biaxial
nematics, meaning that in addition to orienting their long axis, they also
orient along a secondary axis. Nematic LC have fluidity similar to that of
ordinary (isotropic) liquids but they can be easily aligned by an external
magnetic or electric field. Common examples are p-azoxyanisole (117–
137°C) and p-azoxy phentole (137–167°C).

p-azoxyanisole — (PAA, $CH_3O — C_6H_4-NO — N — C_6H_4 — OCH_3$)

Smectic phase

The term "smectic" is derived from the Greek word for soap (owing to the fact that smectic liquid crystals have mechanical properties similar to those of concentrated aqueous soap solutions). In the smectic phases, the molecules have more order than molecules existing in the nematic phase. Just as in the nematic phase, the molecules have their long axes more or less parallel to the director. Additionally, the molecules are more or less confined to layers. The smectic phases are divided into classes based on degree of molecular order; the smectic A phase (SmA) and the smectic C phase (SmC) are the most studied ones. In the SmA phase, the molecules are perpendicular to the smectic layer planes, whereas in the SmC phase they are tilted. Substances assuming these phases have some fluidity, but their viscosities are much higher than that of a nematic phase substance.

Example: p-n-octyl oxy benzoic acid (108–147°C), ethyl p-azoxy-benzoate, ethyl p-azoxy cinnamate,

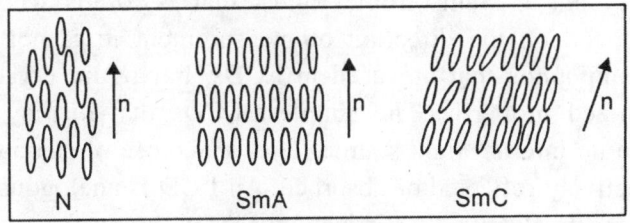

Fig. 13.16: Rodlike molecules in the nematic phase (N), the smectic A phase (SmA) and in the smectic C phase (SmC). The director is denoted as n.

CHIRAL (CHOLESTERIC) PHASE

The chiral nematic phase exhibits chirality (handedness). This phase is often called the *cholesteric* phase because it was first observed for cholesterol derivatives. Only chiral molecules (i.e., those that lack inversion symmetry) can give rise to such a phase. Cholesteric phase is also characterized by its colour. They show strong colour effects in polarised light. This phase exhibits a twisting of the molecules perpendicular to the director, with the molecular axis parallel to the director. The finite twist angle between adjacent molecules is due to their asymmetric packing, which results in longer-range chiral order. In the smectic C* phase (an asterisk denotes a chiral phase), the molecules have positional ordering in a layered structure (as in the other smectic phases), with the molecules tilted by a finite angle with respect to the layer normal. The chirality induces a finite azimuthal twist from one layer to the next, producing a spiral twisting of the molecular axis along the layer normal. For example, Cholestryl benzoate (145.5–178.5°C).

APPLICATIONS

Examples of liquid crystals can be found both in the natural world and in technological applications. Most modern electronic displays are liquid crystal based. Lyotropic liquid-crystalline phases are abundant in living systems. For example, many proteins and cell membranes are LCs. Other well-known LC examples are solutions of soap and various related detergents, as well as the tobacco mosaic virus.

Displays: By far the most important application of liquid crystals is display devices. Liquid crystal displays (LCDs) are used in watches, calculators, and laptop computer screens, and for instrumentation in cars, ships, and airplanes. Several types of LCDs exist. In general their value is due to the fact that the orientation of the molecules in a nematic phase substance can be altered by the application of an external electric field, and that liquid crystals are anisotropic fluids, that is, fluids whose physical properties depend on the direction of measurement. It is not pure liquid crystalline compounds that are used in LCDs, but liquid crystal mixtures having optimized properties.The simplest LCDs that display letters and numbers have no internal light source. They make use of surrounding light, which is selectively reflected or absorbed. An LCD is analogous to a mirror that is made nonreflective at distinct places on its surface for a certain period. The main advantage of an LCD is low energy consumption. More advanced LCDs need back light, color filters, and advanced electronics to display complex figures. The best-known LCD is the so-called twisted nematic display. A liquid crystal display (LCD) is a thin, flat electronic visual display that uses the light modulating properties of liquid crystals (LCs).

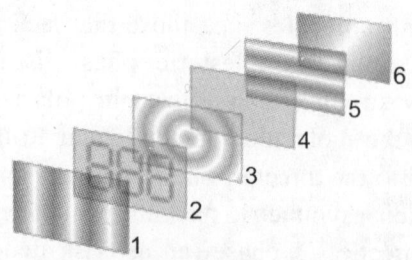

Fig. 13.17: Reflective twisted nematic liquid crystal display (LCD)

LCs do not emit light directly. LCDs are more energy efficient and offer safer disposal than CRTs. Its low electrical power consumption enables it to be used in battery-poweredelectronic equipment.

1. Polarizing filter film with a vertical axis to polarize light as it enters.
2. Glass substrate with ITO electrodes. The shapes of these electrodes will determine the shapes that will appear when the LCD is turned ON. Vertical ridges etched on the surface are smooth.
3. Twisted nematic liquid crystal.
4. Glass substrate with common electrode film (ITO) with horizontal ridges to line up with the horizontal filter.
5. Polarizing filter film with a horizontal axis to block/pass light.
6. Reflective surface to send light back to viewer. (In a backlit LCD, this layer is replaced with a light source.)

LIQUID CRYSTAL THERMOMETERS

The use of liquid crystals as temperature sensors is possible because of the selective reflection of light by chiral nematic (cholesteric) liquid crystals. A chiral nematic liquid crystal reflects light having a characteristic wavelength determined by its pitch and by the viewing angle (the angle between the eye of the observer and the surface of the liquid crystal). Because the pitch of a chiral nematic compound is temperature-dependent, observed color is a function of temperature. Liquid crystals can therefore serve as thermometers. By mixing chiral nematic compounds, thermometers can be customized to be effective in a desired temperature range. The color variation of some liquid crystal thermometers extends across the entire visible light spectrum within changes of a few tenths of a degree centigrade. For use in devices, microcapsules containing chiral nematic mixtures are mixed with binder materials. Liquid crystal thermometers find application in medicine (medical thermography). A liquid crystal thermometer attached to the skin can measure temperature variations of the skin. This can be useful in the detection of skin cancer, as tumors have different temperatures than surrounding tissues. In electronics, liquid crystal temperature sensors can pinpoint bad connections within a circuit board by detecting the characteristic local heating. The colour changes of gadgets such as "mood rings" are a manifestation of chiral nematic mixtures.

QUESTIONS

1. Differentiate between thermotropic and lyotropic crystals.

2. Define liquid crystal and their classification with application.

3. Differentiate between nematic and schematic liquid crystals.(UTU 2010)

4. Differentiate between nematic and cholesteric liquid crystals.(UTU-2012)

FULLERENE
Introduction, Preparation, Properties and Application

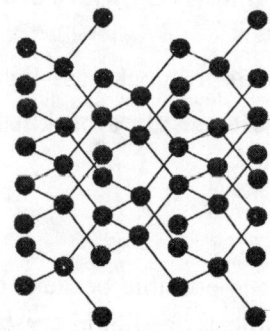
Fig. 13.18: Diamond

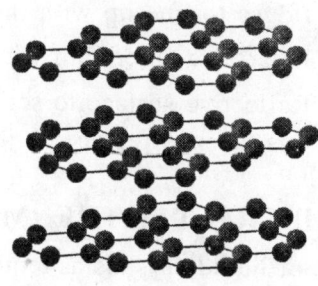
Fig. 13.19: Graphite

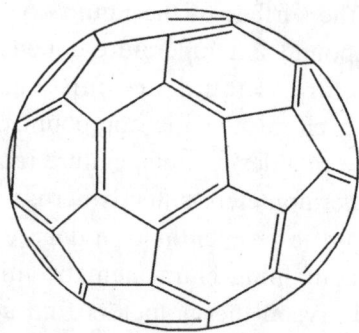
Fig. 13.20: Fullerene C-60

INTRODUCTION

Fullerene is the third allotropic form of carbon, diamond and graphite are other two known allotropic forms. A **fullerene** is any molecule composed entirely of carbon, in the form of a hollow sphere, ellipsoid, or tube. Spherical fullerenes are also called **buckyballs**, and cylindrical ones are called carbon nanotubes oɪ buckytubes. Fullerenes are similar in structure to graphite, which is composed of stacked graphene sheets of linked hexagonal rings;

but they may also contain pentagonal (or sometimes heptagonal) rings. Buckminster fullerene (C_{60}, Fig. 13.20) was fullerene to be discovered, its name was based on popular architect Buckminster Fuller who designed geodesic dome structures based on pentagon and hexagon. It was prepared in 1985 by Richard Smalley, R.Curley, James Health, S.O Brien, and Harold Kroto at Rice University. Fullerenes have since been found to occur in nature. More recently, fullerenes have been detected in outer space. Now a days fullerenes with various number of carbon atoms ranging from C_{20} to C_{500} have been discovered but with 72, 76, 84 and even up to 100 carbon atoms are commonly obtained.

Preparation

Fullerene is prepared by vaporising a graphite rod in a Helium atmosphere. Mixture of fullerenes is obtained,which are separated by solvent extraction (toluene solvent mainly) and chromatographic methods.

Structure

The structure of C_{60} is a truncated icosahedrons (Fig. 13.20), which resembles a soccer ball of the type made of twenty hexagons and twelve pentagons, with a carbon atom at the vertices of each polygon and a bond along each polygon edge. The diameter of a C_{60} molecule is about 1.1 nanometers (nm). The nucleus to nucleus diameter of a C_{60} molecule is about 0.71 nm.The C_{60} molecule has two bond lengths. The 6:6 ring bonds (between two hexagons) can be considered "double bonds" and are shorter than the 6:5 bonds (between a hexagon and a pentagon). Its average bond length is 1.4 angstroms.

Carbon nanotubes (Fig. 13.21) are cylindrical fullerenes. These tubes of carbon are usually only a few nanometres wide, but they can range from less than a micrometer to several millimeters in length. They often have closed ends, but can be open-ended as well

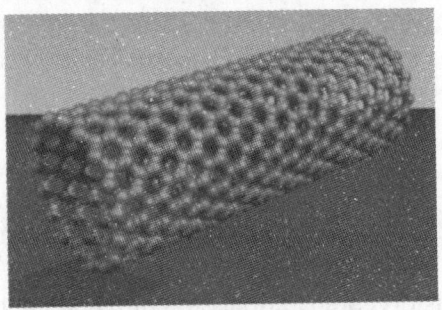

Fig. 13.21: Nano tube

Properties and application

Fullerene is blackish powder smooth material. It is thermally stable before sublimation (600°C). It forms deep magenta solution with benzene. It has been reported that by mixing C-60 with electron donating ions such as Pottasium leads to super conducting material. Fullerene is also used as solid lubricant in space-aircrafts. C-60 is insulator but K_3C_{60} (Potassium buckide) is a stable metallic crystal which is a super conductor below 18Kelvin. The October 2005 issue of *Chemistry and Biology* contains an article describing the use of fullerenes as light-activated antimicrobial agents. Other properties of fullerene are shown by using Fig. 13.22.

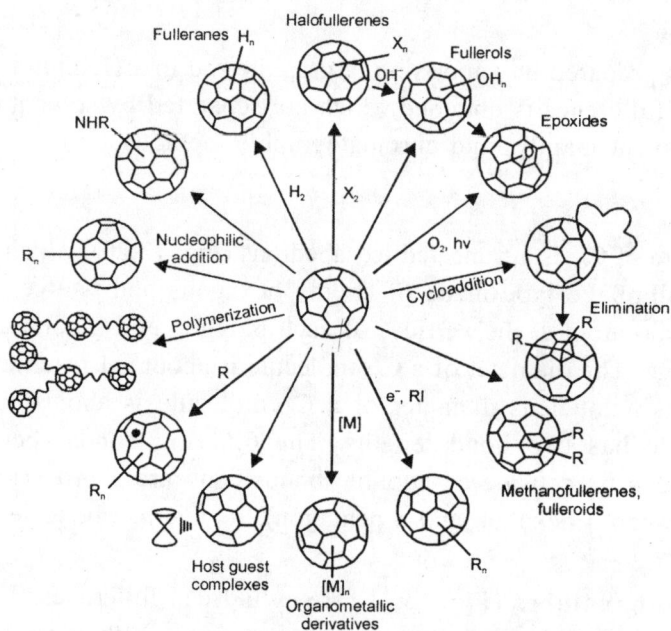

Fig. 13.22: Properties of fullerene

In the field of nanotechnology, heat resistance and superconductivity are some of the more heavily studied properties. One proposed use of carbon nanotubes is in paper batteries.Some properties with reactions are given in the above diagram.

QUESTIONS

Q.1. Describe the structure of fullerene with its application

(UTU-2009, 2012).

Q.2. Describe history, preparation, structure and application of fullerene.

Chapter 14
ORGANIC CHEMISTRY REACTIONS

> ➤ **Electronic Effects**
> ➤ **Reaction Intermediates**
> ➤ **Attacking Reagents**
> ➤ **Organic Reactions Types**
> ➤ **Some Special Reactions**
> ➤ **Mechanism**

ELECTRONIC EFFECTS

An **electronic effect** influences the structure, reactivity, or properties of molecule but is neither a traditional bond nor a steric effect. . Inductive effect, electromeric effect, hyperconjugation, resonance are common electronic effects.

Inductive Effect

When a covalent bond is formed between two dissimilar atoms then shared pair of electrons are slightly shifted towards more electronegative atom, which creates a partial negative charge (δ^-) on more electronegative atom and a partial positive charge (δ^+) on other atom, this phenomenon is called Inductive effect. This is permanent effect and only sigma electrons are involved. To understand this, consider a chain of carbon atoms having Cl atom at one end: C—C—C—C—Cl.

Since chlorine (Cl) is more electronegative than C, the electron pair shared between C and Cl is displaced towards the Cl atom, due its larger electronegativity. A partial negative charge (δ^-) is thus acquired by Cl and C acquires a partial positive charge (δ^+). The displacement is, not limited to C_1–Cl bond but is transmitted to other carbons along the chain. This happens due to the small positive charge on C, which attracts the electrons of C_1-C_2 bond towards it. This displacement results in the positive charge on C_1 being partially neutralized while a small positive charge is developed on C_2. The charge on C_2 is less than that on C_1 ($\delta^{+'}+ < \delta^+$).

Similarly, C_3 will acquire a small positive charge $\delta^{+''} < \delta^{+''} < \delta^{+'}$). ($\delta$ = delta means small)

This process of electron displacement of electrons along the chain of carbon atoms is called negative inductive effect (or I-effect). This is a permanent effect and results due to the presence of a polar covalent bond at one end of the chain. An arrow as shown generally represents this effect:

$$\delta^{+'''} \quad \delta^{+''} \quad \delta^{+'} \quad \delta^+ \quad\quad\quad \delta^-$$
$$-C \rightarrow -C \rightarrow\!\!\!\rightarrow -C \rightarrow\!\!\!\rightarrow\!\!\!\rightarrow -C \rightarrow\!\!\!\rightarrow\!\!\!\rightarrow\!\!\!\rightarrow -Cl$$
$$(\delta^{+'''} < \delta^{+''} < \delta^{+'} < \delta^+)$$

It may be noted that this effect decreases sharply as we move away from the atoms involved in the initial polar bond. From the fourth atom onwards, the effect becomes negligible.

For comparing the relative effects, hydrogen is taken as the standard and atoms or groups are classified into the following two categories:

Atoms or groups of atoms that have a greater electron-attracting capacity than hydrogen are referred to as having-I (electron attracting) effect. For example,

$$NO_2 > CN > COOH > F > Cl > Br > I > OH > OCH_3 > C_6H_5 > HI$$

Atoms or groups of atoms, having smaller electron attracting power than hydrogen are referred to as having +I (electron repelling) effect. Alkyl groups are +I groups.

$$(CH_3)_3C \rightarrow (CH_3)_2CH \rightarrow CH_3CH_2 \rightarrow CH_3-$$

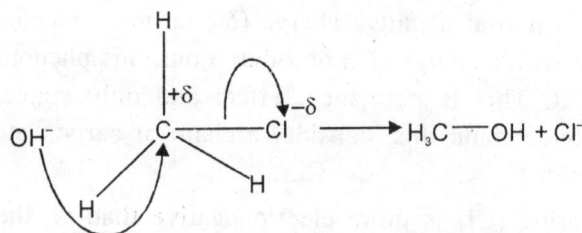

Inductive effect plays very significant role in understanding reactions of organic chemistry. Carbon of methyl chloride, for example, acquires partially positive charge due to shift of electrons towards chlorine and provides a site for attack by a negatively charged species (say OH^-).

Electromeric effect

This is a temporary effect and takes place between two atoms joined by a multiple bond, i.e., a double or triple bond. It occurs at the requirements of the attacking reagent, and involves instantaneous transfer of a shared pair of electrons of the multiple bond to one of the linked atoms. It is temporary in nature because the molecule acquires its original electronic condition upon removal of the attacking reagent

For example, consider the carbonyl group, >C=O, present in aldehydes and ketones. When a negatively charged reagent say $:\overset{..}{X}:^-$ approaches the molecule seeking positive site, it causes instantaneous shift of electron pair of carbonyl group to oxygen (more electronegative than carbon). The carbon thus becomes deprived of its share in this transferred-pair of electrons and acquires positive charge. In the meanwhile oxygen takes complete control of the electron pair and becomes negatively charged. Therefore, in the presence of attacking reagent, one bond is lost and this negatively charged attacking reagent links to the carbon having positive charge.

Attacking
species

This phenomenon of movement of electrons from one atom to another at the demand of attacking reagent in multibonded atoms is called electromeric effect, denoted as E effect. The electromeric shift of electrons takes place only at the moment of reaction. Like the inductive effect, the electromeric effect is also classified as +E and E:

When the transfer of electrons takes place towards the attacking reagent, it is called + E (positive electromeric) effect. For example,

When the transfer of electrons takes place away from the attacking reagent, it is called, -E (negative electromeric) effect. For example,

RESONANCE AND RESONANCE (MESOMERIC) EFFECT

Resonance

The phenomenon in which two or more structures can be written for the true structure of a molecules, but none of them can be said to represent if uniquely, is referred to as resonacne or mesomerism. The true structure of the molecule is said to be a resonance hybrid of the various possible alternative structures which themselves are known as resonating structures or canonical structures. Every two adjacent resonating structures are represented by inserting a double headed arrow between them. Thus the actual structure of benzene may be represented in the following two ways.

Necessary conditions for resonance are:

1. All resonating structures must have the same arrangement of atomic nuclei.

2. The resonating structures must have the same number of paired and unpaired electrons. However, they may differ in the way of distribution of electrons.

3. The energies of the various limiting structures must be sane or nearly the same.

4. Resonating structures must be planar.

All the resonating structures do not contribute equal to the real molecule and hence only the major contributing forms are used while representing a resonance hybrid.

The **mesomeric effect** may be defined as the permanent effect in which p electrons are transferred from a multiple bond to an atom, or from a multiple bond to a single covalent bond or lone pair(s) of p-electrons from an atom to the adjacent single covalent bond. Like inductive effect, the mesomeric effect (denoted by M) may be +M and –M. It is +M when the transference of electron pair is away from the atom and –M when transference of electron pair is toward the atom. In general.Some common atoms or groups which cause +M and -M effect are given below

+ M groups: $-Cl$, $-Br$, $-I$, $-NH_2$, $-NR_2$, $-OH$, $-OCH_3$

– M groups: $-NO_2$, $-CN$, $> C = O$

Conjugation is a redistribution of electron density similar to induction but transmitted through interconnected pi-bonds. Conjugation is not only affected by electro negativity of the connected atoms but the position of electron lone pairs with respect to the pi-system. Electronic effects can be transmitted throughout a pi-system allowing their influence to extend further than induction

Hyperconjugation: The alkyl groups with at least one hydrogen atom on the α-carbon atom, attached to an unsaturated carbon atom, are able to release electrons by a mechanism similar to that of the electromeric effect, the delocalization involves s and p bond orbital (or p orbitals in case of free radicals); thus it is also known as s-p conjugation or σ − π conjugation as sigma as well as pi electrons are involved in conjugation. This type of electron release due to the presence of the system H − C − C = C is known as hyperconjugation.

REACTION INTERMEDIATES

Fission of a covalent bond

Breaking of a Covalend Bond: Generation of reaction intermediates in a reaction depends upon the breaking or fission of a bond present in the molecules. A covalent bond may be broken in two ways.

(a) **Homolytic fission or homolysis:** In homolytic bond fission one electron of the bonding pair goes with each of the departing atom or group resulting in two electrically neutral fragments or atoms generally known as **free radicals**. e.g. alkyl free radicals like CH_3^0, chlorine Cl^0. **Free radicals**: A free radical is a species which has as odd or unpaired electron. Free radicals themselves are electricially neutral, however, due to the presence of odd electron, these are paramagnetic in nature. Again because of the presence of odd electron, free radicals are in constant search for another electron to pair up and hence these are highly reactive species. Carbon free radicals are named after the parent alkyl group and adding the word free radical. A free radical may have an sp^2 hybridized carbon in which odd electron remains in the p orbital, the shape of this type of free radical will be planar. Alternatively, free radical may have sp3 hybridized carbon atom. Now since the homolytic fission always results in the formation of free radicals, the reactions involving such (homolytic) fission are known as free radical reactions and are said to proceed via a free radical mechanism. This fission is favoured by high temperature(above 500°C), presence of non polar solvent,presence of UV radiation, ozone etc.Stability order of free radicals is: 3^0 (tertiary) is more stable than 2^0 (secondary) more stable than 1^0 (primary).

(b) Hetereolytic fission or heterolysis: In this type of fission the electrons pair forming the covalent bond goes to a single atom or group and thus electricity charged fragments (ions) are formed. Thus the reactions involving heterolytic fision are known as ionic reactions and are said to proceed via ionic (polar) mechanism. This fission is favoured by presence of polar solvent and presence of ions.The heterolytic fission of the covalent bond can occur in either of the following two ways.(i) When the electrons pair between C and X leaves the organic group and remains with the departing substituent X and thus the latter attains a negative charge (due to gain of electrons) while the former attains a positive charge (due to loss of electrons)Such organic species which has only six paired electrons (i.e. three pairs of electrons) and a positive charge at its carbon centre is known as carbonium ion or **carbocation (R^+).** Reactions in whcih carbocations are formed as intermediate are said to proceed by carbocation mechanism.Tertiary(3^0) carbocation is most stable.(ii) When the electrons pair between C and X remains with the organic group and the substituent X is devoid of its bonding electron and thus gets positive charge while the organic group (which has gained electrons) is negatively charged. Such organic species which has eight paired electrons (i.e. four pair of electrons) and a negative charge on one of its carbon centre is known as **carbanion.** Carbanions are generally symbolized as **(R^-).** Reactions in which carbanions are formed as intermediate are said to proceed by a carbanion mechanism. Primary (1^0) carbanion is most stable.

Attacking Reagents—Attacking reagents can be divided in two types viz electrophiles and nucleophiles.

Nucleophiles or nuceophilc—Nucleophilic means nucleus + philic (attracting) **i.e** a nucleophile is a species (an ion or a molecule) which is strongly attracted to a region of positive charge in something else. Nucleophiles are either fully negative ions, or else have a strongly δ-charge somewhere on a molecule. Common nucleophiles are hydroxide ions, cyanide ions, water and ammonia. Neutral molecules are electron rich i.e these species contain at least one lone pair of electron. These are also known as lewis base.

$$:\ddot{O}\!\!\vdots\!-H \qquad \bar{:}C\!\equiv\!N \qquad \overset{\delta-}{:\ddot{O}}\!\!\vdots\!\overset{\delta+}{-H} \qquad \overset{\delta+}{H}\!-\!\overset{\delta-}{\vdots\ddot{N}}\!\vdots\!\overset{\delta+}{-H}$$

$$\underset{\delta+H}{} \qquad \underset{\overset{|}{\underset{\delta+}{H}}}{}$$

Notice that each of these contains at least one lone pair of electrons, either on an atom carrying a full negative charge, or on a very electronegative atom carrying a substantial δ-charge.

Electrophile or Electrophilic

Electrophilic means electron attracting i.e an electropile is a species (an ion or a molecule) which is strongly attracted to a region of negative charge. So electrophilics are either positively charged or neutral molecule which is electron deficient somewhere on a molecule. Common electrophilic are like H^+, all cations, or neutral molecule like BF_3, $ZnCl_2$ which are electron deficient and can accept lone pair of electrons.

ORGANIC REACTIONS

Organic reactions are chemical reactions involving organic compounds. In organic synthesis, organic reactions are used in the construction of new organic molecules. The production of many man-made chemicals such as drugs, plastics, food additives, fabrics depend on organic reactions.

Fundamentals

Factors governing organic reactions are essentially the same as that of any chemical reaction. Factors specific to organic reactions are those that determine the stability of reactants and products such as conjugation, hyperconjugation and aromaticity and the presence and stability of reactive intermediates such as free radicals, carbocations and carbanions.

Types of reactions

The basic organic chemistry reaction types are addition reactions, elimination reactions, substitution reactions and rearrangement reactions

1. **Addition Reaction**—The reaction in which a molecule is added across the double or triple bond is known as addition. Degree of saturation increases. Hybridisation is changed from sp – sp^2- sp^3. Unsaturated compounds give such types of reactions. It includes such reactions as halogenation and hydrogenation of alkene. On the basis of mechanism, its subtypes are electrophilic addition reaction, nucleophilic addition reaction and free radical addition. In the addition reaction attacking reagent is attached in the form of electrophile (E^+) or nucleophile (Nu^-), If E^+ is attached first then reaction is electrophilic addition, similarly reaction will be nucleophilic addition.

An addition reaction is the opposite of an elimination reaction. For instance the hydration reaction of an alkene and the dehydration of an alcohol are addition-elimination pairs. Addition reactions are also encountered in polymerizations and called addition polymerization.

2. **Elimination reactions:** The reactions in which some molecules or group of atoms are eliminated from the same molecule are known

$$\begin{array}{c} \diagdown \quad \diagup \\ C=C \\ \diagup \quad \diagdown \end{array} \xrightarrow{E^+} \begin{array}{c} \diagdown \quad \diagup \\ E-C-C\oplus \\ \diagup \quad \diagdown \end{array} \xrightarrow{N^-} \begin{array}{c} \diagdown \quad \diagup \\ E-C-C-N \\ \diagup \quad \diagdown \end{array}$$

$$\begin{array}{c} \diagdown \quad \diagup \\ C=O \\ \diagup \end{array} \xrightarrow{Nu^-} \begin{array}{c} \diagdown \quad \diagup \\ Nu-C-O\ominus \\ \diagup \quad \diagdown \end{array} \xrightarrow{H^+} \begin{array}{c} \diagdown \quad \diagup^H \\ Nu-C-O \\ \diagup \end{array}$$

$$\begin{array}{c} \diagdown \quad \diagup \\ C=C \\ \diagup \quad \diagdown \end{array} \xrightarrow{X} \begin{array}{c} \diagdown \quad \diagup \\ X-C-C\bullet \\ \diagup \quad \diagdown \end{array} \xrightarrow[-X]{H-X} \begin{array}{c} \diagdown \quad \diagup \\ X-C-C-H \\ \diagup \quad \diagdown \end{array}$$

as elimination reaction. Degree of saturation decreases. Hybridisation is changed from $sp^3 - sp^2$- sp. Generally saturated compounds give such types of reactions. It includes such as dehydration, dehalogenation.

An important class of elimination reactions are those involving alkyl halides, or alkanes in general, with good leaving groups, reacting with a Lewis base to form an alkene in the reverse of an addition reaction. When the substrate is asymmetric, regioselectivity is determined by Zaitsev's rule. The one and two-step mechanisms are named and known as **E2 reaction** and **E1 reaction**, respectively.

E 2 mechanism

In the 1920s, Sir Christopher Ingold proposed a model to explain a peculiar type of chemical reaction: the E2 mechanism. E2 stands for **bimolecular elimination** and has the following specificities.

-   ♣ It is a one-step process of elimination with a single transition state.
-   ♣ Typical of primary or secondary substituted alkyl halides.
-   ♣ The reaction rate, influenced by both the alkyl halide and the base, is second order.
-   ♣ Because E2 mechanism results in formation of a pi bond, the two

leaving groups (often a hydrogen and a halogen) need to be coplanar. An antiperiplanar transition state has staggered conformation with lower energy and a synperiplanar transition state is in eclipsed conformation with higher energy. The reaction mechanism involving staggered conformation is more favourable for E2 reactions.

♣ Reaction often present with strong base.

♣ In order for the pi bond to be created, the hybridization of carbons need to be lowered from sp^3 to sp^2.

♣ The C-H bond is weakened in the rate determining step and therefore the deuterium isotope effect is larger than 1.

♣ This reaction type has similarities with the S_N2 reaction mechanism. The reaction fundamental elements are

♣ Breaking of the *carbon-hydrogen* and *carbon-halogen* bonds in one step.

♣ Formation of a $C = C$ *Pi bond*.

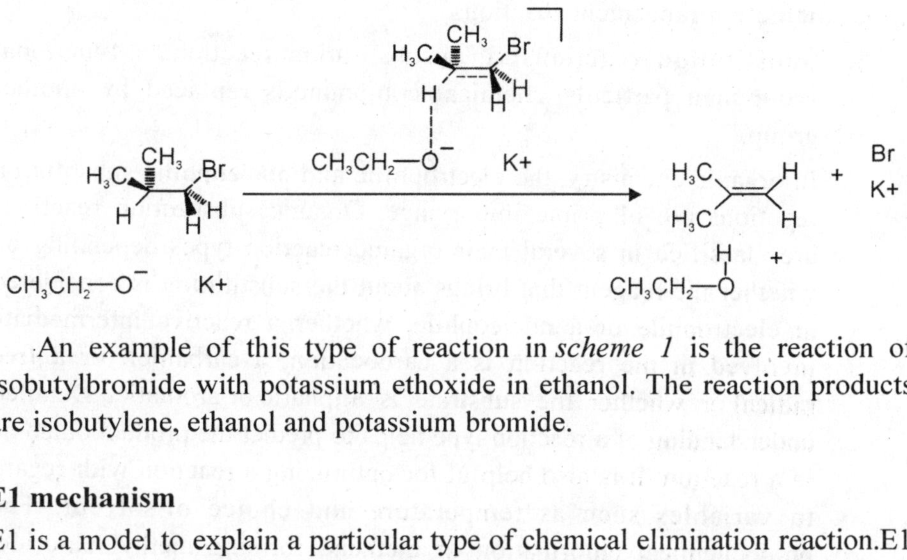

An example of this type of reaction in *scheme 1* is the reaction of isobutylbromide with potassium ethoxide in ethanol. The reaction products are isobutylene, ethanol and potassium bromide.

E1 mechanism

E1 is a model to explain a particular type of chemical elimination reaction. E1 stands for **unimolecular elimination** and has the following specificities.

♣ It is a two-step process of elimination: *ionization and depro-tonation*.

♣ Ionization: the carbon-halogen bond breaks to give a carbocation intermediate.

♣ Deprotonation of the carbocation.

♣ Typical of tertiary and some secondary substituted alkyl halides.

♣ The reaction rate is influenced only by the concentration of the alkyl halide because carbocation formation is the slowest, rate-determining step. Therefore first-order kinetics apply.

♣ Reaction mostly occurs in complete absence of base or presence of only a weak base.

♣ E1 reactions are in competition with S_N1 reactions because they share a common carbocationic intermediate.

♣ A deuterium isotope effect is absent.

♣ No antiperiplanar requirement. An example is the pyrolysis of a certain sulfonate ester of menthol:

Only reaction product **A** results from antiperiplanar elimination, the presence of product **B** is an indicator for a E1 mechanism. Accompanied by carbocationic rearrangement reactions

3. **Substitution reactions:** In a substitution reaction, a functional group in a particular chemical compound is replaced by another group.

   In organic chemistry, the electrophilic and nucleophilic substitution reactions are of prime importance. Organic substitution reactions are classified in several main organic reaction types depending on whether the reagent that brings about the substitution is considered an electrophile or a nucleophile, whether a reactive intermediate involved in the reaction is a carbocation, a carbanion or a free radical or whether the substrate is aliphatic or aromatic. Detailed understanding of a reaction type helps to predict the product outcome in a reaction. It is also helpful for optimizing a reaction with regard to variables such as temperature and choice of solvent. The photochemical chlorination of methane forming methyl chloride, hydrolysis of alkyl halide (RX) by aqueous KOH, etc are good examples of substitution reactions.

Mechanism of Nucleophilic Substitution

The reaction in which atom or group of atoms is replaced by nucleophile, the reaction is known as nucleophilic substitution (SN). It may be SN^1 or SN^2.

SN^{1}- Unimolecular substitution

1st Order

Rate = K. (substrate)

It takes place in two steps

No inversion

Mainly in 3^0 alkyl halide
(most preferred)

SN^2 Bimolecular substitution

2nd order

Rate = K. (substrate) (attacking reagent)

It takes place in one step

Inverted product

Mainly in 1^0 alkyl halide
(most preferred)

The term S$_N$2 means that two molecules are involved in the actual transition state:

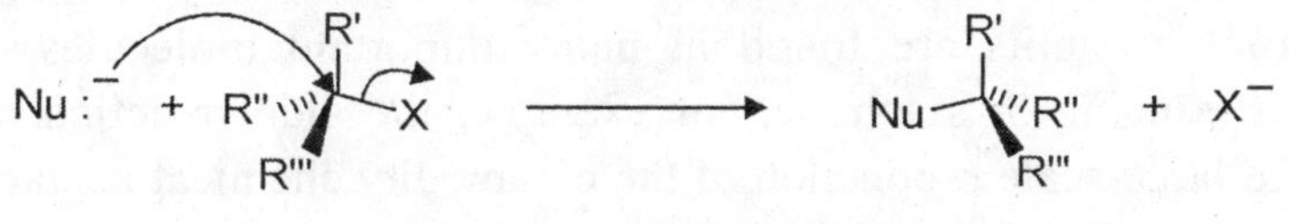

$$\text{Rate = K [Substrate] [Nucleophile]}$$

The departure of the leaving group occurs simultaneously with the backside attack by the nucleophile. The S$_N$2 reaction thus leads to a predictable configuration of the stereocenter-it proceeds with inversion (reversal of the configuration).

In the S$_N$1 reaction, a planar carbenium ion is formed first, which then reacts further with the nucleophile. Since the nucleophile is free to attack from either side, this reaction is associated with racemization.

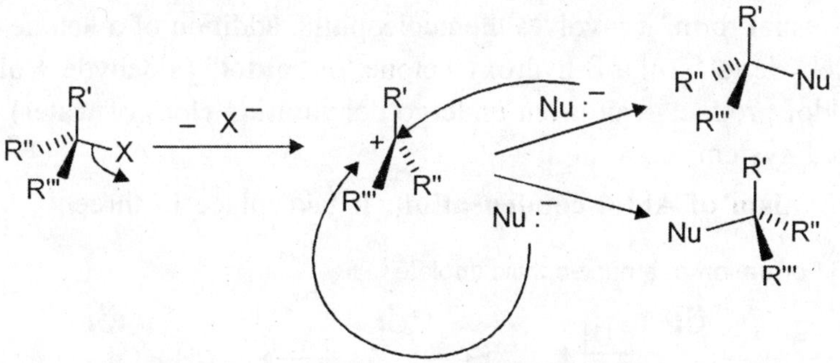

4. **Rearrangement reactions:** A **rearrangement reaction** is a broad class of organic reactions where the carbon skeleton of a molecule is rearranged to give a structural isomer of the original molecule. Often a substituent moves from one atom to another atom in the same molecule. In the example below the substituent R moves from carbon atom 1 to carbon atom 2:

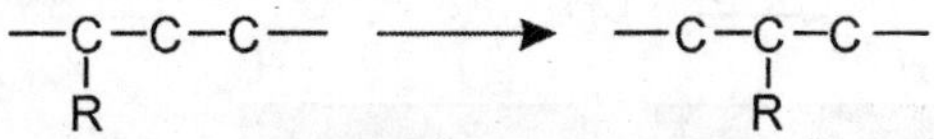

Some rearrangement reactions are Beckmann rearrangement, Curtius reaction, Hoffman reaction etc.

SPECIAL NAME REACTIONS

Aldol Condensation

The **aldol reaction** is a powerful means of forming carbon–carbon bonds in organic chemistry. It was discovered independently by Charles-Adolphe Wurtz and Alexander Porfyrevich Borodin in 1872, the reaction combines two carbonyl compounds (the original experiments used aldehydes) to form a new β-hydroxy carbonyl compound. These products are known as *aldols*, from the *ald*ehyde + alcoh*ol*, a structural motif seen in many of the products. Aldol structural units are found in many important molecules, whether naturally occurring or synthetic. For example, the aldol reaction has been used in the large-scale production of the commodity chemical pentaerythritol and the synthesis of the heart disease drug Lipitor (atorvastatin). Aldol condensation is given by the aldehydes or ketone containing **at least one alpha H atom.**

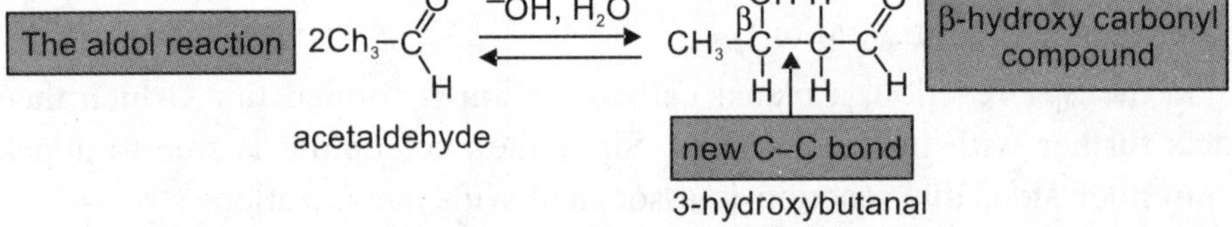

The aldol reaction

acetaldehyde

β-hydroxy carbonyl compound

new C–C bond

3-hydroxybutanal

In its usual form, it involves the nucleophilic addition of a ketone enolate to an aldehyde to form a β-hydroxy ketone, or **"aldol"** (aldehyde + alcohol), These Aldol products can often undergo dehydration (loss of water) to give conjugated systems

Mechanism of Aldol condensation: It takesplace in three

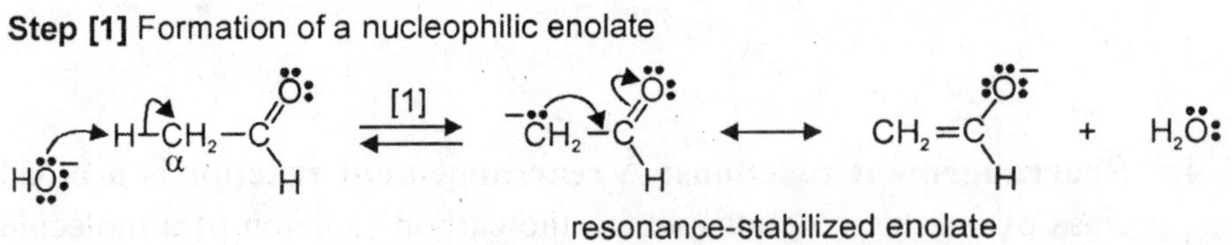

Step [1] Formation of a nucleophilic enolate

resonance-stabilized enolate

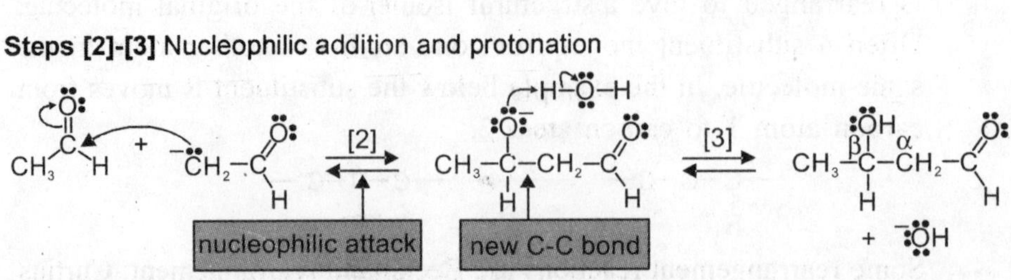

Steps [2]-[3] Nucleophilic addition and protonation

nucleophilic attack

new C-C bond

Cannizzaro reaction

The **Cannizzaro reaction**, named after its discoverer Stanislao Cannizzaro, is a chemical reaction that involves the base-induced disproportionation of an aldehyde lacking a hydrogen atom in the alpha position. Cannizzaro first accomplished this transformation in 1853, when he obtained benzyl alcohol and benzoic acid from the treatment of benzaldehyde with potash (potassium carbonate). In this reaction one molecule of aldehyde (containing no alpha H atom) is oxidised and another is reduced.

$$2HCHO + KOH \rightarrow CH_3OH + HCOOK$$
$$2C_6H_5CHO + NaOH \rightarrow C_6H_5CH_2OH + C_6H_5COONa$$

The oxidation product is a carboxylic acid and the reduction product is an alcohol. For aldehydes with a hydrogen atom alpha to the carbonyl, i.e. $RCHR'CHO$, the preferred reaction is an aldol condensation, originating from deprotonation of this hydrogen.

The first reaction step is nucleophilic addition of the base (for instance the hydroxide anion) to the carbonyl carbon of the aldehyde. The resulting alkoxide is deprotonated to give a di-anion, known as the **Cannizzaro intermediate**. Formation of this intermediate requires a strongly basic environment. This reaction is self oxidation-reduction reaction. Alcohols are formed in the result of reduction and salts of carboxylic acid in the result of oxidation.

Both intermediates can react further with aldehyde to transfer a hydride, H^-. The hydridic character of the $C-H$ is enhanced by the electron-donating character of the alpha oxygen anion. This hydride transfer simultaneously generates an alkoxide anion (RCH_2O^-) and a carboxylic acid, which is rapidly deprotonated to form the carboxylate. Further evidence for the hydridic character of the Cannizzaro intermediate is provided by the formation of H_2 by its reaction with water.

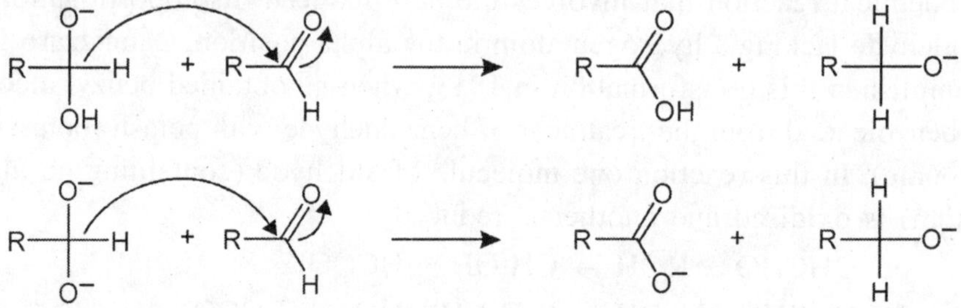

Only aldehydes that cannot form an enolate ion undergo the Cannizzaro reaction. The aldehyde cannot have an enolizable proton. Under the basic conditions that facilitate the reaction, aldehydes that can form an enolate instead undergo aldol condensation. Examples of aldehydes that can undergo a Cannizzaro reaction include formaldehyde and aromatic aldehydes such as benzaldehyde.

Beckmann rearrangement

The **Beckmann rearrangement**, named after the German chemist Ernst Otto Beckmann (1853–1923), is an acid-catalyzed rearrangement of an oxime to an amide. Cyclic oximes yield lactams.

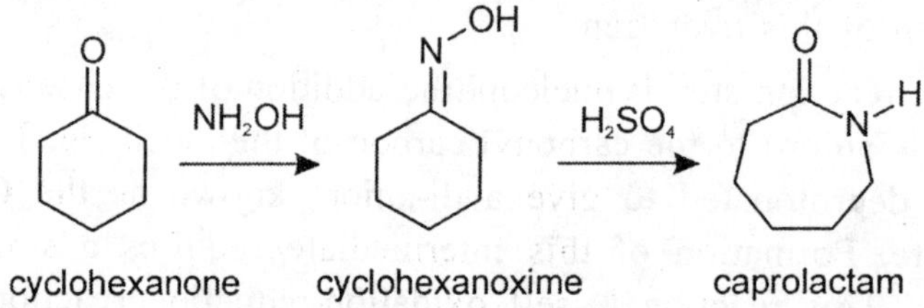

cyclohexanone   cyclohexanoxime   caprolactam

The above reaction starting with cyclohexanone, forming the reaction intermediate cyclohexanonoxime and resulting in caprolactam is one of the most important applications of the Beckmann rearrangement, as caprolactam is the feedstock in the production of Nylon 6.

The **Beckmann solution** consists of acetic acid, hydrochloric acid and acetic anhydride, and was widely used to catalyze the rearrangement. Other acids, such as sulfuric acid or polyphosphoric acid, can also be used sulfuric acid is the most commonly used acid for commercial lactam production due to its formation of an ammonium sulfate by-product when neutralized with ammonia. Ammonium sulfate is a common agricultural fertilizer providing nitrogen and sulfur.

Reaction mechanism

The reaction mechanism of the Beckmann rearrangement is generally believed to consist of an alkyl migration with expulsion of the hydroxyl group to form a nitrilium ion followed by hydrolysis.

In one study, the mechanism is established taking into account the presence of solvent molecules and substituents. The rearrangement of acetone oxime in the Beckmann solution involves three acetic acid molecules and one proton (present as an oxonium ion). In the transition state leading to the iminium ion (σ - complex), the methyl group migrates to the nitrogen atom in a concerted reaction and the hydroxyl group is expulsed. The oxygen atom in the hydroxyl group is stabilized by the three acetic acid molecules. In the next step the electrophilic carbon atom in the nitrilium ion is attacked by water and the proton is donated back to acetic acid. In the transition state leading to the N-methyl acetimidic acid, the water oxygen atom is coordinated to 4 other atoms. In the third step, an isomerization step protonates the nitrogen atom leading to the amide.

Pinacol rearrangement

The pinacol rearrangement or pinacol-pinacolone rearrangement is a method for converting a 1,2-diol to a carbonyl compound in organic chemistry. This rearrangement takes place under acidic conditions. The name of the reaction comes from the rearrangement of pinacol to pinacolone.

In the course of this organic reaction, protonation of one of the –OH groups occurs and a carbocation is formed. If both the –OH groups are not alike, then the one which yields a more stable carbocation participates in the reaction. Subsequently, an alkyl group from the adjacent carbon migrates to the carbocation center. The driving force for this rearrangement step is believed to be the relative stability of the resultant oxonium ion, which has complete octet configuration at all centers (as opposed to the preceding carbocation). The migration of alkyl groups in this reaction occurs in accordance with their usual migratory aptitude, i.e. hydride > Ph— > tertiary > secondary > methyl.

Hofmann's bromamide reaction or degradation

By this method the amide (–$CONH_2$) group is converted into primary amino (– NH_2) group.

$$R \mid CO \mid NH_2 + Br_2 + 4KOH \rightarrow R - NH_2 + 2KBR + K_2CO_3 + 2H_2O$$

  Amide   Pri-amine

This is the most convenient method for preparing primary amines. This method gives an amine containing one carbon atom less than amide.

The reaction is named after its discoverer: August Wilhelm von Hofmann. This reaction is also sometimes called the **Hofmann degradation**, and should not be confused with the Hofmann elimination.

Mechanism

The reaction of bromine with sodium hydroxide forms sodium hypobromite *in situ*, which transforms the primary amide into an intermediate isocyanate. The intermediate isocyanate is hydrolyzed to a primary amine giving off carbon dioxide.

Chapter 15
STEREOCHEMISTRY OF CARBON COMPOUNDS: ISOMERISM

➤ **Introduction**
➤ **Isomerism**
➤ **Optical Isomerism**
➤ **RS nomenclature**
➤ **Geometrical Isomerism**
➤ **E-Z system**
➤ **Conformational isomerism**

ISOMERS

Isomers are molecules that have the same molecular formula, but have a different arrangement of the atoms in space. That excludes any different arrangements which are simply due to the molecule rotating as a whole, or rotating about particular bonds and this phenomenon is known as Isomerism.

Isomerism is of broadly two types:

1. Structural Isomerism and
2. Stereoisomerism

Structural Isomerism

Structural isomerism, or constitutional isomerism (per IUPAC), is a form of isomerism in which molecules with the same molecular formula have bonded together in different orders, as opposed to stereoisomerism. There are multiple synonyms for constitutional isomers. This isomerism arises due to difference in the simple structure of the compounds. It may be of various types viz Chain isomerism, position isomerism,functional isomerism, metamerism etc

Chain or Skeletal isomerism

If compounds have same molecular formulae but there is difference in the chain of C atoms, then this phenomenon is known as Chain isomerism. C_5H_{10} shows 3 chain isomers.

n-Pentane	Isopentane	Neopentane

Position isomerism

In position isomerism a functional group or other substituent changes position on a parent structure. In the table below, the hydroxyl group can occupy three different positions on an n-pentane chain forming three different compounds.

Example of position isomerism

1-Pentanol	2-Pentanol	3-Pentanol

Functional isomers are structural isomers that have the same molecular formula but different functional groups, are functional isomers. For example, C_2H_6O shows ethanol (C_2H_5OH) and ether CH_3OCH_3 functional isomers.

STEREO-ISOMERISM

Stereoisomers have identical molecular formulas and arrangements of atoms. They differ from each other only in the spatial orientation of groups in the molecule. This phenomenon is known as stereo-isomerism. It is of two types, Geometrical and Optical isomerism.

Geometrical Isomerism

Geometrical isomerism is a kind of stereoisomerism. The isomerism due to the difference in spatial arrangements of groups about the doubly bonded carbon atoms is known as **Geometrical Isomerism.** The simplest forms of this isomerism are *cis* and *trans* isomers, both of which are created by the restricted rotation about a double bond or ring system. Butene, C_4H_8, exists in both *cis* and *trans* forms.

cis-butene-I   trans-butene-II

The two CH_3 groups lie on the same side in I and on the opposite sides in II. When two similar atoms or groups lie on the same side, the isomerism is called cis isomerism and the isomers are called cis isomers (cis means "on same side" in Latin). When two similar atoms or groups lie on opposite sides, the isomerism is called trans isomerism and the isomers are called trans isomers (trans means "across" in Latin). Geometrical isomerism is also called Cis-trans isomerism.

Similarly, maleic and fumaric acids exhibit geometric isomerism or they are geometric isomers.

Maleic acid (cis form)   Fumaric acid (transform)

Just as the compounds containing carbon-carbon double bond can't rotate freely and hence exhibit geometric isomerism, those containing carbon nitrogen double bonds also exhibit geometrical isomerism. For e.g., alpha benzaldoxime and beta benzaldoxime are geometrical isomers.

alpha benzaldoxime   beta benzaldoxime
syn or cis form   anti or transform

E-Z system in Geometrical isomers

The traditional system for naming the geometric isomers of an alkene, in which the same groups are arranged differently, is cis or trans. However, it is easy to find examples where the cis-trans system is not easily applied. IUPAC has a more complete system for naming alkene isomers. The priority rules are often called the Cahn-Ingold-Prelog (CIP) rules, after the chemists who developed the system. According to this rule, priority is given to the groups attached to the double bonded carbon atom on the basis of atomic number.

The general strategy of the E-Z system is to analyze the two groups at each end of the double bond. At each end, rank the two groups, using the CIP priority rules (given with optical isomerism). Then, see whether the higher priority group at one end of the double bond and the higher priority group at the other end of the double bond are on the **same** side (Z, from German zusammen = together) or on **opposite** sides (E, from German entgegen = opposite) of the double bond.

Example:

The Figure below shows the two isomers of 2-butene. We should recognize them as cis and trans. Let's analyze them to see whether they are E or Z. Start with the left hand structure (the cis isomer). On C2 (the left end of the double bond), the two atoms attached to the double bond are C and H. By the CIP priority rules, C is higher priority than H (higher atomic number). Now look at C3 (the right end of the double bond). Similarly, the atoms

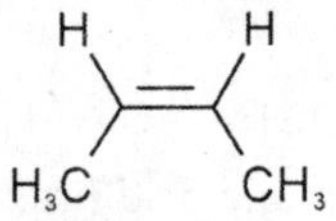

cis-2-butene
(z)-2-butene

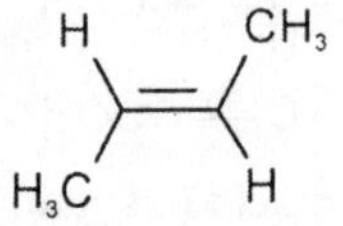

trans-2-butene
(E)-2-butene

are C and H, with C being higher priority. We see that the higher priority group is "down" at C2 and "down" at C3. Since the two priority groups are both on the **same** side of the double bond ("down", in this case), they are zusammen = together. Therefore, this is (Z)-2-butene. Now look at the right hand structure (the trans isomer). In this case, the priority group is "down" on the left end of the double bond and "up" on the right end of the double bond. Since the two priority groups are on **opposite** sides of the double bond, they are entgegen = opposite. Therefore, this is (E)-2-butene.

In the next example below, at the left-hand end of the bond, it turns out that bromine has a higher priority than fluorine. And on the right-hand end, it turns out that chlorine has a higher priority than hydrogen.in the 1st figure higher priority groups are on the same side about double bond hence this is Z form and second form is E form.

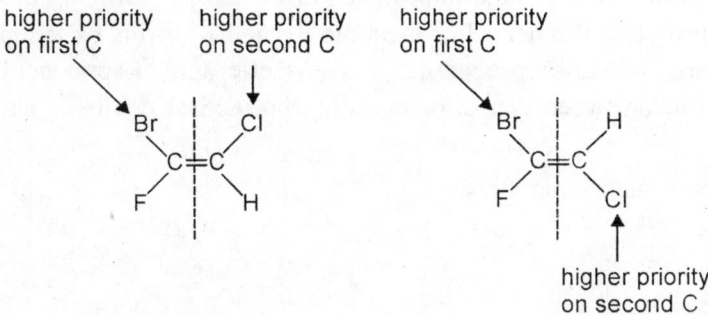

OPTICAL ISOMERISM

Optical isomerism is a form of stereoisomerism. **Optical isomers** are molecules that differ three-dimensionally by the placement of substituents around one or more atoms in a molecule. **Optical isomers** were given their name because they were first able to be distinguished by how they rotated plane-polarized light. These molecules are not necessarily locked into their positions, but cannot be converted into one another, even by a rotation around a single bond.

Optical isomers are named like this because of their effect on plane polarised light. The compounds which can rotate the angle of plane polarized light are known as optically active compounds or **Optical isomers**. If it rotates the light clockwise (as seen by a viewer towards whom the light is traveling), that enantiomer is labeled (+). Its mirror-image is labeled (−). The (+) and (−) isomers have also been termed $d+$ and $l-$, respectively (for *dextrorotatory* and *levorotatory*). The plane polarized light has vibration in one plane only, as shown below.

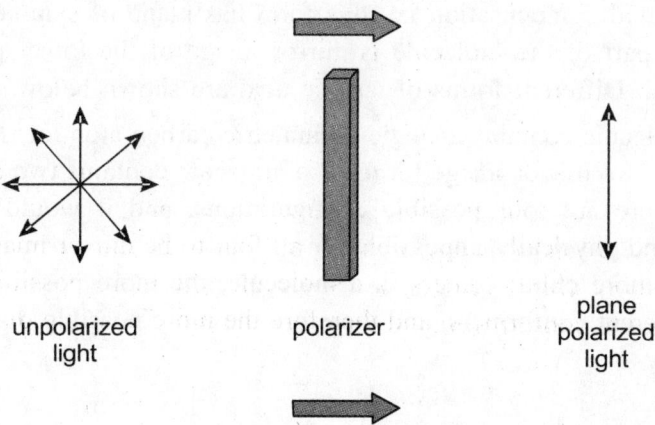

Enantiomers: Non-superimposable mirror images forms of a compound are known as Enantiomers. For example d+ and l– forms of lactic acid are enantiomers. 2-hydroxypropanoic acid is lactic acid. Lactic acid has one chiral centre or stereo centre or chiral carbo. Chiral centre is shown by a star.

The two enantiomers are:

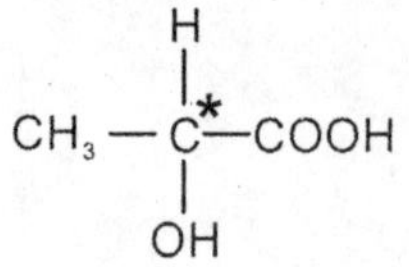

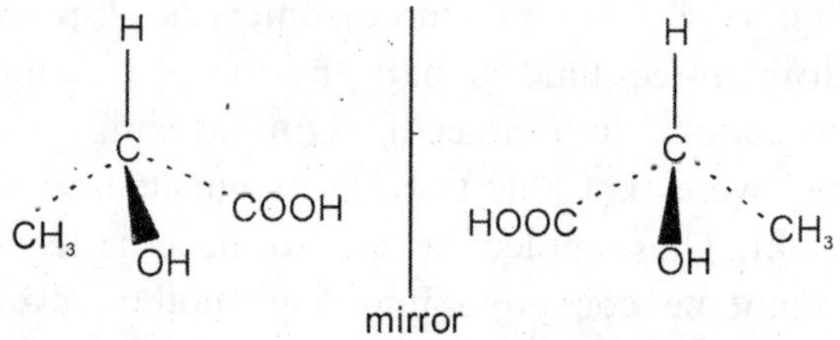

$$CH_3 - \overset{\overset{\displaystyle H}{|}}{\underset{\underset{\displaystyle OH}{|}}{C}} \overset{*}{-} COOH$$

Only one of these isomers occurs naturally: the (+) form.

Diastereomers are stereoisomers that are not enantiomers (mirror images) of each other. Due to their different shape, diastereomers can have different physical and chemical properties. This is perhaps especially true of diastereomers involved in biological systems.

Racemic mixture: This is the equimolar mixture of d+ (dextro) and l-(laevo) forms of same compound .This is optically inactive due to external compensation.

Meso form: This is the form of a compound which is optically inactive due to internal compensation i.e. this form has plane of symmetry so that upper half part of the molecule is mirror image of the lower part like in tartaric acid. Different forms of tartaric acid are shown below.

If a molecule contains a single asymmetric carbon atom or *stereocenter*, it will have two mirror image forms. If a molecule contains two asymmetric carbons, there are four possible configurations, and it would be mathematically and physically impossible for all four to be mirror images of each other. The more chiral centers in a molecule, the more possibilities there are for different conformers, and therefore the more possible diastereomers exist.

As an example, tartaric acid contains two asymmetric centers, but two of the configurations of the tartaric acid molecule are equivalent to one another — and together they are called meso compounds. This configuration is not optically active, while the remaining two configurations are D- and L-mirror images. For this reason, the meso form of tartaric acid is a diastereomer of the other forms.

COOH	COOH	COOH	COOH
H—OH	HO—H	H—OH =	HO—H
HO—H	H—OH	H—OH	HO—H
COOH	COOH	COOH	COOH

HO COOH	HO COOH	HO COOH	HO COOH
HO COOH	HO COOH	HO COOH =	HO COOH

(natural) tartaric acid	D–(–)–tartaric acid	mesotartaric acid
L–(+)–tartaric acid	levotartaric acid	

(1:1)

DL-tartaric acid "racemic acid"

The meso form of tartaric acid (right) is a diastereomer of the other forms

Examples of carbohydrates

The families of 5 and 6 carbon carbohydrates contain many diastereomers because of the large numbers of asymmetric centers in these molecules. Since each carbon in the primary chain of an aldose (one type of carbohydrate) and all but one of the carbons in in the primary chain of a ketose (another type of carbohydrate) have both a hydrogen and a hydroxyl group attached, most of the carbons in any given sugar are actually chiral. Since the number of possible conformers for a chiral molecule is 2 raised to the n power (2^n), where n is the number of chiral centers, this makes for a great deal of variability in carbohydrates and a large number of diastereomers.

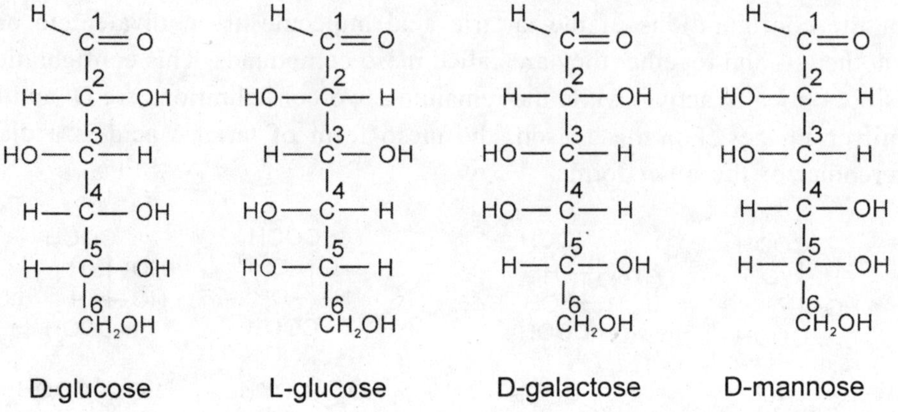

D-glucose   L-glucose   D-galactose   D-mannose

D-glucose and L-glucose are enantiomers. Other pairs of sugars
(e.g. L-glucose and D-mannose) are diastereomers.

Glucose adopts a ring structure in solution. This is awkward to show with a Fischer projection so a Haworth projection is usually used instead:

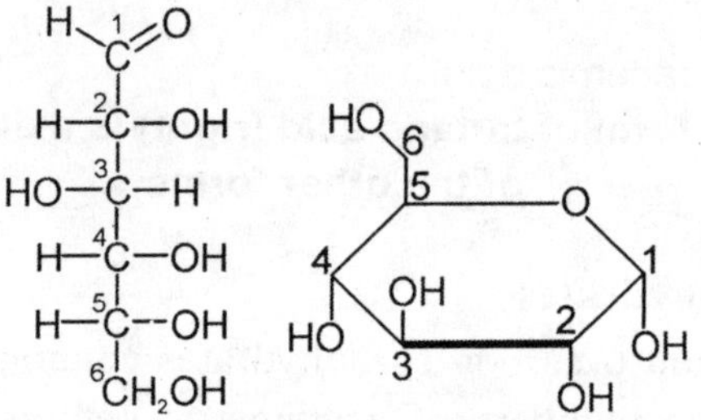

Theoretical concept of Optical Activity: Chirality

Necessary conditions to show optical activity is that the molecule should not have any type of symmetry viz , axis or plane or centre of symmetry. The molecule should be unsymmetrical i.e chiral. The term **chiral** (pronounced as 'kairel') in general is used to describe an object that is non-superimposable on its mirror image. Only chiral molecules have optical isomers. In other words, if one isomer looked in a mirror, what it would see is the other one. The two isomers (the original one and its mirror image) have a different spatial arrangement, and so can't be superimposed on each other. If an *achiral* molecule (one *with* a plane of symmetry) looked in a mirror, you would always find that by rotating the image in space, you could make the two look identical. It *would* be possible to superimpose the original molecule and its mirror image.

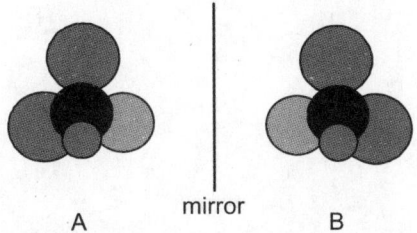

A   mirror   B

Let us take example of *Butan-2-ol*-optical isomers

$$CH_3-\overset{\underset{|}{H}}{\underset{\underset{|}{OH}}{C^*}}-CH_2-CH_3$$

It's extremely important to draw the isomers correctly. Draw one of them using standard bond notation to show the 3-dimensional arrangement around the asymmetric carbon atom. Then draw the mirror to show the examiner that you know what you are doing, and then the mirror image, Notice that you don't literally draw the mirror images of all the letters and numbers! It is, however, quite useful to reverse large groups-look, for example, at the ethyl group at the top of the diagram It doesn't matter in the least in what order you draw the four groups around the central carbon. As long as your mirror image is drawn accurately, you will automatically have drawn the two isomers

```
    CH₂CH₃              CH₃CH₂
       |                   |
       C                   C
  CH₃  ⁞  ⁞H        H⁞   ⁞   CH₃
       ▲                ▲
      OH                OH
              mirror
```

2-aminopropanoic acid (alanine)

This is typical of naturally-occurring amino acids. Structurally, it is just like the last example, except that the –OH group is replaced by $-NH_2$

$$CH_3-\overset{\underset{|}{H}}{\underset{\underset{|}{NH_2}}{C^*}}-COOH$$

The two enantiomers are:

mirror

Only one of these isomers occurs naturally: the (+) form. You can't tell just by looking at the structures which this is. It has, however, been possible to work out which of these structures is which. Naturally occurring alanine is the right-hand structure, and the way the groups are arranged around the central carbon atom is known as an **L-** configuration. Notice the use of the *capital* L. The other configuration is known as **D-**. So you may well find alanine described as *L–(+)alanine*. That means that it has this particular structure and rotates the plane of polarisation clockwise. Even if you know that a different compound has an arrangement of groups similar to alanine, you still can't say which way it will rotate the plane of polarisation. The other amino acids, for example, have the same arrangement of groups as alanine does (all that changes is the CH_3 group), but some are (+) forms and others are (–) forms.

R/S NOMENCLATURE

The *R /S* system has no fixed relation to the (+)/(–) system or D/L system. An *R* isomer can be either dextrorotatory or levorotatory, depending on its exact substituents. R/S is assigned by using a system for ranking priority of the groups attached to each stereocenter. Stereocentre is also known as chiral centre, a chiral center is characterised by an atom that has four different groups bonded to it in such a manner (*e.g.* tetrahedral) that it has a non-superimposable mirror image. Terms such as an asymmetric, or stereogenic are used. The procedure, often known as *the sequence rules*, is the heart of the CIP system.

In order to assign the configuration as R or S:

- Identify each of the chirality centers (most commonly an sp³ C with 4 different groups attached).
- Priority to each group attached to chiral carbon as per CIP rules.
- Assignment of R/S configuretion

Cahn-Ingold-Prelog (CIP) rules : Steps for naming

1. Compare the atomic number (Z) of the atoms directly attached to

the stereocenter; the group having the atom of higher atomic number receives higher priority.

2. If there is a tie, we must consider the atoms at distance 2 from the stereocenter as a list is made for each group of the atoms bonded to the one directly attached to the stereocenter. Each list is arranged in order of decreasing atomic number. Then the lists are compared atom by atom; at the earliest difference, the group containing the atom of higher atomic number receives higher priority.

3. If there is still a tie, each atom in each of the two lists is replaced with a sub-list of the other atoms bonded to it (at distance 3 from the stereocenter), the sub-lists are arranged in decreasing order of atomic number, and the entire structure is again compared atom by atom. This process is repeated, each time with atoms one bond farther from the stereocenter, until the tie is broken.

Then at each chirality center....

- Assign the priority (high = 1 to low = 4) to each group attached to the chirality center based on atomic number.
- Reposition the molecule so that the **lowest priority group** *is away from you* as if you were looking along the C-(4) ó bond. If you are using a model, grasp the lowest priority group in your fist.
- Determine the relative direction of the priority order of the three higher priority groups (1 to 2 to 3)
- If this is **clockwise** then it is the **R**-stereoisomer (Latin; *rectus* = right handed)
- If this is **counter-clockwise** then it is the **S**-stereoisomer (Latin; *sinister* = left handed)
- If there is more than one stereocenter, then the location needs to be included with the locant,

Subrules:

- Isotopes: H vs D? Since isotopes have identical atomic numbers, the mass number is used to discriminate them so D > H
- If the same atom is attached, then look for the first point of difference by moving out **one atom** at a time, locate the first point of difference and apply rules there.
- If a multiple bond is encountered, treat it as if the atoms are attached by the same number of single bonds *e.g.* C = C is treated a 2 C – C and C = O is 2 C – O

Another way for R/S

Determining *R/S* Nomenclature **at a Glance in** Three Easy Steps

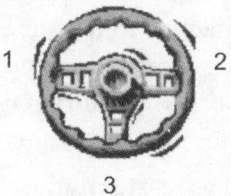

With this method you never **have to switch** groups to see what the stereochemistry is. Using the "drive-the-car" analogy, what we are doing here is defining the steering wheel in relation to the steering column (which is normally **behind** the steering wheel):

1. **Determine the priorities of the four attached groups from highest (1) to lowest (4).**

    This is the same as in previous.

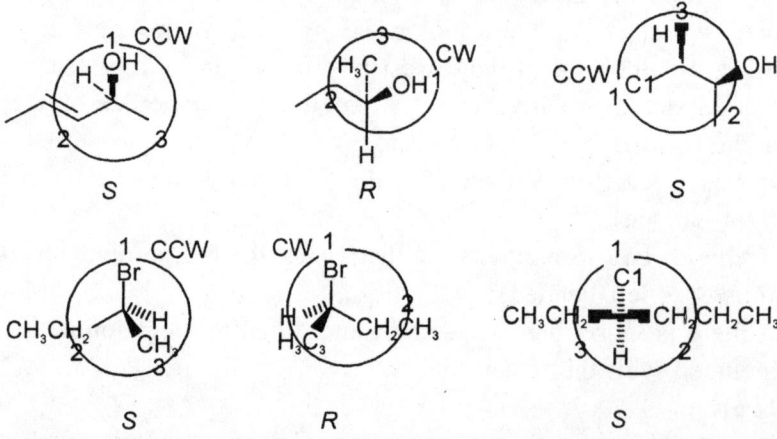

2. **Draw the steering wheel.** Draw a curved arrow around from 1 to 2 to 3 and back to 1 and note which direction this arrow goes, clockwise (cw) or counterclockwise (ccw).

    The distinct feature of this method is that you make a full circle, from 1 to 2 to 3 to 1, completely ignoring the lowest priority group.

3a. If the lowest priority group is *behind* the steering wheel, then *this is the standard orientation:* **clockwise is *R*** and counter-clockwise is *S*.(Turning the steering wheel **clockwise** turns the car to the **right—R.**)

Note that Fischer projections are best depicted as "bow ties" with horizontal groups coming out and vertical groups going back from the central carbon atom.

3b. If the lowest priority group is *in front of* this curved arrow, then the assignment is reversed: clockwise is *S* and counterclockwise is *R*. (Basically, we are looking at the steering wheel from the perspective of the engine compartment). Some examples are given below.

In this compound after giving priority, rotation 1 → 3 is counter (or anti) clockwise, but lowest priority group is in front of us, so this will be reverse of S i.e. it **is R.**

This compound has1 → 3 counter clockwise (simultaneously lowest priority is away from us, so it will be as counter clockwise = S.

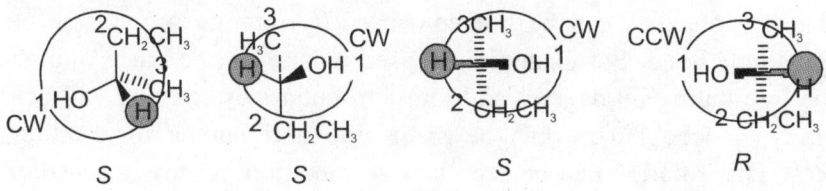

S	*S*	*S*	*R*

CONFORMATIONAL ISOMERISM

In chemistry, **conformational isomerism** is a form of stereoisomerism in which the isomers can be interconverted exclusively by rotations about formally single bonds and are often rapidly interconverting at room temperature. Such isomers are generally referred to as **conformational isomers** or **conformers** and specifically as **rotamers** when they differ by rotation about only one single bond. Conformational isomers are thus distinct from the other classes of stereoisomers for which interconversion necessarily involves breaking and reforming of chemical bonds. The rotational barrier is the activation energy required to interconvert rotamers. Generally saturated hydrocarbons (Alkanes and cycloalkanes) show this phenomenon. **Conformational isomers** are normally best represented by Newman Projections. For example, eclipsed, gauche, and anti butane are all **conformational isomers** of one another.

The Dutch chemist J. H. Van't Hoff based the stereochemical hypothesis he formulated (1874–75) on two principal postulates: (1) the valences of the saturated carbon atom are oriented in space toward the vertices of the tetrahedrons, and (2) the atoms or groups of atoms (substituents) in the molecule can freely rotate about single bonds without breaking them (unlike double bonds whose rigidity causes the formation of geometric isomers).

Eclipsed means that identical groups are all directly in-line with one another, *gauche (or skew)* means that identical groups are 60 degrees or from one another, and *anti* means that identical groups are 180 degrees from one another.) In the skew forms angle may vary hence skew form will be many while eclipsed and anti forms will be one each.

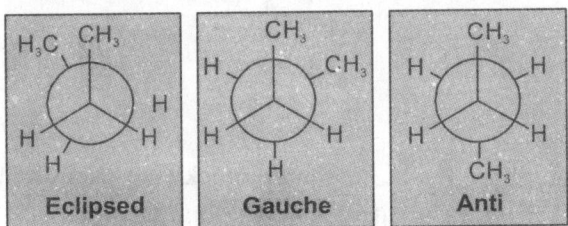

These molecules can be interconverted by rotating around the central carbon single bond. For example, eclipsed butane can be made into gauche butane by rotating 60 degrees and into anti butane by rotating 180 degrees. Similarly, gauche butane can be made into anti butane by rotating 120 degrees. This rotation can be seen in the animation below. Because of this rotational property, eclipsed, gauche, and anti butane are **conformational isomers** of one another.

The simple alkane ethane provides a good introduction to conformational analysis. Here there is only one carbon-carbon bond, and the rotational structures (rotamers) that it may assume fall between two extremes, **staggered** and **eclipsed**. In the following description of these conformers, several structural notations are used. The first views the ethane molecule from the side, with the carbon-carbon bond being horizontal to the viewer.

The hydrogens **are** then located in the surrounding space by **wedge** (in front of the plane) and **hatched** (behind the plane) bonds. If this structure is rotated so that carbon #1 is canted down and brought closer to the viewer, the "sawhorse" projection is presented. Finally, if the viewer looks down the carbon-carbon bond with carbon #1 in front of #2, the Newman projection is seen.

Extreme Conformations of Ethane

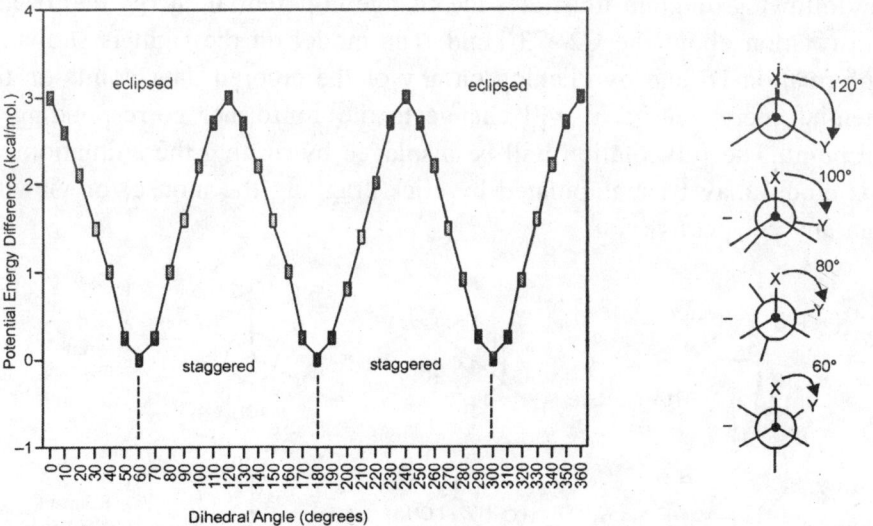

Potential Energy Profile for Ethane Conformers　Dihedral Angle

As a result of bond-electron repulsions, the eclipsed conformation is less stable than the staggered conformation by roughly 3 kcal/mol (eclipsing strain). In the staggered conformation there are six equal bond repulsions, four of which are shown by the blue arrows, and these are all substantially less severe than the three strongest eclipsed repulsions. Consequently, the potential energy associated with the various conformations of ethane varies with the **dihedral angle** of the bonds, as shown in the diagram. Although the conformers of ethane are in rapid equilibrium with each other, the 3 kcal/mol energy difference leads to a substantial preponderance of staggered conformers (> 99.9%) at any given time.

Butane Conformations

The hydrocarbon butane has a larger and more complex set of conformations associated with its constitution than does ethane. Of particular interest and importance are the conformations produced by rotation about the central carbon-carbon bond. Among these we shall focus on two staggered conformers (**A & C**) and two eclipsed conformers (**B & D**), shown below in several stereo-representations. As in the case of ethane, the staggered conformers are more stable than the eclipsed conformers by 2.8 to 4.5 kcal/mol. Since the staggered conformers represent the chief components of a butane sample they have been given the identifying prefix designations **anti** for A and **gauche** for C.

Four Conformers of Butane

The following diagram illustrates the change in potential energy that occurs with rotation about the C2–C3 bond. The model on the right is shown in conformation **D**, and by clicking on any of the colored data points on the potential energy curve, it will change to the conformer corresponding to that point. The full rotation will be displayed by turning the animation on. This model may be manipulated by click-dragging the mouse for viewing from any perspective.

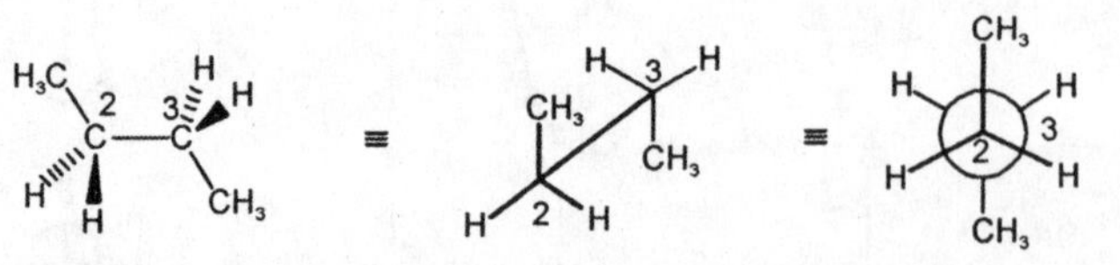

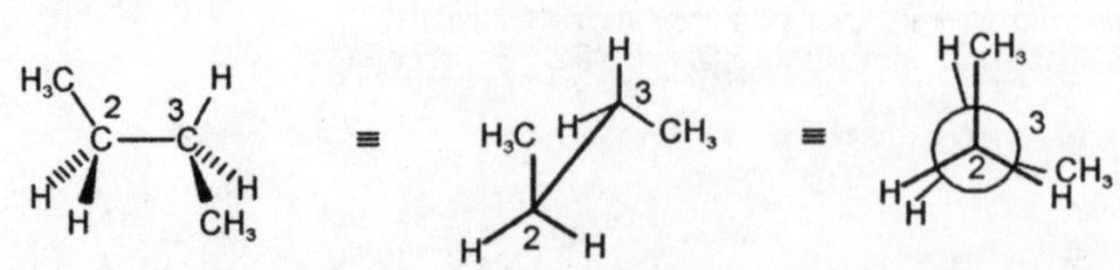

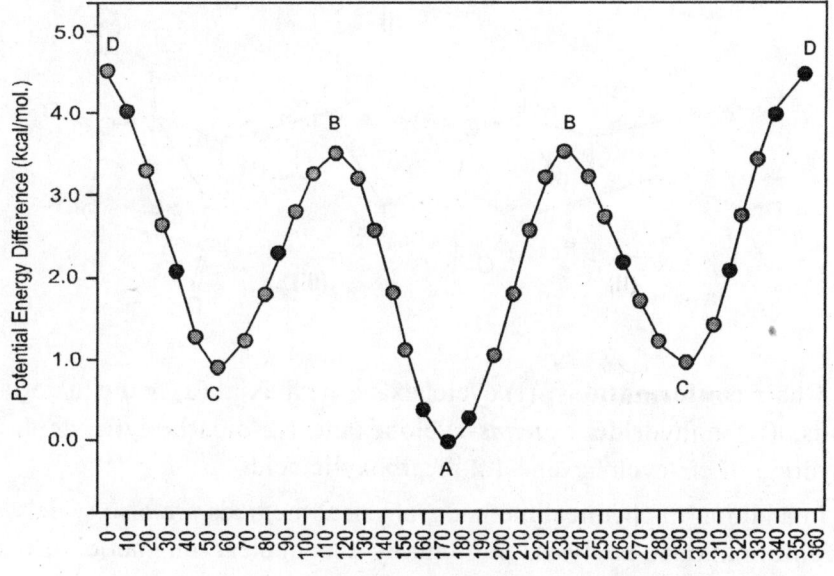

Potential Energy Profile for Butane Conformers

Conformational representations are highly important in explaining the properties of cyclic compounds, especially in the series derived from **cyclohexane**. The last primarily occurs in the chair form, which is particularly favorable since the valency angles are not distorted and the conformations along all the C—C bonds are odd (Figure given below). The remaining two valence bonds of each ring carbon atom are either oriented perpendicularly to the ring (axial bonds—a) or are directed along its periphery (equatorial bonds—e). The equatorial distribution of substituents is more favorable. For example, at room temperature, the conformational equilibrium of chlorocyclohexane e:a = 70:30. When the temperature is lowered to −150°C, the interconversion rate is sharply reduced; under these conditions it is possible to isolate the pure e-form of chlorocyclohexane. A conformational analysis of the cyclohexane ring enables one, for example, to understand the reason why both *cis-* and *trans-* cyclohexane-1,2-dicarboxylic acid can form an anhydride (in both cases the dihedral angle between the bonds leading to the COOH groups is 60°).

(I)

(II)   (III)

Chair conformations: (I) cyclohexane with axial (a) and equatorial (e) bonds, (II) anhydride of *trans*-cyclohexane-1,2-dicarboxylic acid, (III) anhydride of *cis*-cyclohexane-1,2-dicarboxylic acid

In addition to chemical methods, physical methods are also widely used in conformational analysis, particularly the nuclear magnetic resonance method. The data obtained on the conformations of organic compounds serve as an important basis for the interpretation and prediction of the properties of the compounds. Conformational representations have assumed great importance in the chemistry of synthetic and natural macromolecular compounds, as well as in the field of physiologically active substances.

It is useful to summarize some important aspects of conformational stereoisomerism .

    (i) Most conformational interconversions in simple molecules occur rapidly at room temperature. Consequently, isolation of pure conformers is usually not possible.

    (ii) Specific conformers require special nomenclature terms such as *staggered, eclipsed, gauche* and *anti* when they are designated.

(iii) Specific conformers may also be designated by dihedral angles. In the butane conformers shown above, the dihedral angles formed by the two methyl groups about the central double bond are: **A** 180°, **B** 120°, **C** 60° & **D** 0°.

(iv) Staggered conformations about carbon-carbon single bonds are more stable (have a lower potential energy) than the corresponding eclipsed conformations. The higher energy of eclipsed bonds is known as **eclipsing strain**.

(v) In butane the gauche-conformer is less stable than the anti-conformer by about 0.9 kcal/mol. This is due to a crowding of the two methyl groups in the gauche structure, and is called **steric strain** or **steric hindrance**.

(vi) Butane conformers B and C have non-identical mirror image structures in which the clockwise dihedral angles are 300° and 240° respectively. These pairs are energetically the same, and have not been distinguished in the potential energy diagram shown here.

QUESTION BANK

INORGANIC AND ORGANIC CONCEPT

1. What is molecular orbital theory? With the help of molecular orbital diagram, calculate the bond order of (i) O_2 (ii) O_2^2 (iii) He_2 (iv) NO^- (v) N_2 (vi) NO

2. Which of the following is paramagnetic? Explain with MO configuration.

   O_2^-, O_2^{2-}, N_2, CN HF

3. Explain on the basis of molecular orbital theory

   (i) Be_2 molecule is not stable

   (ii) F_2 is diamagnetic while O_2 is paramagnetic

4. Give the essential features of valence bond theory and molecular orbital theories?

5. Explain the terms giving examples:

   (a) bonding molecular orbitals

   (b) anti bonding molecular orbitals

   (c) non bonding molecular orbitals

   (d) bond order

   (e) Give the molecular orbital configuration of CO or NO molecule?

6. Explain band theory of solids? With the help of band theory explain conductors, semiconductors and insulators?

7. What is hybridization? Predict the type of hybridization and geometry of following

   a. (i) XeO_3 (ii) NH_3 (iii) H_2O (iv) PCl_5 (v) SO_2

   b. CH_4, NH_3 H_2O have tetrahedral geometry yet their bond angles are different. Why?

   c. Write hybridization of each C atom of following molecule

   $$CH_3 - CH = C = CH_2$$

8. What are liquid crystals? Classify them? Mention applications of liquid crystals?

9. Derive Bragg's equation for diffraction of X rays by crystals?

10. Explain hydrogen bonding and types. On the basis of hydrogen bonding explain

    a. H_2O is liquid whereas hydrides of this group like H_2Se are gases.

    b. Ethanol has higher B.P. than diethyl ether

11. Write short notes on the following with examples

    (a) Mesomeric effect

    (b) electromeric effect

    (c) Inductive effect

    (d) Hyperconjugation

12. Write a note on carbo-cation and carbanions and which of the following is least stable carbanion?

    a. (i) $(CH_3)_3 \ C^-$ (ii) H_3C^- (iii) $(CH_3)_2CH^-$ (iv) Cl_3C^-

    b. Classify the following into electrophilic and nucleophilic reagents.

    (i) H^+ (ii) Cl^- (iii) NO_2^- (iv) OH^-

13. What are Cannizzaro's reaction & aldol condensation

14. Write two applications of the following with mechanism

    (i) Beckmann's rearrangement

    (ii) Hoffmann's rearrangement

15 (a) Explain optical isomerism of chiral organic compounds and give two examples of organic compounds showing optical isomerism without chirality?

    (b) Which of the following isomeric compounds show optical isomerism:

        (i) 2-aminopentane

        (ii) 3-aminopentane

        (iii) 2, 2-dimethyl propyl amine

        (iv) 1-aminopentane

16. What do you understand by E-Z and R-S configuration

17. Explain why ice floats on water and differentiate between bonding and antibonding molecular orbital?

18. Explain hyperconjugation and on the basis of hyperconjugation explain which one is more stable and why?

    (i) ethene (ii) propene (iii) but-2-ene

19. Arrange the given species in the order of increasing stability and predict their magnetic behaviour by using   molecular orbital theory: NO^+, CO and CN^-

20. Explain why o-nitrophenol is volatile and p-nitrophenol not.

21. Write the Hoffman reaction and Pinnacol-Pinnacolone rearrangement with their application?

22. Write a note on Fullerene with its application.

23. Explain with example – SN_1 and SN_2 reaction.

24. Write the types of elimination reaction. Explain saytzeff rule.

25. Explain electrophilic and nucleophilic substitution reaction with one example of each.

KINETIC, ELECTROCHEMISTRY AND WATER CHEMISTRY

1. Derive the   integrated expression($k = x/t.a.(a - x)$) for IInd order reaction. If half life for Ist order reaction is 15 mins then what % of initial amount will be left after 45 mins.

2. Derive the integrated expression for Zero and Ist order reaction with their half lives.

3. What do you mean by Molecularity and order of the reaction. Derive first order rate expression. Also find out the derivation for half life.

4. Define activation energy. Explain how the rise in temperature will effect the rate of reaction .The specific rate constant for a reaction increases by a factor 4 if the temperature changes from 300K to 327K Calculate the energy of activation for such reaction .

5. Write short notes on

    a. Steady state approximation

    b. Threshold energy and activation energy

    c. Energy barrier

6. Derive the relation ship between half life and average life for Ist order reaction. A first order reaction takes 69.3 minutes for 50% completion. How much time will be needed for 80% completion?

7. A reaction $A_2 + 2B \rightarrow 2AB$ is first order w.r.t both A_2 and B. Derive the rate equation in terms of a, b, x, t and k, where a and b are the initial concentrations of A_2 and B respectively. x is the concentration of AB at any time t and k is the rate constant.

8. If a Ist order reaction is 40% completed in 30mins then how much time it will take to complete 80%.

9. Show that in case of a Ist order reaction, the time required for 99.9% of the reaction to take place is about 10 times that required for half the reaction.

10. What is corrosion. Discuss the types. Explain Electrochemical theory of wet corrosion.

Or

11. Reduction potentials of some elements are given as-

A = +1.2 V

B = –2.21

C = 1.85 and

D = –1.5

   (i) Which can displace hydrogen from its solution.

   (ii) which will be suitable for Cathode and Anode in the electrochemical cell.

   (iii) Arrange elements in the order of increasing corroding nature.

  (b) Define kohlraush law or Nerst distribution law with its application.

  (c) Define Buffer solution. If solubility of $MgCl_2$ is 0.2 mol/litre, calculate its solubility product.

12. Define kohlraush law or molar conductivity. If λ° of weak electrolyte (AB) is 0.036 and λ^c is 0.020 then calculate the degree of dissociation.

13. Explain the anodic method of protection from corrosion.

14. If electrode potentials (V) of elements are given as-

A = + 1.2

B = –2.21

C = 1.85 and

D = –1.5

   (i) Which can displace hydrogen from its solution

   (ii) which is strongest reducing and oxidizing agent

   (iii) Arrange elements in the order of increasing corroding nature.

15. (a) Two copper rods are placed in copper sulphate solution of concentration 0.1M and 0.01M separately in the form of a cell. Write the scheme of the cell and calculate its EMF at 298 K.

(b) Distinguish between degree of corrosion of aluminium (E°_{red} = –1.66V) and magnesium (E°_{red} = – 2.37V)

16. Calculate the hardness of a water sample containing the following and amount of lime and soda required for the treatment of 5000litre water.

$CaSO_4$ = 56 ppm; $Mg(HCO_3)_2$ = 10 ppm; $MgCl_2$ = 9.5 ppm and $CaCl_2$ = 10 ppm

17. Explain the Zeolite process for the removal of hardness of water. A Zeolite softener was exhausted when 10,000 liters of hard water was passed through it. The softener required 200 liters of NaCl solution (50g/l of NaCl solution). What is the hardness of water?

18. What id liquid junction potential. Calculate the cell potential for the cell containing 0.1 M Ag^+ and 4.0 M Cu^{2+} at 298 K .

Given, $E^0_{Ag+/Ag}$ = 0.80 V; $E^0_{Cu+2/Cu}$ = 0.34 V

19. What is Nernst equation. Oxidising potentials of some elements are given as—

$$A = +1.2\ V$$
$$B = -2.21$$
$$C = 1.85\ and$$
$$D = -1.5$$

1. Which can displace hydrogen from its solution.

2. For construction of cell, which should be made Cathode/Anode.

3. Which is the weakest reducing agent.

20. What are the specification for boiler feed water. Discuss the calgon conditioning process for internal treatment of boiler feed water

21. Explain Reverse Osmosis method of water treatment. Calculate the hardness of a water sample containing the following per litre and amount of lime and soda required.

$CaSO_4$ = 16.2 mg; $Mg(HCO_3)_2$ = 1.4 mg; $MgCl_2$ = 9.5 mg

CO_2 = 2mg

22. Explain Ion exchange method of water treatment. A Zeolite softener was exhausted when 10,000 liters of hard water was passed through

it. The softener required 200 liters of NaCl solution (50g/l of NaCl solution). What is the hardness of water?

23. Reduction potentials of some elements are given as-

$$A = +2.2 \text{ V}$$
$$B = -3.21$$
$$C = -2.75 \text{ and}$$
$$D = -1.9$$

   (i) Which can displace hydrogen from its solution.

   (ii) which will be suitable for Cathode and Anode in the electro-chemical cell.

   (iii) Arrange elements in the order of increasing corroding nature.

24. Define Nernst distribution law with its application. If saturated solubility of compound "x" is 2.3 and 3.6 mol/litre between water and benzene solvents then calculate the distribution coefficient.

25. Define Buffer solution. If solubility of $MgCl_2$ is 0.2 mol/litre, calculate its solubility product.

26. Define pH .Calculate the pH of 10^{-8} molar HCl solution.

27. Discuss cathodic and anodic method of protection from corrosion.

28. Define transport number and molar conductivity. If $\lambda°$ of weak electrolyte (AB) is 0.036 and λ^c is 0.020 then calculate the degree of dissociation .

29. Derive the relation ship between conductance and conductivity. What is the effect of dilution on conductance of weak electrolytes.

30. What is Henderson equation.what should be the molar ratio for acetic acid and sodium acetate to get buffer of 5.5 pH. pKa $= 1 \times 10^{-5}$

ENGINEERING MATERIALS

1. Write down the structure/formula for the monomers and polymers of the following:

   Polystyrene   PMMA   Nylon 6,6   PAN

2. Discuss briefly intrinsic conducting polymers and their applications.

3. Discuss the types of polymerization. Explain suspension poly-merization.

4. How will you convert propylene into natural rubber and discuss at least one advantage of vulcanization of rubber. Also differentiate

natural and synthetic rubber.

5. Discuss the monomer and polymer structure of polyurethanes and resins.

6. What do you understand by biodegradable polymers. Write the various types of polythenes and polyamides.

7. Differentiate between bulk polymerization and emeulsion polymerization.

8. What is glass. Write four types of glasses. Explain how toughened glass is made.

9. What are the main constituents in the ceramics. Give example of acid refractory and basic refractory.

10. What do you mean by Refractroy.Discuss the types and applications.

11. Write a note on "Nano composites with application".

12. What is the significance of Protective coating? Discuss cathodic or anodic coating.

13. Write the main 2-alloys of Fe, Al, Cu and Pb with their chemical composition and application.

14. Write a note on organometalics compounds and their application.

15. Write the synthesis of 3-types of organometalics with reaction and application.

16. Write short notes on-Neutral refractory and Grignard reagent.

17. Write the composition of various types of steel. What additives are added to provide hardness, stiffness, mechanical strength and anticorrosive property .

18. Write the composition of the following alloys-Gun metal, type metal, bronze, brass, duralumin and solder wire.

19. Write the names and structures of the polymers made from the following monomers?

    $CH_2 = CHCl$, $C_6H_5 = CH_2$, $CH_2 = CHCN$ and Methylmethacrylate.

20. Discuss the classification of Nanocomposites with their significance.

LUBRICANTS AND FUELS

1. Define lubricant and types of mechanism. Explain one mechanism of lubrication.

2. Write the classification of lubricants. Explain Bio-lubricants and synthetic lubricants.

3. Explain hydrodynamic lubrication and extreme high pressure lubrication with application.

4. Discuss the Thin film or fluid film lubrication mechanism and define Fire point, Flash Point, Consistency and drop point of lubricants.

5. Discuss semisolid or solid lubricants with applications.

6. Write short notes on-Viscosity index, cloud point, pour point and aniline point.

7. Define Bio-fuel. Explain esterification and transesterification with reaction.

8. Write notes on Coal, Bio gas and Biomass.

9. Define GCV and calculate the GCV and NCV of a fuel by using the given data of Bomb Calorimeter. Fuel weight = 1.25 gm, water weight = 3.5 kg, rise in temperature = 21 to 24.3°C, Water equivalent of calorimeter = 2.2 kg, fuse wire correction = 2.5 calories, acid correction = 1.7 calories, cooling correction = 0.8°C.

10. Write the classification of fuels. Calculate the amount of air required for complete combustion of 2kg carbon.

11. The following data is obtained in a Bomb calorimeter experiment :

Weight of crucible = 3.649 gm

Weight of crucible + fuel = 4.678 gm

Water equivalent of calorimeter = 570 gm

Water taken in the calorimeter = 2200gm

Observed rise in the temperature = 2.3°C

Cooling correction = 0.047°C

Acid correction = 62.6 calories

Fuse wire correction = 3.8 calories

Cotton thread correction = 1.6 calories

Calculate the Gross calorific value of the fuel sample. If the fuel contain 6.5% H determine the Net calorific value

12. Calculate the mass of air needed for complete combustion of 5Kg coal containing 80% C, 15 % H and rest oxygen.

13. Derive the relationship between GCV and NCV of a fuel. Bomb Calorimeter. Fuel weight = 2.05 gm, water weight = 2.5 kg, rise in temperature = 25 to 28.5°C, Water equivalent of calorimeter = 2.1 kg, fuse wire correction = 2.5 calories, cooling correction = 0.8°C.

14. Calculate the volume (litres) of air required for complete combustion of 1 kg coal sample containing 60% C, 15% H, 4% S and rest is oxygen.

15. The percentage composition of coal sample is C = 80%, H = 4%, O = 3%, N = 3% S = 2% Ash = 5% moisture 3%, calculate the quantity of air needed for complete combustion of 1kg of coal, if 60% excess air is supplied.

16. Write characteristics of a good fuel. How will you determine the Net calorific value of a fule by Bomb calorimeter?

17. Define Absolute viscosity and kinematic viscosity. How will you determine the kinematic Viscosity of lubricant oil using Redwood viscometer.

18. Discuss one experimental method for determination of viscosity index.

19. Differentiate between Redwood viscometer no1 and 2 with their application.

20. What are the factors which affect the efficiency of Lubricant. Write the criteria for selection of a lubricant.

SPECTROSCOPIC AND ANALYTICAL METHODS

1. Explain basic principle of mass spectrometer with schematic diagram.

2. Write the laws of spectroscopy.Explain bathochromic and hypso-chromic shift.

3. Define chemical shift. Predict the number of **NMR** signals in CH_3CH_2OH, CH_3-CH_3 and $CH_3 - C - (CH_3)_2 - Cl$.

4. Define chromophores and auxochrome.Calculate the λ_{max} for the following compounds. $H_3C - HC = CH - C = C - CH_3$ and

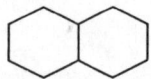

5. Explain various types of electronic transitions with their energy diagram.

6. Write the basic principle of NMR spectroscopy with its diagram.

7. What do you mean by spin active nuclei.How NMR signal get splitted.

8. Discuss the number of NMR signals and their splitting in 2-propanol and 2-propanone.

9. How will you use NMR spectroscopy to distinguish the isomers.

10. What are the ranges of UV, Visible and Radio waves in electromagnetic spectrum. Explain the basic principle of UV spectroscopy.

11. What is m/e ratio in mass spectrum. Discuss the possible fragmentation of methanol .

12. Write the basic principle of titrimetric analysis. Define Normality and Molarity.

13. Explain the principle of Redox titration with suitable example.

14. Discuss iodometric and iodimetric titration with example.

15. What do you mean by chelates. Write the principle of Complexometric titration with example.

16. Explain various types of acid base titration with suitable indicators.

17. How will you determine the strength of a weak acid experimentally? Calculate the Normality and Molarity of 20gpl solution of H_2SO_4.

18. Explain the principle of Precipitation titration with suitable example.

19. How will you determine the alkalinity and acidity in the water sample.

20. How will you determine the temporary and permanent hardness in the water sample.

21. If 3.5 ml of N/10 HCl was used for 25 ml of water sample in the alkalinity sample, calculate the alkalinity of water in ppm and °French.

22. What amount of sodium bicarbonate to be dissolved in 200ml of water to get seminormal solution.

23. Which indicator is used in hardness of water? Calculate the hardness of water sample if 20 ml of water sample required 12 ml of N/30 EDTA solution.

24. How will you differentiate between butane, 2-butene and butadiene by using UV spectroscopy.

25. Write short notes on- spin-spin coupling, up-down field, splitting of signal and coupling constant.

INDEX

1st Order 128

2nd Order 132

Acid-Alkalimetry 8

Activation Energy 140

Alloys 311

Basic Terms 1

Battery and Fuel Cell 215

Biodegradable Polymers 304

Biofuel 378

Biogas 384

Biomass 381

Boiler Problem 248

Bragg's law 436

Buffer Solutions 223

Calorific Value: GCV 374

Ceramics-Glass 326

Classification of Lubricant 343

Classification of Polymers 269

Complexometry 11

Conducting Polymers 306

Conductivity 175

Conformations 477

Corrosion Control 234

Density of unit cell 427

Dry Corrosion 229

Electrochemical Cell 185

Electrochemical series 205

Electrochemical theory 230

Electronic Effects 449

Esterification and Transesterification 380

Fuel: classification 362

Fullerene 446

Functions of Lubricants 340

Gaseous fuel 371

Geometrical Isomerism 466

Hardness of Water 242

Hydrogen Bonding 397

Hydrolysis of Salts 225

Infra-red Spectroscopy 74

Internal Treatment of Water 250

Ion Exchange Process 260

Kohlrausch Law 182

Laws of Electrochemistry 172

Laws of spectroscopy 40

Lime Soda process 252

Liquid Crystal 439

Liquid fuel: Petroleum 369

Mass Spectroscopy 100

Mechanism of Lubricants 353

Metallic Bonding 393

MOT 410

Nanocomposites 317

NMR Principle 53

NMR Signals 62

Numerical Problems 25

One Component System 153

Optical Isomerism 469

Order determination methods 133

Organometallics 334

Phase rule and derivation 148

Polymerisation mechanism 276

Polymerization techniques 282

Polymers 268

Precipitation Titrations 21

Properties of Lubricant 356

Rate of reaction 108

Reaction Intermediates 453

Redox Titrations 18

Refractory 318

Reverse Osmosis 262

Solid fuel: Coal 366

Solubility and Solubility Product 225

Special Name Reactions 460

Structural Isomerism 465

Surface chemistry 141

Synthetic lubricant 351

Two Component System 163

Types of Attacking Reagents 454

Types of Reactions 456

Unit Cell 423

UV-Visible Spectroscopy 41

VBT 400

VSEPR 401

Wet Corrosion 230

Woodword Fieser rules 45

Zeolite process 256

Zero order 126

Reader's Note

Reader's Note